More prai
The Autoimmune Epidemic

"Nakazawa articulates highly complicated medical processes in extremely comprehensible language. Highly recommended."

—*Library Journal*

"Nakazawa's comprehensive heads-up is not all gloom. She discusses scientific studies and breakthroughs that may stem the tide and an assortment of dietary supplements and . . . preventatives that may help."

—*Booklist*

"Provides practical advice about making the personal, political, and economic choices that can help curb this epidemic."

—*Indianapolis Star*

"An insightful exploration of one of the greatest medical mysteries of our time."

—Frederick W. Miller, MD, PhD, Chief, Environmental Autoimmunity Group, National Institutes of Health

"Autoimmune diseases touch millions of Americans. Most of these diseases seem to be increasing in frequency. It is most likely that the environment is a major contributor to this increase. Nakazawa deserves credit for putting this important issue before the public."

—Noel R. Rose, MD, PhD, Director, Johns Hopkins Center for Autoimmune Disease Research

Also by Donna Jackson Nakazawa
· ·

Does Anybody Else Look Like Me?
How to Make the World a Better Place for Women

Donna Jackson Nakazawa

THE

AUTOIMMUNE

EPIDEMIC

A Touchstone Book
Published by Simon & Schuster
New York   London   Toronto   Sydney

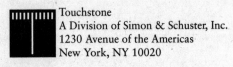

Touchstone
A Division of Simon & Schuster, Inc.
1230 Avenue of the Americas
New York, NY 10020

First Touchstone trade paperback edition February 2009

TOUCHSTONE and colophon are registered trademarks
of Simon & Schuster, Inc.

For information about special discounts for bulk purchases,
please contact Simon & Schuster Special Sales at
1-800-456-6798 or business@simonandschuster.com.

Designed by William Ruoto

Manufactured in the United States of America

10 9 8 7 6 5 4 3 2 1

The hardcover edition of this book was cataloged by the Library of Congress as
follows:

Nakazawa, Donna Jackson
  The autoimmune epidemic : bodies gone haywire in a world out of balance—
and the cutting-edge science that promises hope / by Donna Jackson Nakazawa.
    p. cm.
  "A Touchstone Book."
  Includes biographical references.
    1. Autoimmune Diseases—epidemiology. 2. Autoimmune Diseases—etiology.
    3. Autoimmunity—drug effects. 4. Disease outbreaks—prevention & control.
    5. Environmental Exposure—adverse effects. I. Title.
    RC600.N35 2008
    616.978—dc22
    2007048306

ISBN-13: 978-0-7432-7775-4
ISBN-10:   0-7432-7775-9
ISBN-13: 978-0-7432-7776-1 (pbk)
ISBN-10:   0-7432-7776-7 (pbk)

For Christian, for Claire

Autoimmune disease: Normally the immune system's army of white blood cells helps protect the body from harmful substances, called antigens. Examples of antigens include bacteria, viruses [and] toxins.... But in patients with an autoimmune disorder, the immune system can't tell the difference between healthy body tissue and antigens. The result is an immune response that destroys normal body tissues.

—National Institutes of Health (NIH)

It takes the human body thousands of years to adapt to new environmental stresses—yet in a hundred years we've dumped so many toxic substances into our environment that our immune system is being asked to differentiate between our own body and unrecognizable invaders nonstop. Which makes our body much more likely to make a mistake than it was, say, a century ago. There are just so many more opportunities to make mistakes.

—Ahmet Hoke, MD, PhD

Director, Neuromuscular Division, Johns Hopkins Medical Institutions

We have no other good explanation as to why there should be an increase in autoimmune diseases, except for the things to which we are exposed in the environment. Autoimmunity is our immune system's effort to adapt to all the new environmental agents and shifts that we're being bombarded with. It's an unsuccessful adaptation, but it's our body's way of trying to fight back.

—Noel R. Rose, MD, PhD

Director, Autoimmune Disease Research Center,
Johns Hopkins Medical Institutions

CONTENTS

Chapter Three: Dirty Little Secrets: Cluster Epidemics from Buffalo to Texas

Chapter Four: A Potent Package: Viruses, Vaccines, and Heavy Metals

Chapter Five: The Autoimmune Disease Detectives: Era of the Mavericks

Chapter Six: Shielding Your Immune System: Rethinking Food, Stress, and Everyday Chemicals

FOREWORD

. . . .

by Douglas Kerr, MD, PhD

As a faculty neurologist and neuroscientist at the Johns Hopkins Hospital in Baltimore Maryland, I have spent the last decade evaluating and treating patients with autoimmune disorders of the nervous system. I founded and continue to direct the Johns Hopkins Transverse Myelitis (TM) Center, the only center in the world dedicated to developing new therapies for this paralyzing autoimmune disorder. Increasingly, I see that more and more patients are being felled by this devastating disorder. Infants as young as five months old can get TM and some are left permanently paralyzed and dependent upon a ventilator to breathe. But this is supposed to be a rare disorder, reportedly affecting only one in a million people. Prior to the 1950s, there were a grand total of four cases reported in the medical literature. Currently, my colleagues at the Johns Hopkins Hospital and I hear about or treat hundreds of new cases every year. In the multiple sclerosis clinic, where I also see patients, the number of cases likewise continues to climb.

Autoimmune diseases have not always been this common. The prevalence of autoimmune diseases like systemic lupus erythematosus or lupus, multiple sclerosis, and type 1 diabetes is on the rise. In some cases, autoimmune diseases are three times more common now than they were several decades ago. These changes are not due to increased recognition of these disorders or altered diagnostic criteria. Rather, more people are getting autoimmune disorders than ever before.

Something in our environment is creating this crisis. What you will read about in the following pages is a powerful and touching and scholarly exposé of what those things may be.

The immune system in our bodies is charged with an amazingly complex task: to recognize and ignore all the cells and tissues within our body and—at the same time—to attack any and all "invaders," foreign cells, viruses, bacteria, or fungi. Our wondrously complex immune system can successfully protect our bodies while recognizing and eliminating billions of distinct infections with which we come in contact. When functioning well, the immune system immediately recognizes a virus or bacteria that has gotten into our body and initiates a spirited and robust attack on the invader, allowing us to recover from a cold after only a few days. But this precisely choreographed dance between the immune system and the tissues it is designed to protect goes badly awry in autoimmune diseases. In such diseases, the immune system mistakes friend for foe and begins to attack the very tissues it was designed to protect. The soldiers guarding the castle turn and attack it.

But what triggers autoimmunity to occur? Throughout human history, our exposure to such myriad infectious agents has triggered an evolutionary arms race. Our immune system has evolved increasingly sophisticated countermeasures and recognition systems to combat the increasing diversity of the infectious agents with which we come in contact. But this increasing sophistication comes with a cost: an increased chance of the system breaking down. We have evolved right to the edge of the immune system's capacity.

Now, over the last forty years, something has been pushing that system over the edge. Something is causing the immune system to increasingly make mistakes in which the line becomes blurred, the immune system attacks the body itself, and autoimmune disease occurs. In all likelihood, much of the reason for this often catastrophic mistake of the immune system comes from the countless environmental toxins to which we are currently exposed—toxins that interfere with the way the immune system communicates with the rest of the body. To paraphrase W. B. Yeats, when that communication is lost, "things fall apart, the centre cannot hold."

The numbers are staggering: one in twelve Americans—and one in nine women—will develop an autoimmune disorder. And since it is clear that not every patient with an autoimmune disease is correctly diagnosed, the prevalence is certainly higher than that. The American Heart Association estimates that by comparison, only one in twenty Americans will have coronary heart disease. Similarly, according to the National Center for Health Statistics, one in fourteen American adults will have cancer at some time in their life. This means that an American is more likely to get an autoimmune disease than either cancer or heart disease. Yet we hear much more in the press about heart disease and cancer than we do about autoimmunity. And this silence is mirrored in relative funding by the National Institutes of Health, the major funding agency for biomedical research in the United States. Though the NIH has expanded funding for autoimmunity significantly over the last several years, the 2003 expenditure of $591.2 million is still only a fraction of the money spent for heart disease and cancer. The NIH budget for cancer is over 5 billion dollars, ten times that of autoimmune diseases. The NIH budget for cardiovascular disease is over 2 billion dollars, four times that of autoimmune diseases. We have not yet recognized the urgency of the autoimmune epidemic.

Why is the prevalence of autoimmunity increasing at such alarming rates? There is almost universal agreement among scientists and physicians that the environmental toxins and chemicals to which we are increasingly exposed are interfering with the immune system's ability to distinguish self from non-self. Most of the risk of autoimmunity comes from environmental exposures rather than from genetic susceptibilities. So, have those environmental exposures changed over time? The answer is clearly yes. One example of this comes from a 2003 study in which blood and urine samples from Americans were tested for 210 substances, including industrial compounds, pollutants, PCBs, insecticides, dioxins, mercury, cadmium, and benzene. The volunteers, none of whom had any occupational or residential risks for such exposure, had detectable levels of 91 of these. In other words, these are ordinary people with ordinary lives who have numerous toxins in their body from ordinary exposure. In a 2005 study, researchers found 287 industrial chemicals, including pesticides, phthalates, dioxins, flame-retardants, and the breakdown chemicals of Teflon, in the fetal cord blood of ten newborn infants from around the country—transmitted to the infants by their mothers' exposures before and during pregnancy.

We are facing both an increasing prevalence of autoimmunity and an increasing exposure to environmental toxins. Is it clear that the increased exposure of environmental toxins is causing the increase in autoimmunity? Several lines of evidence suggest that this jury, too, has issued the verdict—"guilty." Researchers recently showed that when added to the diets of rats, PFOA (perfluorooctanoic acid, a breakdown chemical of Teflon and one of the chemicals found in the blood panel screenings mentioned above), causes significant impairments in the ability of rats to develop an appropriate immune response. Similarly, other researchers showed that mice given organochlorine pesticides were much more susceptible to getting the autoimmune disease lupus than control mice.

Are these data absolutely definitive? It's not clear that the type of exposure these animals had is the same type that humans have. It's not clear that lupus in animals is the same thing as lupus in humans. It's not clear that a rodent's immune system is the same as a human's. Much more research needs to be done on this subject—in the form of both epidemiologic (human population studies correlated with exposures) and animal studies. Meanwhile, the difficulty in finding the smoking gun/definitive evidence of causality is increased exponentially by the number of chemicals to which we are exposed. Do we have to give animals the 287 compounds found in the fetal-blood-cord study cited above to examine their combinatorial effect on the immune system? Not only is such research impractical, it is unethical and probably still wouldn't be viewed by some as definitive.

There are some who might say that this is nothing more than another case of ranting "the sky is falling" when it's really not. I suspect those might be the same people who believe that the undeniable warming of the planet is simply a geological cycle that has nothing to do with human activity. But taking these positions—that environmental exposures are not adversely affecting our bodies' health or that we are not causing our planet to get hotter—is dangerous. To miss the opportunity to change is to not only deny the evidence and miss what may be a fleeting opportunity to reverse these trends, but also, ultimately, a selfish position. What about our children and their children? If we have the opportunity to make a healthier future for them but fail to act either because of indifference or denial, what will tomorrow hold for them?

What is just as disturbing is that only 5.4 percent of the NIH budget for autoimmunity is dedicated to environmental factors that underlie autoimmunity. We need to recognize the urgency of the autoimmune epidemic. And we need to take steps to combat it. Future research is unlikely to define a single cause for autoimmunity, but rather varied triggers that include environmental exposures and infectious agents interacting in complex ways with an individual's immune system. This research will, in all likelihood, clearly establish the link between these exposures and autoimmunity and will begin to define how these exposures cause autoimmunity. We won't be able to eliminate autoimmunity in the future. Genetic predisposition and infectious triggers will always be with us. But the fight against autoimmunity needs to be fought on several levels: more extensive research, development of better therapies that more effectively treat these diseases, and action to decrease our environmental exposures. The last action will require personal responsibility, political action, and corporate accountability. If we do these things, autoimmunity will be a cluster of rare diseases that we treat with effective medicines. If we don't, autoimmune diseases will increasingly devastate families, including five-month-old babies, and will increasingly tax our health-care system. If we don't act now, it will be too late.

The book that follows is astounding. It is a combination of

touching personal stories about individuals affected by autoimmune diseases and rigorous research of the medical and scientific literature. It is the kind of book that will scare you. It will make you angry. It will amaze you with the courage of some of the people described in the book. Ms. Nakazawa examines all of the theories about autoimmunity in detail, from heavy metals to toxic chemicals to viruses to vaccines and finally to the hygiene hypothesis. *The Autoimmune Epidemic* is every bit as compelling as Upton Sinclair's groundbreaking novel *The Jungle* and every bit as necessary as *An Inconvenient Truth,* the startling movie featuring Al Gore and directed by Davis Guggenheim, that shows us that global warming is upon us and may at some point in the near future be irreversible.

You will leave this book with no reservations about the veracity of the conclusions: put simply, there is no doubt that autoimmune diseases are on the rise and our increasing environmental exposure to toxins and chemicals is fueling this rise. The research is sound. The conclusions, unassailable.

Ms. Nakazawa introduces a term, "autogen," used to describe chemical triggers of autoimmune disease, drawing upon the term "carcinogen," which denotes chemical triggers of cancer. This term, which should become part of our society's lexicon, may serve as the clarion call for change that emerges from this book. The change needs to take the forms of personal responsibility and societal change. Companies should have to determine the effect of chemicals in developing autoimmunity as well as cancer, and state and federal legislation is needed to compel corporations to make this happen. This book will inspire you to want to do something to protect yourselves and your loved ones; to do what you can to restore a healthy balance between our environment and our bodies. What that something is will vary depending on the individual. At a personal level, no single recommendation fits all individuals and the degree to which an individual alters his/her environment will depend on the levels of exposures and his or her susceptibility to autoimmunity. *The Autoimmune Epidemic* ends with a logical and empowering solution to protect yourself and your family and, in so doing, to begin the process of cleaning up our environment in order to help reestablish a balanced immune system in our bodies.

Reading *The Autoimmune Epidemic* is a necessary first step. Reading *The Autoimmune Epidemic* is a life-altering event. It needs to be.

INTRODUCTION

. . . .

This book is about a global health epidemic that threatens to affect each and every one of us. However, the seeds for this book were sown in my own health crisis. Like 23.5 million other Americans, I suffer from autoimmune disease, and it has ravaged my life, placing before me the greatest obstacles I have ever known. Pages of this book were written during different stays in the small white hospital rooms of Johns Hopkins Hospital, and many chapters were drafted during long bedridden months at home.

The greatest of these challenges began one fine spring afternoon as I was celebrating "Carpet Day" with my daughter. Carpet Day is our own personal mother-child holiday, celebrated only by us. On the first great spring day we take an old carpet and unroll it on our suburban drive. We bring pillows, chalk, snacks, and lemonade and lie there, reading and chatting, pretending it's the beach for a whole afternoon. On Carpet Day, you can almost hear the seagulls and feel the breeze from the ocean waves that we still won't visit for months. That day, we brought our golden retriever puppy outside with us. He saw a squirrel, and off he went. I bounded after him, or tried to, only to find that my left leg wouldn't follow my right. I hurtled headlong into the grass.

• • •

Over the next seventy-two hours, my left leg, then my right, then both arms lost all muscle control as my body underwent what was—for me—the all-too-familiar creeping paralysis of Guillain-Barré syndrome, an autoimmune illness in which the nerve's myelin sheaths are destroyed by the body's own immune system.

Guillain-Barré syndrome, or GBS, usually attacks a month or so after a patient has had a common viral or bacterial infection. Just three weeks earlier, I had had a stomach bug. My body's immune fighter cells had mounted a war to eliminate those germs, but once they'd achieved that goal, instead of ceasing their attack they turned on my own body—in a deadly game of self-sabotage. With Guillain-Barré, the immune system gets its wires dangerously crossed and while trying to fight off the infectious agent also damages the myelin sheaths that wrap around all of our nerves like a protective insulation. The damage is so rapid that a patient's myelin sheaths and the axonal nerves they protect can be methodically and painfully stripped away—leaving them entirely paralyzed within weeks, or even days.

It was the second time in four years that I had been paralyzed with GBS. Once before, in the spring of 2001, when my son was six and my daughter two, I had developed this same bizarre and devastating disease after a stomach bug. In 2001, physicians at the local emergency room confidently misdiagnosed my leg weakness and back pain as a back injury and prescribed bed rest. But instead of improving with rest, I lost nerve and muscle control in my legs by steady degrees over a period of nearly two weeks. One day I could stand on my toes, a few days later I couldn't quite manage it. A few days after that I couldn't flex my feet. A week later, I would stand up and try not to crash into the wall, but suddenly the wall would be there to greet me.

A day or two later, I attempted to get to my two-year-old after she bloodied her toe by stubbing it on the leg of my dresser, but I couldn't make it there, even on my knees. The communiqués my brain sent to my body to feel the floor beneath my feet simply didn't connect.

One afternoon my son, then six, tried to rouse me by showing me how competent he'd become overnight at tying his shoes, as if by some magical power he could banish his mom's bizarre inability to budge from bed.

"Look, Mom!" he called to me from downstairs, near the front door where we kept our shoes. "I tied my shoes! On my *own!*" There was a moment's pause, and then—making a decision to ignore the no-shoes-in-the-house rule—he clambered up the stairs to show me his handiwork, pride widening his smile.

"*Great* job, buddy." I tousled his hair and smiled back, ignoring the sneaker prints trailing behind him across the bedroom rug.

"Mom?" he asked, his tone uncertain. "Can you help me tighten the loops?" He put his foot up on the side of the bed. I tried to pull at both laces to make the floppy loops smaller but my fingers weren't strong enough.

"I can't manage it at the moment, buddy," I said. His face grew ashen and tight. I tried to comfort him, repeating a made-up acronym I sometimes used to soothe my children, hoping it would do the trick again. "Remember? My love for you is very FINE—it is Forever, Infinite, Neverending, and *Everywhere* you go." We lay side by side, my words all I had to embrace him with as I struggled to hide my own panic. Why was I losing muscle control in my arms as well as my legs?

Within twenty-four hours, my breathing became shallow and short. It was clear I was facing something other than a back problem. I was admitted to Hopkins, where the neurologist who took my case ordered infusions of immunoglobulin, or other people's healthy immune cells, the standard treatment for GBS. In many first-time cases, but not all, GBS paralysis is 90-percent reversible with treatment, and the myelin sheaths begin to regenerate. It is a remarkable process. If left untreated, GBS can be fatal; the paralysis spreads to the lungs, and patients require intubation—a tube inserted into the airway to prevent them from suffocating to death. In 2001, I recovered well with immunoglobulin treatments followed by months of physical therapy. Although I was left with strange neurological bells and whistles—jingly nerve endings, tired, locked muscles, twitchy connections—it seemed a minuscule price to pay for being able to walk unassisted again.

I was so very fortunate.

Still, other problems emerged. I was told that I also had leucopenia, a dangerously low white blood cell count. Leucopenia and GBS came on the heels of two earlier autoimmune diagnoses that had spanned the previous fifteen years. Small-fiber sensory neuropathy, which leads to a permanent loss of some of the normal sensation in the hands and feet, and hypothyroidism, or an underactive thyroid. In addition, I suffered from vasovagal syncope, a fainting and seizure disorder caused by the heart sending incorrect signals from the brain to the vagus nerve and failing to pump enough blood through the body, "cured" by doctors surgically implanting a pacemaker when I was twenty-eight.

Still, when Guillain-Barré struck a second time in April 2005, it came as a devastating shock. You simply were not supposed to get GBS twice. If you did, your chances of regenerating your nerves went from 90 percent to—well, no one quite knew. Toward the end of my hospital stay in the rehabilitation center, my physical medicine specialist stood at my bedside one day, patting my leg. "You might not get any better than you are right now," she warned, her voice soft for the blow. "But that doesn't mean you should give up hope."

I had no intention of giving up hope. As a child, I had watched my father suffer through a constellation of what I have since learned were autoimmune illnesses: inflammatory bowel disease, rheumatoid arthritis, and leucopenia. By the time my father was forty-two years old, he could barely walk a step without wincing with joint pain, and his bowels were continually inflamed. He died without warning one August morning following routine abdominal surgery to remove inflamed parts of his duodenum. I was twelve. It turned out that the heavy steroids his rheumatologist had prescribed for his arthritis had eaten through the sutures his stomach surgeon had sewn in, and the peritonitis that ensued caused his body to go into shock and his heart to arrest. "Normal courses of antibiotics proved unsuccessful," read his death report.

We knew so little then. Still, thirty years later, when my own frightening journey through autoimmune disease began, it seemed to me that we knew little more than we had in my father's era.

As I lay on that hospital bed with Guillain-Barré for a second time in 2005, I couldn't help but compare my father's odyssey to my own. Like him, it seemed I possessed an irrationally overexuberant immune system. I lay in a hospital bed in the same medical institution, Johns Hopkins, one ward over from where my father had died from autoimmune-related complications at almost the very same age I was now. With a young son and daughter at home yet to raise, the similarities terrified me.

Back home, physical therapy, meditation, and an autoimmune-preventive diet all helped to bring incremental gains in mobility. I would later come to think of that time as a five-month journey around my room, often accompanied by my physical therapist at my side, as I sweated to graduate from wheelchair to walker to cane—with no guarantee that I would improve. As one doctor explained, "You've had several forest fires, and each time it's harder and harder to get healthy regrowth." It was the second time in four years that my work as a journalist came to a sudden halt. Deadline after deadline passed. I was simply too weak to sit in front of a computer, let alone tap out words on the keyboard. I tried to get to the bathroom one night on my own, using my walker, without waking my husband to help steady me, but misjudged my stamina. On the way back I crashed into a window and fell in a heap on the floor, unable to get up on so much as one elbow. When you hear the phrase "and he scraped her up off the floor" and wonder what that really means, it means exactly what my husband did that night. He sat up and called my name out in confusion: where were my cries coming from? When he found me beneath the window he picked me up and laid me back in bed. We lay side by side, both too close to tears to risk words.

A few moments later, our son, ten then, crept silently into our room, having heard the commotion. He laid his head down in the dark beside me, his arm circling my waist from behind.

"Mom?" he said, his voice questioning, as he grasped my hand.

I tried to hide my wet eyes and clear my voice.

He pressed his face into the back of my neck, quietly, tentatively. "Mom?" he asked. "Don't you know that I'm old enough to know that even grown-ups can get scared?" Then he hesitated. "The only time I get really scared is when it gets all quiet at school," he said, his fingers tapping the ends of mine, one at a time, gently, rhythmically. "Like when we're about to take a test, and the only thing I can hear is the rustling of paper. And then I worry . . . what if you die before I get back home to see you again?"

My children had spent three-quarters of a year of their young lives with their mom either in the hospital or bedridden.

Scared? We were all terrified. Autoimmune diseases, which often strike when people are in their prime—making them wonder whether they'll ever be lucky enough to get back on their feet again—tend to have that effect. Like any family in which one member is felled with autoimmune disease, my husband, son, and daughter had been through hell as much as I had.

By the end of July, I got up and down the stairs with a cane for the first time. In August, four months after being discharged from the hospital, I was able to make it with a cane all the way to the mailbox—a few yards down the sloped driveway on which we'd celebrated Carpet Day that April. It was a tremendous milestone, one I had been warned I might never reach. One day my in-home physical therapist and I headed out the door to test my stability walking across the bumpy grass in our wooded backyard. When I'd managed to go twenty or thirty feet he whisked the cane away. In

September, my feet were strong enough to drive, and I drove my children to school for my daughter's first day of first grade and my son's entry into middle school.

A few months later, in December, my six-year-old daughter asked me to dance with her in the kitchen to a funny song we'd danced to together for years—about a cow, funnily enough, who wouldn't listen to anyone who told her what she couldn't do.

"Can you dance, Mommy?" she asked.

"Let's see," I said, curious myself. We cranked the music, held hands, and stomped our feet and turned in circles as we shouted out the refrain, "No one can tell you who you oughta be or what you oughta do!" until we began to laugh with a raucous joy that morphed into tears, before we fell spent on the floor. The relief on my daughter's face was akin to that of Christmas morning—Santa *did* come!

Still, my doctors could not guarantee that I would not plunge into more devastating autoimmune crises. As one told me, "All we can do is wait and see until another shoe drops—then treat you as best we can." Sometimes, the shoe does drop—and hard. In the spring of 2006, I caught a seemingly innocuous, low-grade gastro-intestinal infection that would not go away. Six weeks later I landed in the hospital to treat a bowel neurological dysfunction—a complication that arises in some who have had Guillain-Barré syndrome.

Because I am a journalist by trade, it was in some ways inevitable that my personal journey into autoimmunity would turn into a professional quest. I wanted to know what was being done to investigate autoimmune disease. Why didn't we as a society hear more about these illnesses—both the problems they cause and research under way to combat them? What factors coalesced to cause autoimmune disease? Did environmental components play a role—and if so, what were they? What could a patient do to stem the damage and prevent future crises? Driven by an urgent need for information, I sought out answers from the top researchers in the field.

It quickly became clear in talking to these cutting-edge scientists, however, that the story was far bigger: my own case was but one tiny part of an emerging, global health crisis—one with disturbing and widespread implications for every American. During the same years that I have been waging my own battle with autoimmunity, researchers at dozens of top international institutions around the world have been documenting an alarming rise in autoimmune disease rates. In 2005, the National Institutes of Health (NIH) released a report called *Progress in Autoimmune Diseases Research* in which the director of NIH pronounced that nearly one hundred known autoimmune diseases—such as multiple sclerosis, type 1 diabetes, rheumatoid arthritis, myositis, lupus, scleroderma, thyroiditis, Graves' disease, ulcerative colitis, Crohn's disease, myasthenia gravis, and eighty-some others—now afflict 23.5 million people in the U.S., or one in twelve Americans, and these diseases are now on the rise worldwide—for reasons unknown. The statistics are stark: over the past forty years, rates of lupus, multiple sclerosis, type 1 diabetes, and a range of other autoimmune diseases have doubled and tripled in Western countries around the world. Just as worrisome, rates are rising dramatically among children, as are other related syndromes in which the immune system becomes hypersensitive, such as food allergies and asthma. These growing numbers cannot be attributed to better diagnostic procedures or disease awareness alone. An escalating number of people in the industrialized world are facing diseases in which their immune systems are turning on and damaging their own bodies.

What is propelling this epidemic? Scientists the world over agree that the root cause of this frightening trend is environmental. Twin studies elucidate that two-thirds of the risk of developing autoimmune disease is acquired through some environmental trigger, genetic risk being the smaller part of the equation. Over the past decade, labs around the globe have proven definitive links between a list of commonly used industrial-age chemicals, heavy metals, and toxins and the development of numerous autoimmune diseases. As hundreds of industrial byproducts interact with the immune cells of our bodies, they are sabotaging an extraordinarily complex and fine-tuned blueprint for healthy cellular communication. Facing a dismal picture in which the numbers of people afflicted with autoimmune disease in industrialized countries continue to rise, the race to turn the tide of this worldwide trend has become a race against time.

This book explores this scientific race—the watershed discoveries that are revolutionizing our understanding of the way the immune system functions and the complex, interlocking factors that cause it to go haywire; what role genes and environmental toxins play in who will be struck by disease; why scientists now believe that even people who are *not* genetically predisposed to autoimmunity may fall ill with these diseases; the groundbreaking interventions emerging out of today's top labs that promise to help halt the disease process; and ways in which we can each lessen the multitude of exposures that threaten our immune systems and our health.

Four decades ago, writer Rachel Carson, author of *Silent Spring*, demonstrated how our chemical age has altered our environment to the degree that the fertility and survival of many of the species with which we coexist are threatened. Then, as now, there is great resistance to the idea that environmental contamination can alter the health of both animals and people. Indeed, it has taken several decades for many researchers in the autoimmune-disease field to come to the conclusion that our contaminated environment is causing the human immune system to run amok. But the consensus is rapidly building. These pages lay bare this "inconvenient truth"— one as disturbing to today's top scientists as global warming. My hope is that the chapters you are about to read will awaken a deep understanding about how the environmental changes of the industrial age and our twenty-first-century lifestyles are wreaking havoc with the immune cells of our own bodies.

We *are* our environment. What we put into it, we also put into ourselves. What we do to it, we also do to ourselves. The way in which our bodies are turning against themselves when autoimmune disease strikes serves, sadly, as a disturbing modern analogy for what we are doing to ourselves as a society as we continue to dump thousands of chemicals into the soil, water, and air that surround us. Our mass dependence on chemically manufactured home and lifestyle products and our diet of chemically processed foods, in many ways, constitute a great societal health experiment, as we continue to surround ourselves with thousands of chemicals whose properties we do not yet fully understand.

With our eyes open to that knowledge we can begin to make critical and profound choices, embarking on a journey of small steps that will slowly start to make all the difference between health and disease. As we educate ourselves about the consequences of our day-to-day lifestyles and strive to make the personal, political, and economic choices to counter those ill effects, we will be taking back our environment, our bodies, and our future.

CHAPTER ONE

THE RED FLAG DISEASE

Between them, Jan Pankey and David Calhoun shared four decades of experience as physicians. Yet in the quiet dark of one August night in 2003, all that experience seemed to count for nothing. Something was going terribly wrong inside Jan's body, and neither husband nor wife could make sense of what was happening, or why.

It was shortly after midnight on the first night of a long-anticipated vacation in Montana when Jan awoke to a burning ache that encircled her upper chest. It was all she could do to draw in a breath. If Jan hadn't known better she might have thought she'd been pummeled with an iron rod across both front and back while she slept. Fumbling in the pitch black of their Idaho hotel room, where they had stopped en route to their final destination, Jan switched on the bedside lamp and stood for a moment in the circle of reassuring yellow light. Her legs felt unsteady. She couldn't feel the carpet beneath the soles of her feet. It took a blink or two for her mind to register that she was about to faint.

A minute later Jan came around to find herself staring at the coarse hotel rug, struggling to take in a full breath—trying to piece together where she was and why her upper body was in so much pain. In that split second every nerve ending inside Jan Pankey's body stood on full alert, signaling that something ungodly was happening. She crawled to the bed to wake her husband.

David quickly shook off sleep along with his bewilderment as to why his wife of twenty-eight years suddenly was writhing uncontrollably beside him—in a hotel room a thousand miles from home and an hour from the nearest metropolitan hospital. Together they struggled to diagnose. Jan and David were well versed in the medical school mantra "When you hear hoofbeats, think horses, not zebras," and so they stuck to Jan's prior, known medical history rather than coming up with exotic could-be's. Recently, Jan, who was forty-nine, had started taking birth-control pills to help even out hormonal fluctuations and irregular periods. But that seemed of little consequence here. She'd also been plagued by bouts of indigestion, which her doctor had chalked up to gastritis, a chronic inflammation of the stomach and intestinal tract, due to a fairly common condition known as gastroesophageal reflux disease, or GERD. In GERD, the stomach overproduces gastric acid and the esophagus spasms, causing excess acid to rise into the fragile lining of the throat. It can be quite painful.

Jan and David concurred that Jan must be experiencing spasms in her esophagus due to her GI problems. David felt that Jan's asthma must be acting up, too; recent forest fires had plagued Montana's wooded areas and some neighborhoods, and the noxious smoke clouds had grown closer and more visible as the couple had neared the Idaho-Montana border. Still, severe chest pain was not usually indicative of asthma. Could asthma coupled with esophageal spasms produce so much pain? That was their best educated guess at one o'clock in the morning in the middle of nowhere.

Jan and David had left home early the day before with the goal of cycling more than a hundred miles of Montana's Glacier National Park, an expedition they had spent the past year planning. Jan had been feeling well enough—you'd certainly never know that she suffered from any health issues to look at her. Slim and vitally active in the middle of life, she had already biked more than 3,300 miles in the previous twelve months. She held down a demanding professional schedule, commuting by plane from rural New Mexico to downtown Oakland, California, every two weeks to work long hours as a pediatric and neonatal anesthesiologist at Oakland's Children's Hospital. She was also a regular team member on physician-run medical missions overseas, helping children in third-world countries obtain lifesaving operations they might never otherwise receive.

The first night after departing for their big Montana trip—fourteen hours in the car after they'd left behind the rural farming village where they lived near New Mexico's Rio Grande—the couple had stopped at their Idaho motel just shy of the Montana border. Once settled in their room Jan and David had turned on the air-conditioning to help filter out the polluted soot from the smoking Montana fires that had drifted in behind them and hoped for a good night's rest. It was a few hours later that Jan's chest pain suddenly and inexplicably set in.

Then, just as unexpectedly, a few hours before dawn, the wrenching pain began to lift. Jan could take in a deep breath again. She told David she was feeling some relief. David felt reassured by Jan's slowly returning calm. He would later realize that it was a veneer Jan had perfected all too well after decades of reassuring parents with critically ill infants and soothing children who were about to undergo surgery.

That morning they crossed the border into southern Montana, where ash from the fires hung so thick in the air that you couldn't see across the street. Neighborhoods were being evacuated. As they got out of their Legacy station wagon to stretch their legs and survey the situation, Jan was seized again by debilitating chest pain and shortness of breath. She dropped to a crouch, gasping for air, unable to stand up.

Half an hour later David was wheeling Jan into the local hospital in Missoula. The emergency-room doctor reassured them that Jan's X-rays looked fine, except for a small, barely distinguishable anomaly: a slight shading along the lungs above the left half of her diaphragm, deemed insignificant. The doctor surmised that Jan's discomfort—and she was now twisting in pain on the hospital gurney—might be a kidney stone. Urinalysis ruled that out. Nor was Jan displaying signs of wheezing. The ER doctor, stumped, concluded that Jan and David's initial hunch had to be right: Jan was suffering from severe spasms in her esophagus due to her gastroesophageal reflux disease. In addition to the spasms themselves, Jan was experiencing muscle strain caused by the spasms along her chest wall. Or so the doctor thought.

The ER physician ordered an intravenous drip to be inserted in Jan's right forearm and dosed her with Demerol for pain as well as a sedative to help her relax. Afterward, Jan was given Prilosec for her gastritis and reflux, and was released. She felt she could and should go on with the trip.

Jan explained her feelings to David. "We've paid the money," she told him. "And I don't want to waste an opportunity we've been looking forward to all year because of stomach problems." Beneath her words David heard Jan's characteristic determination not to be a "wimp."

By the time the bike tour began later that afternoon, Jan wasn't so game, and she stayed behind at the hotel. But when the riders headed out again the next morning, she was resolute: she would ride the "sag wagon"—for lagging bikers—up the mountain a thousand feet, then coast down on her bike so that she could see the stunning vistas of glacier and rock she had driven so far to view. She was a veteran biker; what in the world could happen to her as she coasted down a mountain road? She donned her bike jersey, choosing one that would turn out to be all too fitting. Her jersey material was dotted with small red blood cells and sported the logo of the whimsical company that had made it, the Republic of Anaerobia—literally meaning "the state of insufficient oxygen." Beneath the logo were the words *Veni Vidi Vomiti*. A twist on Julius Caesar's *"Veni, vidi, vici"* ("I came, I saw, I conquered"), *Veni, vidi, vomiti* was a hardcore no-sissy bike-til-you-drop insiders' joke: "I came, I saw, I vomited."

Jan began her glide down the mountain only to find that smog drifting from the fires nearly obliterated the view of the icy gorges and glaciered valleys. But that would turn out to be the least of Jan's worries. She had coasted another half mile in her red jersey when the now familiar vise of pain returned with a vengeance, nearly jolting her from her seat. She found it hard to pull in a breath. The scenery grew blurry. Colors turned to shades of black and white. She was close to passing out.

David discovered Jan crouched by her bike alongside the narrow mountain pass. All they could think of was getting back to the Albuquerque, New Mexico, medical center near their home where David was on staff, as fast as he could drive them.

Meanwhile, neither of them had a clue that in their empty pink adobe house near the Rio Grande the phone was ringing over and over again as the Missoula hospital's radiologist—who had finally reviewed Jan's X-rays—tried in vain to locate the couple.

They were halfway home—still assuming the pain was due to a wicked combination of reflux and gastritis—when Jan noticed a new problem. A hot, angry red line was moving up the vein in her right arm from where her IV needle had been. As a physician she knew a blood clot on sight. She knew that if it progressed it could easily block the flow of oxygen to her heart or lungs, causing a heart attack or even a life-threatening heart infection known as endocarditis. Jan took a dose of the antibiotics that she and David always carried in their first aid kit when traveling, and they stopped at a pharmacy for a heating pad to wrap around her arm to help disperse the clot—both standard protocol. They passed a road sign pointing to a local hospital along the deserted highway. David looked at Jan questioningly.

She shook her head no. "I want to get home to medical care I know we can count on," she told him. With Jan's eyes locked on the crimson line to make sure it wasn't progressing, they headed home.

Eight hours later Jan Pankey lay prone on a gurney inside the Albuquerque Regional Medical Center ER in severe pain, breathing through an oxygen mask while a technician performed a scan of her chest. Jan watched from across the X-ray room as the picture of her lungs began to register on the machine. She didn't have her glasses on, but even so she could see the clots as they appeared on the scan. The technician stared at the screen in stunned silence, then turned to Jan and said, "Honey, I don't think you're going anywhere tonight."

The X-ray was startling. It looked as if someone had taken inch-sized bites out of several areas of each lung. Blood clots, or pulmonary emboli, had proliferated out of nowhere. Large clots were blocking several large arteries. Three of the five lobes in Jan's lungs weren't getting any blood at all, while the other two had been damaged by smaller clots. Together, clots had cut off 50 percent of the oxygen flow to Jan's lungs. The state of anaerobia indeed. It was a wonder Jan was still alive.

The ER physician on call later explained to Jan and David that the area above Jan's diaphragm that had appeared tinted in that first Missoula X-ray had been, no doubt, the first lung tissue to be injured.

The red line on Jan's arm hadn't progressed, so clearly the clots weren't originating from there. Additional ultrasounds revealed, however, that Jan's entire right leg vein was blocked from ankle to groin with a huge clot known as a deep vein thrombosis, or DVT. It was from this larger clot that smaller ones were traveling up to block the major arteries of her lungs. From torso to toes, Jan's blood was clotting up like sludge and no one could explain why.

Without knowing exactly what was causing Jan's condition, the ER physicians put her on the blood thinner Coumadin with the understanding that she would need to stay on it for several months to avert further crises. She stayed six days in the hospital before being discharged. But the second day home it didn't seem to matter that she was taking the full recommended dose of anticoagulants. Jan bent over to pick up a leaf that had fallen from a neglected plant in their foyer and felt "a hard thunk" in her chest that nearly toppled her. She called 911 and David, who was fifteen minutes away at work. The twenty-minute ride alone to the hospital in the back of the ambulance was terrifying.

"Even though I was wearing an oxygen mask I was gasping for every breath," Jan recalls. When David met the ambulance crew at the hospital, they confirmed what he already feared. Jan's situation was deteriorating.

The hospital was so full that day that they turned a U-shaped, curtained area of the emergency room into a temporary critical care unit to treat Jan. Kwaku Osafo-Mensah, a young lung specialist from Ghana who'd come to Albuquerque five years earlier after medical training at UCLA and Stanford, was rushed in to consult on Jan's case. Drawing the beige hospital curtains closed around her makeshift room in the busy ER, Osafo-Mensah quickly explained to Jan and David that even though Jan had been on blood thinners, X-rays showed that she had lost two *more* areas of lung. Her EKG had as many spikes and valleys as the Swiss Alps. Jan and David were terrified.

It was as if someone had punched a hidden self-destruct button inside Jan's lungs and there was no shutoff switch to be found. She knew that if they couldn't stop the clots from forming, she would lose all the pathways by which oxygen entered her bloodstream. What was unfolding inside her body was petrifying; it was as if she were being suffocated to death by her own blood cells.

Osafo-Mensah shook his head as he talked to his new patient, trying to nudge the pieces together. Jan's first embolisms had developed during a long, two-day car ride to Montana. And she was often sitting on airplanes commuting from New Mexico to Oakland. Perhaps both sedentary activities had led to exacerbated clotting. On top of that, anesthesiology is a pretty sedentary job, he explained to Jan. Still, it didn't add up. Not for someone like Jan Pankey who biked 150 miles a week.

Regardless of the diagnosis, Osafo-Mensah knew what he had to do if he was going to save Jan's life, and he knew there wasn't much time. He decided to immediately place a filter in the vein at the top of Jan's leg, known as the inferior vena cava, which pumps blood up from the lower two-thirds of the body. The filter would stop any clots before they traveled up to Jan's heart or lungs. That, along with an intravenous infusion of the blood thinner heparin, would prevent more clots from rising toward her lungs.

It worked. Jan went home again. But a disquieting mystery still lingered in the air. Why weren't blood thinners working for Jan as they did for other patients? Jan scheduled an appointment with her local internist and posed the question to her, only to be brushed off with the words, "Well now, *that's* chasing a real zebra." Jan never went to her again.

Still, the insertion of the blood filter had made some difference for Jan; she was no longer living in a state of full-out perpetual crisis. The clots blocking the pathway to her arteries had dispersed, allowing oxygen to flow into her lungs again—except for the small percent of lung tissue that had died. Nevertheless, she felt so wiped out that she couldn't walk down a hall without pausing to catch her breath. Stairs were out of the question. Twelve hours of sleep did nothing to relieve her weariness. Many days, it was all she could manage to get out of her bathrobe and make a cup of tea by noon.

Despite the residual severe fatigue, weakness, and shortness of breath, she managed to attend a medical conference six weeks later. At the conference, as serendipity would have it, Jan met a dynamic young physician by the name of Alex Spyropoulos, whose passion was deciphering unusual clotting disorders. As the medical director and founder of the Clinical Thrombosis Center at Lovelace Sandia Health Systems in Albuquerque, Spyropoulos was presenting his research on designing new ways to use blood-thinning drugs. He also happened to be the author of a case report in a medical journal on a newly emerging autoimmune disease that dangerously altered clotting factors.

Reeling from what she calls a kind of "mortal exhaustion," Jan approached Dr. Spyropoulos after his hour-long lecture and put forth the question, "How could an active woman like me have recurring clotting even on blood thinners? What's *happening* to me?"

• • •

Two weeks later, Jan sat on an examining table inside Alex Spyro-poulos's office, relaying to him a medical history that had stumped half a dozen physicians. In addition to all that she had been through physically, she told him, she'd also been experiencing some cognitive problems—a kind of recurring brain fuzziness and forgetful-ness that deeply concerned her. Hearing this, Spyropoulos looked up over his notes at Jan, one thick, black brow furrowed. It was his dedication to tough cases that had earned Alex the nickname of "Dr. Spy" among patients who were grateful for his detective-like zeal on their behalf. He had a hunch, he told Jan, that she was not yet on a high-enough dose of anticoagulants. Rather than worry her by playing out possibilities, he ordered extensive blood work and, for added insurance, wrote her a prescription on the spot, upping her dose of medication. "If you have what I think you have, the anticoagulants you're taking will not be sufficient to do the job," he told her, ripping the script off the pad and handing it to Jan.

One week later, Dr. Spyropoulos received Jan's blood work and found his earlier suspicions confirmed. He immediately called Jan's office at Oakland's Children's Hospital where she was work-ing late. It was well into the evening and most of the hospital office lights were out. Jan still remembers hearing her line ring and rush-ing in to pick it up.

"I think I know what you have, Jan," Dr. Spyropoulos told her, excitement accelerating his delivery. Spyropoulos had already treated a number of patients with mysterious clotting problems who'd also reported the onset of "brain fog" as a debilitating symp-tom. When Jan's blood work hit his desk, so did Alex's eureka mo-ment. Jan's blood showed the precise biomarkers for an autoimmune disease known as antiphospholipid antibody syndrome, or APS, an illness he'd seen too often of late in other thrombotic patients.

"I had no idea what he was talking about," Jan recalls. "I had never even heard of APS." She fumbled for pen and paper in her darkened office. The three other doctors who shared her workspace had already gone home, and the hospital was unusually quiet.

Spyropoulos explained to Jan that APS, also known as "sticky blood," or Hughes syndrome, was an autoimmune disease in which the body produces antibodies, or immune fighter cells, that mistakenly disable the very proteins in the blood that the body needs to prevent excessive clotting. Without these proteins, called phospholipids, your blood begins to clot and has no mechanism by which to *stop* clotting.

As Dr. Spy talked, Jan began to put the pieces together. One of the functions of the immune system is to act like a rapid-response SWAT team, reacting to any invading microorganism, such as viruses or bacteria, by producing antibodies—fighter cells—which seek out and destroy those unhealthy and often life-threatening organisms.

But in a wide range of autoimmune diseases, the body's immune cells lose their ability to read the difference between your own healthy cells and the foreign bacteria or viruses—or other unrecognizable microscopic organisms from the environment around you—that enter your body. They don't stop at merely disabling these invading foreign agents, they go on to destroy the body's own healthy tissue in deadly rounds of friendly fire. For reasons scientists are only now beginning to understand, the immune system goes on an erratic rampage, disabling the body itself.

In Jan's case, antibodies that were supposed to keep her healthy were instead attacking the very phospholipids that were instrumental to keeping her blood from clumping like cottage cheese in her veins.

Antibodies that turn on one's own tissue are known as autoantibodies—*antibodies* meaning "fighter cells," *auto* literally meaning "self." As with many of the more newly recognized autoimmune diseases, isolating and testing for specific autoantibodies that point to the diagnosis of APS can be tricky to perform, and new blood tests for APS, in particular, are hard to compare from one lab to the next. At Jan's office visit several weeks later, Dr. Spyropoulos explained to her that her screening test was "positive for autoantibodies that show you have APS." Although a second follow-up blood test didn't confirm as high a level of those autoantibodies, nevertheless, Spyropoulos told Jan, "I think it fits. Your body is certainly acting like you have APS." In 2003, antiphospholipid antibody syndrome was a recently discovered disease; physicians had only known of its existence for twenty years. "There may be other antibodies involved that we don't yet understand or know how to test for," he admitted to Jan. "But that doesn't mean that we can't name and treat your disease."

Dr. Spy started Jan on much higher than usual doses of the heavy-hitting anticoagulant Coumadin, which is often required for patients with sticky blood. He also set her up on a constant home blood-monitoring program so that she could keep tabs on her coagulation levels around the clock. When Jan failed even on this regimen, he started her on long-term self-injections of an anticoagulant known as low-molecular-weight heparin, which had only recently been used to treat patients with APS who had not responded to Coumadin therapy.

Today, Jan has expert supervision of her case and is better able to manage her disease. But myriad threats still lurk in her future. Patients with APS have a dramatically increased risk of migraine, sudden stroke, multiple sclerosis (MS), and lupus, the latter a disease in which the immune system develops antibodies that can mistakenly attack a range of organs in the body, including the joints, kidneys, heart, lungs, brain, and skin. Like all autoimmune patients, Jan is statistically three times more likely than others to be struck with more autoimmune diseases down the road.

Meanwhile, four years after her diagnosis, the side effects from the drugs Jan takes pose additional problems. She lives with constant bruising that she describes as "permanent bands of discoloration across my abdomen." Recently, she knocked her foot against the side of a swimming pool, and what started as a tiny bruise morphed into a black and blue hematoma from heel to toe, requiring a trip to the ER.

Those kinds of crises are commonplace for her now. But Jan

doesn't just worry about what might happen if she were to be insufficiently anticoagulated again. She worries, she says, "about uncertainties like how long will I be able to stay in medicine?" Already, Jan has opted to retire early from the operating room, concerned that the damage APS has done to areas of her brain and her resulting brain fog might jeopardize her ability to keep "the promise I make to all my kids' parents that I will do my best to take care of them in the operating room." Having stepped out of anesthesiology she has decided, instead, to work with children in palliative and hospice care.

She and David also want to backpack again, but she asks, "Will we be able to? What if I bleed and we're too far from help?" She also dreams of rejoining overseas medical missions to help children. But she's not willing to risk falling sick far from U.S. borders. "U.S. doctors don't know much about autoimmune diseases in general and APS in particular," she explains. "What about doctors in the remote parts of India or Belarus or Kenya or Brazil or the other places I have worked?"

Despite all this, she pushes herself to ride her bike, swim, and even run as often as she can. She pushes herself, she says, "because I'm afraid if I stop, I'll never get going again."

In a certain light, it makes sense that six out of the seven doctors whom Jan saw completely missed her disease. Healthy women in the prime of life rarely have lung clots, much less APS. Still, doctors didn't miss Jan's disease just because blood clots seem a counterintuitive diagnostic call in a hard-core cyclist, or because APS is a relatively rare disease. Statistically, Jan's chances of having APS at the age of forty-nine were greater than her risk of having ovarian cancer or leukemia—uncommon cancers that physicians routinely test for when telling symptoms appear. In fact, recent studies reveal that antiphospholipid antibodies are found in 2 to 5 percent of the population. As many as a quarter of women with recurrent miscarriages end up being diagnosed with the autoimmune disease APS, and one in five women who've suffered blood clots in the legs or strokes in the prime of life test positive for APS, making it more prevalent in women than leukemia and ovarian cancer combined.

No, the real reason doctors missed Jan's syndrome is because APS falls into the category of one of nearly one hundred autoimmune diseases that doctors have only in the last decade begun to recognize and understand. Almost every one of Jan's physicians failed to see that she was suffering from an autoimmune condition because, like most day-to-day practitioners, they remain uninformed about how to recognize patients who are suffering from these diseases in the first place. Because Jan's disease was autoimmune in nature, they missed the call.

THE COLD, HARD NUMBERS

Most of us, at some juncture in our lives, have played out in our minds how devastating it would be to have our doctor hand down a cancer diagnosis or to warn us that we are at risk for a heart attack or stroke. Magazine articles, television dramas, and news headlines all bring such images home. But consider an equally devastating health crisis scenario, one that you rarely hear spoken about openly, one that receives almost no media attention. Imagine the slow, creeping escalation of seemingly amorphous symptoms: a tingling in the arms and fingers, the sudden appearance of a speckled rash across the face, the strange muscle weakness in the legs when climbing stairs, the fiery joints that emerge out of nowhere— any and all of which can signal the onset of a wide range of life-altering and often debilitating autoimmune diseases.

Imagine, if you can: the tingling foot and ankle that turns out to be the beginning of the slow paralysis of multiple sclerosis. Four hundred thousand patients. Excruciating joint pain and inflammation, skin rashes, and never-ending flu-like symptoms that lead to the diagnosis of lupus. One and a half million more. Relentless bouts of vertigo—the hallmark of Ménière's. Seven out of every one thousand Americans. Severe abdominal pain, bleeding rectal fissures, uncontrollable diarrhea, and chronic intestinal inflammation that define Crohn's disease and inflammatory bowel disease. More than 1 million Americans. The incapacitating weakness and burning pain that accompany the inflammation of the joints and other organs and lead to the crippling effects of rheumatoid arthritis. More than 2 million patients. Dry mouth so persistent eight glasses of water a day won't soothe the parched throat and tongue and the mysterious swallowing difficulties that are the first signs of Sjögren's. Four million Americans. And, with almost every autoimmune disease, intolerable, life-altering bouts of exhaustion. If fatigue were a sound made manifest by the 23.5 million people with autoimmune disease in America, the roar across this country would be more deafening than that of the return of the seventeen-year locusts.

And yet, despite the prevalence of autoimmune disease, surveys show that more than 90 percent of people cannot summon the name of a single autoimmune disease when asked to name one specifically. Think of it—other than walkathons for multiple sclerosis, how many fundraising walks or lapel ribbons have you seen for autoimmune disease in general? Nearly 24 million Americans are suffering from an autoimmune illness, yet nine out of ten Americans cannot name a single one of these diseases. It boggles the mind.

Each of these nearly one hundred autoimmune diseases derails lives. Taken collectively, these diseases, which also include type 1 diabetes, Graves' disease, vasculitis, myasthenia gravis, connective tissue diseases, autoimmune Addison's disease, vitiligo, rheumatoid arthritis, hemolytic anemia, celiac disease, and scleroderma (see the appendix for full list) are now the number-two cause of chronic illness in America and the third leading cause of Social Security disability behind heart disease and cancer. (Acquired immune deficiency syndrome, or AIDS, by contrast, is *not* an autoimmune disease; in fact, it is entirely different. In AIDS a virus attacks the immune system and destroys it, whereas in autoimmune disease, the immune system leads the attack, mistaking the body's tissue for an invader and turning on the body itself.) Autoimmune diseases are the eighth leading cause of death among women, shortening the average patient's lifespan by fifteen years. Not surprisingly, the economic burden is staggering: autoimmune diseases represent a yearly health-care burden of more than $120 billion, compared to the yearly health-care burden of $70 billion for direct medical costs for cancer.

To underscore these numbers, consider: while 2.2 million women are living with breast cancer and 7.2 million women have coronary disease, an estimated 9.8 million women are afflicted with one of the seven more common autoimmune diseases: lupus, scleroderma, rheumatoid arthritis, multiple sclerosis, inflammatory bowel disease, Sjögren's, or type 1 diabetes, almost all of which can lead to potentially fatal complications. Or, slice these statistics another way: while one in sixty-nine women below the age of fifty will be diagnosed with breast cancer, according to estimates, as many as one in nine women of childbearing years will be diagnosed with an autoimmune illness, which strike three times as many women as men—and most often strike patients in their prime. According to the National Institutes of Health, autoimmune disease affects far more patients than the 9 million Americans who have cancer and the 16 million with coronary disease.

"THE WESTERN DISEASE": A RISING EPIDEMIC

Even as autoimmune diseases remain underrecognized and underaddressed, the number of patients afflicted with these illnesses has been steadily growing. Yet few of today's practicing physicians are aware of the escalating tsunami of epidemiological evidence that now concerns top scientists at every major research institute around the world: evidence that autoimmune diseases such as lupus, MS, scleroderma, and many others are on the rise and have been for the past four decades in industrialized countries around the world:

• Mayo Clinic researchers report that the incidence of lupus has nearly tripled in the United States over the past four decades.

Their findings are all the more alarming when you consider that their research has been conducted among a primarily white population at a time when many researchers believe lupus rates are rising most significantly among African Americans.

- Over the past fifty years multiple sclerosis rates have tripled in Finland, corroborating data reported in Scotland, England, the Netherlands, Denmark, and Sweden, where rates of MS have been rising at nearly 3 percent a year. Multiple sclerosis rates in Norway have risen 30 percent since 1963, echoing trends in Germany, Italy, and Greece, where MS rates have doubled over the past thirty to forty years.

- Rates of autoimmune thyroiditis have risen steadily over the past several decades.

- Rates of type 1 diabetes are perhaps the most telling. Data over the past forty years show that type 1 diabetes, a disease in which immune cells attack the insulin-producing beta cells in the pancreas, has increased fivefold. The story regarding childhood-onset type 1 diabetes is more disturbing. Studies show that the number of children with type 1 diabetes is sky-rocketing, with rates increasing 6 percent a year in children four and under and 4 percent in children aged ten to fourteen.

- Rates of numerous other autoimmune diseases—scleroderma, Crohn's disease, autoimmune Addison's disease, and poly-myositis—show the same alarming pattern.

As with all epidemiological research, it can be more art than science to tease out what percentage of these rising rates is the result of more people being diagnosed with a disease because physicians are more aware of it, versus the increase from a genuine rise in the number of people falling ill. Yet the researchers behind these epidemiological studies hold that something more than an improved ability among doctors to diagnose autoimmune diseases is driving these numbers upward.

Norwegian epidemiologists, for instance, argue that rising rates are "due to a real biological change of the disease" rather than being caused solely by better diagnostics and are concerned by the higher occurrence of autoimmunity in urban than in rural areas. Swedish and German researchers concur that enhanced diagnostics alone cannot explain today's significant increases in MS. Type 1 diabetes researchers insist that today's rapid rise in this disease cannot be explained by either better diagnostics or by more people suddenly becoming genetically susceptible to type 1 diabetes; rather, a change in environmental factors is the "more plausible explanation." At the Mayo Clinic researchers are beginning to ask if rising rates of lupus are the result of an increased exposure to environmental triggers of some unknown origin. Because autoimmune disease is spreading in almost every industrialized nation, scientists the world over have dubbed it "the Western disease."

A GROWING AUTOIMMUNE PATIENT LOAD

While epidemiological studies provide a global portrait of an autoimmune-disease crisis in the making, it is through patients' eyes that it takes on more personal meaning. And nowhere is this more evident than at the offices of Dr. Michelle Petri, clinical director of the Johns Hopkins Lupus Center, at the Johns Hopkins Outpatient Center in downtown Baltimore, Maryland. Dr. Petri is a heavy hitter in the field of rheumatology and a nationally known speaker on lupus. Many of the people she treats have waited months for an appointment in order to confirm a diagnosis or gain better treatment for such rheumatic autoimmune diseases as lupus and antiphospholipid syndrome. Some of them are local residents who live merely a few blocks away from her office, while other patients fly thousands of miles to see her.

On one recent Thursday evening, Dr. Petri has just finished seeing the last of her forty patients for the day. Outside the glass-paneled hallways that stretch along the clinic's waiting area, the afternoon light has long disappeared into the bank of gray clouds that seem to settle at dusk over this downtrodden part of Baltimore. But Petri shows no signs of flagging. A small powerhouse of a woman, Petri's freckled, youthful face and boyish cropped hair contrast with strands of newly appearing gray and gold-framed glasses that hint at years spent bent over medical texts, papers, and lab work. She pushes her glasses up as she peers down at her watch, noting with little surprise that she has clocked another thirteen-hour stint between patients, paperwork, and rounds. Petri missed the first of several of our telephone interviews, scheduled to take place at eight-thirty p.m. one night, because she'd been working such late hours she hadn't been home long enough to realize that her phone was out of order.

Over the course of her thirty-year career, Petri has witnessed a dramatic rise in patients with lupus. In the 1960s there were only 150 to 200 lupus patients registered in the Hopkins Rheumatology Clinics. Today, there are 1,700 lupus patients registered from the immediate neighborhood alone. "The population in Baltimore is going down, and yet the number of people coming to our clinic from Baltimore with autoimmune disease is going up," she says. In an administrative building nearby sits the lupus clinic records room. In the twenty-by-twenty-foot space loom four walls of filing cabinets—enough to easily fill up the four walls in your local 7-Eleven—packed with patient files that, twenty years ago, would have fit neatly into a few metal drawers. Although Petri has no way of conducting formal epidemiologic research through her clinic, the continued rise in the percent of patients afflicted in her own small urban area is, she says, a "very disturbing" sign.

Certainly, some of the increase that Petri and other clinicians are seeing in lupus is due to the improved treatment many patients receive through kidney dialysis and transplants, which help them live longer (the longer patients survive, the larger the overall patient number). And the skill with which physicians diagnose lupus has improved somewhat in many large metropolitan hospital centers. However, this increase in lupus "is so enormous," says Petri, part of it can only be explained by an increase in the incidence of lupus itself.

Petri's emphatic tone reveals her concern for her patients' well-being as well as her frustration over how little physicians understand about why so many people's immune systems are attacking their own healthy tissue. In hopes of helping other doctors catch autoimmune disease earlier in their patients, before irreversible tissue damage has already occurred, Petri spearheads an international task force to rewrite the symptom list and lab criteria for diagnosing lupus.

The fact that so many front-line practitioners are ill trained in how to diagnose these diseases can result in patients facing costly delays—both physically and emotionally—in getting the help they need. As Dr. Ahmet Hoke, associate professor of neurology and neuroscience at Johns Hopkins Medical Institutions and a colleague of Petri's who treats numerous patients with autoimmune neurological disorders, explains, "Most of the autoimmune patients we see here have already been to several doctors and often they've been struggling for diagnoses for years. We see those patients who slip through their doctors' diagnostic fingers."

PATIENTS ON THE SIDELINES

Patients like Jan often feel they pay a high price for the fact that so many doctors remain ignorant of the autoimmune-disease epidemic. "I saw a total of six doctors before I got the diagnosis of APS," Jan says. "And yet relatively speaking I consider myself lucky. I was diagnosed within months of becoming ill. It takes most patients with autoimmune disease years to find a doctor who has enough faith in them to really listen to what they're experiencing." Even then, as we shall see in subsequent chapters of this book, few doctors are well versed in piecing together the moving-target symptoms and in interpreting the complex biomarkers in lab tests that are necessary to accurately diagnose autoimmunity.

Jan pauses as we talk over tea at her kitchen table, the three dogs that she and David have rescued over the past decade settled on the floor around her. As we talk, she glances out the window past the cacti garden she and David have painstakingly planted. For a moment, her short, sandy curls catch sparks of sun reflecting off a truck traversing the dirt road in front of her New Mexico home, and her expression shifts from that of an incredulous patient to steely physician. "The time devoted to autoimmune diseases in medical education is dismally small," she says. "I learned more about syphilis than autoimmune diseases in medical school, and in the twenty years since not much has changed for med students. The sad thing is that there is a huge number of patients out there who are completely off the radar screen of most docs."

For years, one of these patients was Kathleen Arntsen, a forty-four-year-old sales professional from Verona, New York. After five years of searching for a diagnosis for what would turn out later to be myasthenia gravis, a disease in which sufferers develop severe muscle fatigue and disabling weakness, Kathleen was told by a doctor she'd been to eight times, "We've given you every test known to man *except* for an autopsy. Would you like one of those too?" For half a decade, she says, "I was treated like an absolute fruitcake. No one could tell me what was wrong with me, much less treat me."

Arntsen's story is not unusual. The average patient with autoimmune disease sees six doctors before attaining a correct diagnosis. Recent surveys conducted by the American Autoimmune Related Diseases Association reveal that 45 percent of patients with autoimmune diseases have been labeled hypochondriacs in the earliest stages of their illnesses. Some of this, no doubt, has to do with the fact that 75 percent to 80 percent of autoimmune disease sufferers are women, who are more easily dismissed by the medical establishment when hard-to-diagnose symptoms arise. In half of all cases, women with autoimmune disease are told there is nothing wrong with them for an average of five years before receiving diagnosis and treatment. Patients—most especially women—are often left feeling both confused and marginalized, or worse, labeled as psychosomatic malingerers.

Arntsen was fortunate to find her way eventually to Johns Hopkins University's neuromuscular clinic and later to Michelle Petri for confirmation, consultation, and validation regarding her polyautoimmune disorders, which include lupus, Sjögrens, Graves' thyroid disease, APS, psoriasis, Raynaud's disease, and myasthenia gravis. Yet despite having an accurate set of diagnoses, Arntsen's autoimmune illnesses have forced her to give up almost everything she once equated with normal life in order to preserve the stamina to get through each day. Once a healthy young woman on a full scholarship to Colgate University, where she was captain of the women's rugby team, Arntsen now has to stop and pick up each knee as she goes up the stairs. "I coexist," she says, "with bone-gnawing pain." For years, her long flame of red hair, which once reached her tailbone, turned scarce and thin, the fallout of her autoimmune thyroiditis, coupled with drug side effects. In the past decade she has spent almost a year and a half in the hospital during her most severe lupus flares. Although she is carefully monitored, there is little the medical establishment can offer Kathleen for her lupus and myasthenia gravis other than steroids, a healthy diet, and boatloads of rest—especially since no new U.S. Food and Drug Administration–approved drugs have been developed for lupus in more than forty years.

Kathleen's debility and exhaustion, which have taken a permanent toll on her life and career, will never go away. A top-performing sales rep for an insurance company while in her thirties, Arntsen, who used to run three miles a day, now lives on Social Security disability—which, she says ruefully, allows time for "my new full-time job—seeing specialists." She gets going each day by around noon and spends what stamina she has left volunteering at the Lupus Foundation of Mid and Northern New York, which has become her "baby," although it can hardly begin to make up for the fact that "the chance to be a mother has been stolen from me." The best Kathleen and her husband of fifteen years can hope for is that with the careful monitoring of diet, stress, and sleep, she will have more good days than bad.

To look at Kathleen, however, you would never guess what she has been through or what she faces each morning at the start of her day. Like many people who suffer from autoimmune diseases, Kathleen's symptoms remain largely invisible. And as was the case with cancer several decades ago, those who have the disease tend not to talk about it.

"People don't see what lies behind the scenes in most autoimmune diseases," she says. "Because we go through ups and downs, you might see us on a good day, between severe flares, when we seem to be perfectly fine. You don't know that we've just spent six weeks in hell." Few can imagine, she adds, that behind her bedroom door even on one of these good days, Kathleen has to take twenty-two medications about an hour before she tries to get up, just so she can handle the pain when her feet hit the floor. "By the time you run into me at the grocery store at two o'clock in the afternoon and say hello to me, I'm ready to nod and say, 'Oh, I'm fine, how are you?' " Kathleen worries, she says, that because autoimmune disease so often remains hidden from public view, she and other women like her will continue to be stigmatized as malingerers.

A CASE OF BLINDED SCIENCE

How is it that autoimmune diseases have remained so obscure? Why do so many of these diseases go undiagnosed for so long, and why do we have so little comfort and treatment to offer the patients who suffer from them? The answers to these questions require a step back in time, to half a century ago.

The medical age of wonders began seventy years ago, and what an age of miracles it was. When my own grandfather, C. Donald Larsen, a research biochemist and founding member of the National Cancer Institute, served as head of the cancer research grants program at the National Institutes of Health in 1955, he walked into medical laboratory settings every day that, world over, boasted little more than test tubes, microscopes, and Bunsen burners. As a young thirty-eight-year-old scientist in 1939, he had already become world renowned for being the first to demonstrate that cancer-causing chemicals could pass through the placenta and later cause tumors in offspring. Yet his was only one small speck of discovery in the burgeoning age of miracles.

In the span of the next thirty to forty years scientists discovered a range of antibiotics, invented vaccines that would wipe out polio and prevent hundreds of thousands of deaths from rubella and typhus, and America began the war on cancer. Heart surgeons were opening up chest cavities in living patients and transplanting hearts, pacemakers were invented, and neonatal care began to save infants so small it seemed God's hand had reached down from heaven itself and snatched them from death.

Yet, ironically, during the same time span in which cures for ancient scourges were tumbling out of laboratories, the medical establishment had no idea that autoimmune diseases even existed. Scientists, in general, were clinging to an erroneous presumption that the body's immune system could not turn on itself; researchers were convinced that an autoimmune response was simply not possible. This presumption—set forth in the early 1900s by Nobel laureate Paul Ehrlich, a charismatic German immunologist who termed this theory *horror autotoxicus*—stood as dogma across the immunology domain for more than half a century.

It would take a young PhD and dedicated medical student to slowly begin to turn the theory of *horror autotoxicus* upside down. In 1951, as a newly minted twenty-three-year-old PhD from the University of Pennsylvania, Noel Rose and his pregnant wife, Deborah, packed all their meager belongings into the back of an ancient, rear-dragging Oldsmobile station wagon and journeyed north from Philadelphia to the State University of New York at Buffalo. Back then, the little-explored and poorly understood domain of immunology—the study of how the immune system functions in the body—was hardly a bustling field, and few labs existed where a young PhD could go to complete his medical studies in the field, much less support a new wife and coming child.

Today Rose, a genteel seventy-nine-year-old whose generous smile spreads nearly as wide as his signature bow tie, serves as director of the Center for Autoimmune Disease Research at the Johns Hopkins School of Medicine and Bloomberg School of Public Health. Back then, Rose considered himself fortunate to receive an invitation from Ernest Witebsky and his immunology team at the University of Buffalo to serve as a junior faculty member. Part of the appeal of moving to Buffalo was the fact that Witebsky was the scientific grandson of Nobel laureate Paul Ehrlich. Ernest Witebsky was a student of Hans Sachs, who, in turn, had been one of Paul Ehrlich's principal protégés. Witebsky was the inheritor of the Ehrlich mantle and was universally recognized as a vigorous champion of the *horror autotoxicus* theory.

Assigned one part-time assistant and a ten-by-ten office that also served as his lab, Rose set to work. At Witebsky's request, Rose was seeking to prepare a pure form of thyroglobulin, the major protein of the thyroid gland, in a natural, unadulterated form for use in other experiments Witebsky was busy conducting at the time. Rose had worked with rabbits for years, and all those long hours spent amidst rabbit cages had led him to develop a severe allergy to rabbit fur. He often had to wear a mask in order to help circumvent an asthma attack. Nevertheless, Rose quickly succeeded.

In one of the final steps involved in creating this pure thyroglobulin and assuring it was not altered, Rose injected that thyroglobulin—derived from rabbit thyroids—back into his rabbits. Later, however, when he examined the rabbit thyroids, he was shocked by what he saw. The rabbit thyroids were inflamed—and that should not have happened. They had produced antibodies to the thyroglobulin and developed lesions in their thyroids. Thyroid lesions signaled that the presence of an antigen—a foreign invader that is capable of causing the production of an antibody—had caused the rabbits' immune systems to turn on and destroy their own thyroid tissue. Almost all of the rabbits had slowly developed a disease that mimicked the human disorder known as Hashimoto's thyroiditis. Although Hashimoto's was already a recognized disease in 1951, its cause had remained unknown. That Hashimoto's might be caused by the immune system attacking the cells of the thyroid was a concept that stood completely at odds with *horror autotoxicus*. Yet in that small postdoc lab, fifty years ago, Rose was staring at proof positive of autoimmune disease—a completely revolutionary idea at the time.

"I sat there for a long time, looking at the results with a mixture of awe and fear," Rose recalls. "It was one of those marvelous and rare eureka moments in science when you realize that you're on the edge of an important new discovery. But I was also afraid. I realized that it would be difficult to convince my mentor as well as the world that I was right."

For the next several years, Rose worked, at Witebsky's urging, to run his experiments again and again to correct for any possible errors. Finally, Witebsky too became convinced: when an antigen from the thyroid gland was introduced into the body, the body's fighter antibodies could mistakenly damage the patient's own cells in devastating blasts of self-sabotage, resulting in thyroid diseases such as Hashimoto's and hypothyroidism. Together, Rose and Witebsky published their findings.

By 1957, the concept of autoimmune disease was born—though it would be another ten years or more before it was accepted. Yet despite Rose's startling discovery—and despite the growing number of scientists whose quiet work would, over the next several decades, substantiate his findings—medical schools continued to churn out specialists who were taught *horror auto-toxicus*: the body's immune system could *not* develop an autoimmune response. For Rose, it was a train wreck in the making: while fellow scientists could and should have been ferreting out potential causes for autoimmune disease, no one was even on the case.

It was a classic case of what twentieth-century scientific philosopher Thomas Kuhn once termed "normal science." Science is conservative in nature, unwilling to abandon ideas without persuasive evidence. The overwhelming majority of scientists accept a single scientific ideology as the starting point from which they form their own viewpoint—the pathway from which they view the entire scientific landscape—to the degree that they cannot overturn that ideology, even if research begins to show that it is blatantly leading them astray.

It wasn't for another decade that scientists around the country began to wake up—at first one by one, and then in droves—to what Rose and his colleagues had long known: autoimmune responses could be triggered to affect virtually every organ and system of the body. Meanwhile, as this startling autoimmune connection came to light, different groups of specialists quickly scrambled to claim whole sets of diseases as their own. Rheumatologists, discovering that the root cause of rheumatoid arthritis was the body attacking and inflaming its own tissue, claimed arthritis, lupus, and all other joint-related autoimmune illnesses as rheumatologic disorders. Neurologists, discovering that in a whole host of diseases—MS, myasthenia gravis, myositis, Guillain-Barré syndrome—the body was destroying parts of its neuromuscular system, became designated specialists in those diseases. Likewise, bowel disorders—Crohn's disease, ulcerative colitis, and inflammatory bowel disease—were farmed out to the gastroenterologists.

By the early 1970s autoimmunity was finally an accepted precept—and yet there was no one standing on the mountaintop, looking down at these various specialists' fiefdoms and seeing how the roads leading to them intersected or asking what the common biological origins or treatments for these diseases might be.

Certainly no one was asking what triggered these diseases. What was wreaking havoc with the intricate inner workings of the human immune system in populations throughout the industrialized world?

In fact, up until the mid 1990s, no one had bothered to figure out how many Americans had an autoimmune disease. Numbers on how many Americans have each type of cancer in each state have been collected by the National Cancer Institute since 1973; the National Center for Health Statistics and the Centers for Disease Control have collected data on cancer since the early 1900s. Yet it was only a decade ago that scientists first began to cast about for a general sense of how many Americans might be afflicted with autoimmune disease. In 1995, Noel Rose approached Virginia Ladd, president of the then fledgling American Autoimmune Related Diseases Association (AARDA), the only autoimmune advocacy organization that encompasses all of the autoimmune diseases, and said, "We have *got* to find the numbers." Ladd, a small but determined gray-haired dynamo who had founded the organization, was able to come up with only five thousand dollars to fund the project, a paltry sum in the high-roller arena of scientific research. With that, Rose hired a PhD candidate, giving her about a month to ferret out how many patients had each of the twenty-five autoimmune diseases they would be counting. Two years later, Rose's student came up for air with the astounding statistic that 9 million patients were suffering from those twenty-five autoimmune diseases alone—as many patients as had cancer.

In what is called the epidemiology of epidemiology, Rose and his PhD candidate were able to take those figures and extrapolate to the fifty-five other recognized autoimmune diseases that had not yet been included in their study. They arrived at the figure of 22 million—one in twelve people—who were being taken down by an enemy within. Twenty-two million, for a set of diseases no one was looking at, was a startling statistic.

Since that time, NIH has revised that number to be as high as 23.5 million as more diseases are recognized as autoimmune and are added to the tally. Still, say many advocates, the actual number of patients may be far higher: a recent NIH report states that many autoimmune patients are never properly diagnosed. And existing epidemiological studies on how many individuals have each autoimmune disease have been sparse at best.

One of the more interesting diseases that is not yet officially under the autoimmune umbrella lies in the field of cardiology, where researchers have recently shown that the autoimmune process is deeply implicated in atherosclerosis—the narrowing and hardening of the arteries from the slow buildup of plaque—which is implicated in 1.2 million heart attacks a year. In 2005, Mayo Clinic researchers reported that rheumatoid arthritis patients carry twice the risk of heart failure as other patients. Other studies show similar elevated risk of heart disease among patients with lupus, diabetes, and MS. Researchers believe that some of the genetic variants that predispose a patient to autoimmune disease are the same genetic variants that predispose a patient to heart disease.

Although the exact means by which autoimmune disease is

linked to atherosclerosis is only now becoming clear, significant evidence suggests that somewhere in the disease sequence—the cascade of plaque building up on the arterial wall, inflammation, the rise of C-reactive protein levels, and the atherosclerotic plaque erupting—an immune response against the self is involved, just as in autoimmune disease in other parts of the body. Researchers believe that the triggering event may be viral. Recent studies show that in artherosclerosis the body's immune cells mount an attack against the proteins in a common virus, cytomegalovirus, and in the process become confused, mistakenly attacking the arterial walls themselves.

Michelle Petri, who is involved in a trial to treat lupus patients prophylactically with Lipitor, a potent anticholesterol drug thought to lower the risk of heart attack, says that "the risk is fifty times greater of having a heart attack if you have lupus."

The concern here extends beyond the autoimmune patients who may develop heart disease. It encompasses those with atherosclerosis who do not know that autoimmunity is involved in their disease and who may be unaware that they are more susceptible to other autoimmune diseases as well.

THE POSTWAR CHEMICAL EXPLOSION: A NEW PLAGUE OF AUTOGENS

During the four or five decades that science lingered at the side-lines—at best, underinvestigating autoimmune disease, at worst, ignoring it—another cultural drama was unfolding in America, the portentous ramifications of which were also slipping under the national radar. Throughout the exact same decades that science was dismissing autoimmunity, the wheels of big industry were moving into high gear across the American landscape, augmenting the greatest industrial growth spurt of all time.

All across America, production plants were starting to spring up in town after town, as corporations ramped up production of thousands of novel products manufactured through brilliantly efficient new chemical processes. New pesticides were being introduced to boost crop yields, prolong the shelf life of produce, keep lice, fleas, roaches, and termites out of the home, and zap dandelions from the lawn. Ingenious new chemicals were starting to be employed to help manufacture everything Americans demanded to make their lives easier, simpler, and more luxurious—from plastics to hair shampoo, detergents, brake linings, carpet pads, cold creams, dry cleaning fluid, foam cushions, paint strippers, household cleansers and bleaches, and bigger, grander cars. Almost overnight, Americans began to find themselves inundated with and clamoring for the suburban home products, packaged goods, and manufactured foods churned out by mega-industry. Over four short decades—between 1940 and 1980—factory plumes came to shroud small towns, fleets of trucks spewed diesel exhaust as they transported a myriad of newly manufactured goods from coast to coast, and the ChemLawn truck began to circle the cul-de-sacs in neighborhood after neighborhood.

The coincidence in timing—between a medical community turning a blind eye to a mysterious, growing set of diseases with an unknown set of triggers and a society's rapid swell in production of everything from SUVs to Teflon pans to furniture stuffed with flame-retardant foam—would turn out to be an ominous one, altering the well-being of millions of Americans.

Together, these two seemingly unrelated trends would set in place two of the key factors that would establish a "perfect storm" enabling an autoimmune epidemic to gather force and take hold. And both would go far in explaining not only why millions of autoimmune sufferers like Jan Pankey and Kathleen Arntsen would be underdiagnosed, undertreated, and marginalized once they did become ill, but why their bodies were so much more likely to turn against their own healthy tissue in an autoimmune reaction in the first place.

For nearly half a century, as big industry flourished, scientists sat idle in the lull of a gathering storm, not only missing today's autoimmune disease epidemic in the making but blinded to its possible causes.

During these same decades, the idea that chemicals from our industrial age could trigger cancer would become so widely accepted that the term "carcinogens" would emerge as a household word by the 1970s. But science would be sluggish to accept the idea that chemicals could have similar effects on the human immune system. So slow that, even to this day, there still exists no comparable word to "carcinogens" in the world of immunology. The best we can do to describe the notion that environmental chemicals might be linked to autoimmunity is to use the clunky phrase "environmental autoimmune disease triggers," which is analogous to saying "environmental cancer disease triggers" instead of, simply, "carcinogens." The term "autogen," I believe, might prove useful for this purpose, and I will use that term to describe chemical triggers to autoimmune disease throughout the remainder of this book.

It would, in fact, be 2005 before the head of one of the most prestigious research institutes in the country would herald the call, stating that the link between autoimmune disease and environmental contaminants from our manufacturing age had become "the next tobacco and cancer." Research results would begin to mount, showing that it is the very chemical by-products of the goods we demand to live more convenient lives that are sabotaging the blueprint of how our bodies are meant to interact with Mother Nature. But getting this claim to be taken seriously was going to prove a very tough sell.

CHAPTER TWO

THE INVISIBLE INVADERS:
THE DRIVING FORCE BEHIND
THIS EPIDEMIC

A light is going on in the upstairs bedroom window of a small yellow Cape Cod on Pine Street in the suburbs of Richmond, Virginia. Becky Sandler's* newborn, Zachary, is awake again, his high-decibel cry filling the house. Becky rolls over and lifts him from his bassinet to nurse, and Zachary's wails subside as he moves toward total satiation, suckling in the healthiest food source on the planet.

Becky considers trying to sleep for a few more seconds but the day has begun. Rising from the queen-size mattress with the "comfort sleep" foam padding on top that she and her husband purchased over the weekend, Becky gets up to face an array of domestic tasks. She is aided in these by a range of twenty-first-century products and conveniences that help to simplify her life.

This particular Tuesday is a fairly typical day for the Sandlers. Rick Sandler is traveling on business. Becky, on maternity leave, is home with the kids. She whips up pancakes on her nonstick Teflon

---

* In order to retain their privacy, Becky Sandler, her family, and their experiences are a composite of interviews of two families.

griddle for her four-year-old daughter, Selena, then slices strawberries and cantaloupe on top and squeezes on a dollop of syrup. A piece of cantaloupe, she notes, has fallen from Selena's plate to the tile floor, and a small line of ants—the same ants that have plagued her kitchen all summer—are veering in that direction. The house is sprayed yearly for termites, but she hasn't yet called their pest-control company about the ants. Spraying means leaving the house with the kids for the day, to be on the safe side, and she can't figure out when a good day for that might be.

A burning chemical smell suddenly assails her nostrils: the pancakes. A thin wisp of gray smoke rises up from the Teflon pan's edges, emitting a chemical stench so intense that Becky throws open the kitchen window, batting the air with her hands.

Half an hour later they arrive at Selena's preschool. Becky stands holding Selena's hand, with Zach strapped to her chest in a baby carrier, at the crosswalk, waiting for the light to change. A bus pulls out in front of them, spewing a blast of diesel exhaust. A few seconds later a delivery truck rumbles by, letting out another diesel belch.

Inside the classroom, Becky waves as Selena races outside onto the playground, eager to clamber on a new wooden pirate ship climber that has just been built. On the way back out of the preschool, Zachary drops his pacifier and begins to fuss. An advocate of the five-second rule, Becky brushes it off on her shirt and gives it to him, hoping to stave off his hunger until she can breastfeed him again in the car.

After drop-off, there are errands to run, first to the dry cleaners, then to the mall to pick up Becky's moisturizer, which she has been out of for days. Then to her hairdresser, to have her roots dyed auburn, as she does by rote every six weeks. On the way back to pick up Selena she stops to fill up the tank of her hybrid SUV, then on to McDonald's to pick up a Happy Meal with the newest Happy Meal toy for Selena's lunch. As she pulls into her driveway, the lawn company is pulling away, having just sprayed weed killer on the crabgrass and dandelions that threaten to ruin the lawn.

Later, after lunch, both children take a midday nap, Zach in his bassinet, Selena on Becky's bed. The dry-cleaned garments hang on the bedroom closet door a few feet away, the cosmetics have been bought, and Becky's roots are a sleek red-brown again. She has called the dentist because one of her mercury fillings has been aching whenever she drinks something cold or hot. And she has also managed to microwave a cup of noodle soup for her lunch in its disposable bowl, throw a load of baby clothes in the dryer, put tick and flea killer on the dog's neck, and scour out the toilet and shower tiles with a foaming bathroom cleaner she doesn't like to use when the children are up and about because the label carries a warning that reads "hazardous to humans and domestic animals" and the fumes make her feel woozy.

Next, she turns to stripping the paint off a child-sized chair and table she found in a thrift shop, which she is refinishing for her daughter's birthday. When the job is done she takes advantage of the children's nap to fix a broken plastic horse with a bottle of contact cement that boasts of being "the strongest glue on the planet." Just as she is putting the horse's leg back on, the children wake up. Becky sits down to feed Zach while Selena plays Reader Rabbit Preschool on the computer. Zach is cooing at the sounds emitting from the monitor, or maybe it's the sight of the bottle of breast milk—which Becky pumped the night before in anticipation of a moment just like this, when her milk might run low, and then warmed up in the microwave—that's making him so excited. It is, by and large, a happy scene. All in all, from Becky's point of view, her Tuesday with her children has been pretty great.

If you were to view Becky Sandler's life from the vantage point of the cells of her immune system, however, which are working diligently to distinguish Becky from everything "not-Becky" in order to protect her against foreign invaders and infections, her Tuesday with her children would not appear so idyllic. From the perspective of Becky's immune cells, it is one more day of bombardment by chemical and industrial agents, forcing her immune system to stay poised on high alert. Each time Becky came into contact with a new irritant, her body engaged in an exquisite chain reaction of cellular events, making split-second decisions as to whether it needed to fight these foreign invaders or not. Throughout this Tuesday, like every day, Becky's body labored to keep her tissue and organs from being adversely affected by all the external substances that she came into contact with.

Becky and Rick are more environmentally minded than most—they recycle, drive a hybrid, and avoid fumigating for pests around their children. They are also healthier than most, except perhaps for the fact that Becky has Raynaud's disease, a quite mild autoimmune disorder that causes her fingers to turn white and cold from lack of circulation. But Raynaud's does not affect her except when she's exposed to sudden changes in temperature or to emotional stress. Selena, like nearly a fifth of her preschool class, has eczema and food allergies (dairy and tree nuts), but other than that, the Sandlers are all quite healthy.

Becky would no doubt be surprised, then, to learn how many noxious, invisible chemicals are quietly entering her family's bloodstreams every day, silently lodging in their cells, fat tissue, and, in Becky's case, her breast milk. Many of these contaminants—the by-products of our modern manufacturing chemical age—are familiar to immunotoxicologists, who study the effects of chemicals on the immune system, and are known to interfere with the intricately calibrated workings of our immune cells.

THE BURDEN OF CHEMICALS WE ALL CARRY IN OUR BODIES

For decades, scientists have been studying pollutants in the air, water, and on land. But over the past five years, they have begun studying pollution in people, and the findings are causing many researchers to reevaluate their assumptions about how successfully our bodies interface with the chemical-laden world in which we live. The most telling work detailing what contaminants are entering our bodies and how much toxicity accumulates in our cells and bloodstreams over time comes from a 2003 study by the Mount Sinai School of Medicine in New York City, in collaboration with the Environmental Working Group (EWG), an advocacy organization in Washington, D.C. Their findings reveal the "body burden" of environmental chemicals and heavy metals carried by the average American. After testing the blood and urine of nine representative Americans from around the country for 210 substances (sample groups are small as these tests are prohibitively expensive), these scientists discovered that each volunteer carried an average of 91 industrial compounds, pollutants, and other chemicals—including PCBs, commonly used insecticides, dioxin, mercury, cadmium, and benzene, to name just a few. This plethora of chemicals had accumulated in these individuals through the common and minute exposures that we all experience in our daily lives. None of the test participants had worked with chemicals on the job; none had lived near an industrial facility. Yet the average participant had detectable levels of 53 known immune system–suppressing chemicals in their bloodstreams and in their urine.

In 2004, the Centers for Disease Control and Prevention (CDC) in Atlanta conducted a similar study testing blood and urine samples of 2,500 people across the country. The CDC found traces of all 116 chemicals they looked for. Then, in 2005, a set of findings emerged that shocked toxicologists around the world. Researchers working through two major laboratories found an alarming cocktail of 287 industrial chemicals and pollutants in the fetal cord blood of ten newborn infants from around the country, in samples taken by the American Red Cross. These chemicals included pesticides, phthalates, dioxins, flame retardants, and breakdown chemicals of Teflon, among other chemicals known to damage the immune system. Shortly after, investigators in the Netherlands turned up similar findings: they discovered an array of chemicals commonly found in household cleaners, cosmetics, and furniture in the cord blood of thirty newborns.

OUR AUTOGEN-FILLED WORLD: HOW DID WE BECOME SO CONTAMINATED?

How do these chemicals creep into our bodies? The process occurs through the simple exposures to contaminants in our world that most of us rarely think twice about. Consider the substances that Becky came into contact with in just one day.

Becky wakes up on her new mattress—with the luxurious foam pad on top—both of which have been manufactured, as have all U.S. bedding materials, with a flame-retardant known as poly-brominated diphenyl ethers, or PBDEs. PBDEs are chemicals that manufacturers use to mix or coat almost every single product that surrounds you. Consider what you sit on throughout your day: your chairs, mattresses, pillows, the foam cushions in your cars and sofas. Airline seats and airplane plastic and fabric interiors are drenched in flame retardants to meet safety standards. Add to these exposures the ones from your footwear, the insulation in your walls, and the plastic in your computer, video monitor, BlackBerry, and TV. All these have been made with plastics or furniture parts soaked in and manufactured with PBDEs.

In the 1950s, during the heyday of the American industrial revolution, a singular new invention, polyurethane, began beefing up manufacturing profit margins as it scaled up the comfort level of the American home. Polyurethane, a thermoplastic polymer, was both inexpensive and malleable. It began to be used in novel ways in resins, coatings, insulation, adhesives, foams, and fibers—from refrigerator and wall insulation to upholstered foam chairs and sofas. But there was one drawback: it was also highly flammable. Starting in the 1970s, consumer protection laws were put in place to treat all polymer products with flame retardants. PBDEs began to be used liberally in manufactured goods as the chemical indus-try's insurance policy that your furniture, bedding, pajamas, and carpet—all of which are highly flammable—would not go up in a burst of flame if there happened to be an electrical short while you slept or if you should mistakenly knock over a candle while doing your crossword puzzle in bed. But PBDEs had their own downside. They are not molecularly bound to anything in the products into which they're manufactured. As a result, they continually leach out from the plastics that make up our computers, TVs, and wire insulation, the insides of our window frames, the upholstery, carpets, and clothing we buy, and the lint from the clothes dryer into the air around us. From there they do not waft away in the breeze or disappear; instead, they fall to the floor and attach to the minuscule bits of dust in our homes. One recent study found PBDEs in every single sample of dust evaluated from seventy homes across seven states from New York to California. A separate study of seventeen homes conducted by the National Institute of Standards and Technology found disturbingly high concentrations of PBDEs in household dust and dryer lint.

From our floors, this chemical-laden dust is then kicked up into the air, where it is inhaled into our bodies. Babies and toddlers, who have the highest levels of PBDEs, ingest even greater levels because they chew on plastic toys, drop them in that invisible household dust, and then pick them up and mouth on them again (think of Zachary's dropped pacifier, and suddenly the five-second rule loses its appeal).

Thirty years ago, Swedish researchers decided to start testing nursing women to find out whether these ubiquitous chemicals could be found in women's breast milk, and, if so, whether levels of flame retardants in breast milk were rising. They discovered, to their alarm, that levels of PBDEs in nursing moms have doubled every five years. In 2003, a study of twenty first-time American mothers found that PBDE levels in U.S. women are much higher than those found in Swedish women, indicating that Americans' exposures to PBDEs may be particularly worrisome. Overall, levels of PBDEs in the general population of the United States are ten to one hundred times higher than levels found in individuals living in Europe. Other recent studies show that levels of PBDEs are rising in humans at an alarming rate, doubling every two to five years.

In 2004, U.S. manufacturers agreed with the Environmental Protection Agency to stop making and selling two potent forms of

PBDEs known as penta-BDEs and octa-BDEs. However, these continue to leach out from goods manufactured prior to that time, as well as circulate into the air, soil, and sediment, which is why they continue to be commonly detected in our fruits, vegetables, meats, and dairy products. Deca-BDEs, the most commonly used subgroup of PBDEs, remain in wide use because they were thought to be less easily absorbed into the body. Recently, however, investigators have found that even deca-BDEs turn into the more easily absorbed and toxic penta-BDEs as they degrade in the environment around us.

Meanwhile, we know far less than we need to about the direct effect of these chemicals on the immune system. While chemical companies have to divulge information if their chemicals have been found to be carcinogenic in lab testing, no such testing and reporting are required on whether chemicals act as autogens and damage the human immune system. While debates brew between the chemical industry, which argues that these exposures are safe for humans, and the growing number of scientists investigating their damaging effects, recent published studies on PBDEs have not been reassuring. The CDC's website now informs concerned consumers that PBDEs may indeed impair the cells of the immune system in animal studies.

Let's look at some of the other culprits Becky encountered in her day, such as Teflon, pesticides, and plastics. At breakfast, Becky's favorite no-hassle, stick-free Teflon pan is sending up gaseous fumes. Teflon is manufactured with a chemical known as perfluorooctanoic acid, or PFOA—as are other nonstick cookware, car parts, flooring, computer chips, phone cables, Stainmaster carpet guard, upholstery, clothing, grease-resistant french fry boxes, and disposable coffee cups like the ones you get at your local coffee shop. PFOA can also now be found in blood samples of 96 percent of people in the United States. It does not break down in the environment and has a half-life of 4.4 years in humans.

A chemical's half-life is important because it is the measure of how long it takes a pollutant to break down to half of its initial amount. Because we are constantly exposed to PFOA, it always resides within us—we never have a chance to break down, metabolize, and excrete all that we are exposed to. As with PBDEs, we do not know much about what PFOA does in or to the body. In 2005, the Environmental Protection Agency (EPA) determined that even low-level exposure to PFOA poses "a potential risk of developmental and other adverse effects" on human health. In one recent and provocative paper from Stockholm University's Unit for Biochemical Toxicology, investigators were unable to find a dose that *didn't* alter the function of our immune cells at each major step that the immune system takes in mounting a defense to protect us against foreign antigens. Despite such evidence, manufacturers of the chemical maintain that PFOA does not pose a health risk to humans, citing a lack of sufficient evidence.

Consider now the strawberries and cantaloupe Becky prepares for breakfast. Prior to arriving on her daughter's plate they have been sprayed repeatedly with insecticides to help protect their skins from pests both in the field and during transit to Becky's local grocery store, where she bought them wholly unblemished. Back on the farm, this cantaloupe, like most cantaloupes, was treated with organochlorine pesticides—in this case, a type known as endosulfan. Commonly used today on melons, traces of endosulfan are found in the food we eat more than any other pesticide. In one recent study—which found that 100 percent of pregnant women now carry numerous pesticides in their placentas—endosulfan was found to be present at the highest concentration of any organochlorine pesticide. Like PFOA, organochlorine pesticides such as endosulfan also affect the immune system. Indeed, if you were to do a search on "endosulfan and immune system" on the National Library of Medicine's Internet database, PubMed, you would receive twenty hits detailing the link between endosulfan and immune system dysfunction. While a few well-known organochlorine insecticides that are notoriously injurious to animals—DDT, for example—have been banned in the United States, even these persist for decades in the soil in which our fruits and vegetables are grown and in our water, meanwhile accumulating up the food chain (which is why traces of DDT can be found in the steaks Becky has yet to cook for dinner).

Hundreds of other pesticides and insecticides remain in regular use, including herbicides such as atrazine (which Becky's lawn company sprays on her yard), and termiticides (which the local pest-control company uses to liberally spray the foundation, cracks, and crevices of Becky's house every year). For the dog, there is tick and flea killer: more pesticides. In the Mount Sinai study examining what chemicals are found in the average American, every single participant carried detectable levels of pesticides that have been banned, like DDT, as well as a wide range of pesticides in liberal use today. A mixture of twenty-one pesticides was found in the umbilical cord blood of every single newborn baby tested.

Immunologists, meanwhile, are trying to ascertain what happens to the immune systems of lab mice when they expose them to organochlorine pesticides such as DDT and methoxychlor, the latter having been manufactured as a safer replacement for DDT and now being used widely on food crops, home gardens, and as flea and tick control on pets. They do not like what they see.

In a 2005 study, six researchers at the University of Florida College of Medicine in Gainesville set out to discover whether mice exposed to organochlorine pesticides would be more prone to develop autoimmune disease. Mice have long been known to possess the genetic potential to develop autoimmunity; like some 25 percent of humans, certain mice possess more of the genes that make them susceptible to autoimmune diseases such as lupus—that is, if and when they meet up with the right environmental trigger. Since autoimmune disease primarily affects women, over the past twenty years researchers have used female mice as the litmus-test lab animal for determining whether a chemical pollutant might cause or exacerbate autoimmune disease. The disease most easily distinguishable in mice is lupus—which means that the gold standard in the laboratory for ascertaining whether a pollutant might cause autoimmunity in humans is to see if it causes lupus in genetically-at-risk female mice.

Every single one of the female mice that the Gainsville team exposed to organochlorine pesticides rapidly developed the autoimmune disease lupus, while none of the mice in the control group did. The presence of these pesticides "markedly influenced" the progression of autoimmune disease, resulting in elevated levels of lupus autoantibodies. "It is worthwhile noting," say the study's authors, that the lower dose of the organochlorine pesticide methoxychlor that mice were exposed to was "4-fold lower" than the level set by the Environmental Protection Agency as acceptable. This suggests, say the authors, that the commonly used pesticide methoxychlor might stimulate autoimmunity at a much lower dose than doses necessary to cause other adverse health effects, and is "therefore of particular interest for risk assessment."

Pesticide manufacturers dismiss the idea that pesticides pose health risks, arguing that it is an extrapolation to say that a given exposure that leads to disease in mice will do the same in humans. Yet occupational studies that link groups of people who work with pesticides to higher rates of autoimmune disease tell us that such an association clearly exists. In one 2007 study, researchers studied data from over 300,000 death certificates in 26 states over a 14-year period to examine the association between a person's occupational exposures and their risk of dying from a systemic autoimmune disease such as lupus, rheumatoid arthritis, or scleroderma. Their findings were stark: farmers who worked with crops—and who were therefore more exposed to pesticides—were more likely to die from an autoimmune disease. In another study, rural farmers who had a lifetime exposure to organochlorine pesticides had a greater likelihood of having a high antinuclear antibody, or ANA, count— the telltale diagnostic sign that the immune system is turning against the organs and tissue of the body itself in the autoimmune disease lupus. In yet another research finding, farmers who reported mixing pesticides for agricultural work were significantly more likely to suffer from lupus. Despite such danger signals, in the United States we apply greater quantities of pesticides, such as the weed killer atrazine, to suburban tracts than to agricultural land. Just think back again to Becky, who pulled into her suburban driveway just as the lawn company was pulling away after spraying the crab-grass and dandelions.

Throughout Becky's day, we can trace chemical triggers that tax her immune system and those of her children. As Becky and her children prepare to cross the street in the morning, they are blasted with microparticle bursts of exhaust from a diesel bus, then a truck. Within that diesel exhaust exist a host of extremely small particles that are well absorbed by the body, where they move from the lungs to enter the bloodstream. There is mounting evidence that this air pollution we inhale may cause an erratic response in our immune cells, leading to an elevated death rate of immune cells in some laboratory tests, exacerbating autoimmune disease or leading to immune-system dysfunction in others. Recent studies also show that mice exposed to fine particles of pollution at concentration levels equal to those found in the air in major metropolitan areas are more likely to develop atherosclerosis, which researchers now believe involves an autoimmune response.

One of the most potent by-products of exhaust fumes is dioxin, which is carried into the air by the fuel combustion of diesel trucks and buses. Dioxin is also produced through the industrial manufacturing of bleached fibers for paper and textiles, in the production of wood preservatives, chlorinated pesticides and herbicides, and in the manufacturing process of virtually every type of plastic and bleached or resin-coated food packaging that you can find lining the aisles of your neighborhood supermarket. We each receive some small, additional daily dose of dioxin through our steady diet of seafood, meat, and dairy. Like DDT and PCBs, when dioxins are released into the atmosphere (as they are in manufacturing, as well as through the burning of trash, hospital debris, and trees), they become attached to particles and fall back down to earth, where they are consumed by fish and other animals and concentrated and stored in their fat—before eventually ending up on our dinner plates. All nine people tested by Mount Sinai researchers tested positive for blood levels of dioxin, and every infant's cord blood carried dioxin.

Dioxin is a recognized immune suppressor. It has long been known to cross the placenta from animals to their unborn and is increasingly linked to cancer and developmental effects. But recently researchers have observed that dioxin may work in more complex ways on the immune system as well—not only by suppressing immune cells, but by overcoming control mechanisms that should prevent an autoimmune response. In lab studies, when female rodents are exposed to dioxin during gestation, their offspring go on to develop autoimmune disease after being born. Other research is examining the role everyday exposure to dioxin may play in increasing the likelihood that an autoimmune response will be set in motion in general.

One of the complex aspects of understanding how autoimmunity works—and why chemicals can act as autogens, triggering autoimmune disease—involves comprehending the intricate way in which immune cells are schooled. T cells are made in the bone marrow. From the bone marrow they move to the thymus, a butterfly-shaped organ situated over the heart in the center of the upper chest, right behind your sternum, or breastbone. It is in the thymus that T cells mature before they enter your bloodstream. You might think of the thymus, in fact, as a kind of a military training school—one housing both an undergraduate training school for cadets as well as an officer training school. Millions of T cells are "educated" in your thymus to perform specific roles—such as, say, to recognize and eradicate an infiltrating influenza-A germ or food-borne bacteria like salmonella from your body, as well as hundreds of other antigens with which your body may come into contact. Some of the cells in the thymus, however, undergo a more sophisticated sort of education—a kind of officer training program if you will. They are schooled, instead, in a different class altogether and become regulatory T cells. Regulatory T cells do pretty much what their name implies: they act as the senior officers of the other T cells, in this case ensuring that educated T cells will not mistake the body for a foreign antigen and turn against the body's own organs or tissue as they diligently scour the body for invading agents. You might think of them as the officers who make sure that T cells perform their military training exercises just right.

Scientists aren't completely sure how, in a perfectly healthy immune system, these teacher or regulatory T cells neutralize other

T cells so that they almost never erroneously target your own tissue in an autoimmune response (or, as scientists put it, so that all T cells stay "tolerant" of your body's own cells). They do know, however, that when regulatory T cells lack a proper education, or when regulatory T cells are not formed in sufficient quantity in the thymus, antigen-seeking T cells can be suddenly freed to wreak havoc in the body, turning on both foreign antigens and body tissue at will, with nothing to tell them to stop.

Understanding the way in which T cells work in the body is key to comprehending why chemicals such as dioxin and PCBs, as well as other substances, can be so damaging to the immune system and lead to autoimmunity. There are several things that can cause the thymus to atrophy, or decrease in size, which in turn leads to an insufficient number of these regulatory T cells being educated to keep an eye on other T cells. Pregnancy is one of them—which may be why so many women develop autoimmune disease after the birth of a child. Exposure to a number of contaminants such as dioxin and PCBs is another.

Indeed, environmental exposures to dioxin and PCBs—at amounts as low as five times the average level that most of us come into contact with in our day-to-day lives—can cause the thymus to shrink as much as 80 percent. When that shrinkage happens, the number of regulatory or "officer" T cells decreases, and there are no longer as many of them to keep the "cadet" T cells in line. The immune system becomes unsupervised—which can trigger acts of friendly fire in the systems and organs almost anywhere in the body.

THE DANGER OF TINY DOSES

Dioxin, along with pesticides, insecticides, and plasticizers such as bisphenol A, or BPA, a plastics building block used in everything from safety helmets, dental sealants, and eyeglass lenses to everyday food packaging, are what are also known as endocrine disruptors, a group of environmental contaminants that can affect our immune system and our resistance to disease in another particularly insidious way—and in particularly small doses—by disrupting our bodies' natural hormonal signals.

Animals and humans secrete minuscule amounts of hormones, such as estrogen, that trigger responses when they occupy special receptors made to receive them on the cells of various organs in our bodies. These hormones are secreted into the blood by the endocrine glands that produce them—the thyroid, pancreas, and adrenal glands, as well as the ovaries and testes—in response to signals from the brain. Chemicals like PCBs, plastic additives such as BPA, and common pesticides are among the numerous chemicals that, upon entering our bloodstreams through daily exposure, can mimic estrogen by occupying our cells' estrogen receptors.

You might think of estrogen being secreted in the body as something akin to a radio signal that's being sent out from a station, and its receptor—a protein on the surface of a cell elsewhere in the body—as the antenna. The proper signal has to reach the antenna in order for the signal to be received—and for music, rather than static, to come out of the radio. When endocrine disruptors mimic real estrogen they can wreak havoc in one of two ways: first, they can block the estrogen receptor site altogether, keeping our natural estrogen from triggering the responses it's supposed to so that it can do its normal job in the body. When estrogen signals are blocked, it prevents our hormones from sending out any signal at all. The second way that endocrine disruptors work is not by blocking communication completely, but by sending the wrong signals between cells.

Researchers now understand that a wide array of environmental chemicals can act as endocrine disruptors, affecting us at much lower doses than scientists previously thought possible. A growing body of new science on low-dose exposures suggests to investigators that even minute traces of many common chemicals—at levels that have been touted by industry and some scientists to be biologically safe—can affect our cell activity by sending out artificial messages to the body through our endocrine system.

Endocrine-disrupting chemicals are remarkably adept at traveling through the bloodstream and entering our cells by tricking specific receptors on cells into believing that the chemicals are, in fact, real estrogen being secreted by our own bodies (endocrine literally means "secreting internally"). Once in the cell, these chemical imposters bind with estrogen receptors and begin to set things askew by sending out a false signal to the rest of the body—one that the brain did not intend or command. It is as if the radio waves have been hijacked by a rogue station. Suddenly, instead of music emerging from the radio, these imposters send out scrambled signals—a completely different kind of sound. The cells in the body begin to respond inappropriately, acting as if they've been signaled by real estrogen to cause other cellular interactions to take place when in fact these exchanges are not what the body intended at all. The cells begin to dance to the wrong tune—engaging in precarious missteps.

When this normal cellular interaction begins to go haywire at major phases of development—say, when Becky's son Zachary was developing in her womb, or while his infant brain is maturing, or in eight or so years when Selena comes into puberty—these artificial chemicals usurping the place of natural estrogen can trigger unnatural biological responses. Scientists have worried for decades about data showing endocrine disruptors' effects on the brain and the reproductive system. As we learn more about how these chemicals interfere with cellular signaling in the body, endocrine mimickers have become a grave concern to scientists studying autoimmune disease.

Dr. Allen Silverstone, a professor of microbiology and immunology at the State University of New York Upstate Medical University at Syracuse, has been demonstrating in the lab how endocrine disruptors disturb the regulation of the immune system, given the profound influence the endocrine system has over the workings of our immune cells. When our endocrine system's exquisite communication network goes on the blink, the immune system's network can go haywire as well.

Silverstone, an unassuming sixty-four-year-old immunologist whose own wife has suffered greatly from rheumatoid arthritis, began to investigate the role of endocrine disruptors on the immune system after developing successful target therapies for childhood leukemia. "I thought cancer was messy," he says. "But autoimmunity is so much messier."

One particular endocrine receptor interests Silverstone in particular. In 1979 a new receptor was discovered, called the aryl hydrocarbon receptor, which binds specifically with dioxin and PCB. The aryl hydrocarbon receptor is found in almost every tissue of the body and it is found far down the evolutionary chain, even in fish. Even though we've known about this protein for nearly thirty years, says Silverstone, we "still don't have a good idea of what it normally does." But scientists know this much. When dioxin enters the body and binds with this receptor, says Silverstone, "it's like a bad accident happening in the body. Dioxin and PCB bind very tightly with the aryl hydrocarbon receptor and keep it turned on for way too long." That, in turn, causes the body to turn on other cellular interactions that it shouldn't turn on, which can result in altered immunity, including autoimmune disease. Different chemicals bind with different receptors—be they estrogen receptors, androgen receptors, insulin receptors, and so on—and not only block the receptors, but begin to send out false information to other cells, creating a cascade of misinformation.

At the University of Tokyo, a team of eight Japanese immunotoxicologists recently demonstrated that in mice, endocrine-disrupting chemicals, such as BPA, promote a significantly increased production of autoantibodies—antibodies that set out to destroy one's own tissue. Other lab research confirms that environmental estrogens, including plastic additives, exert a direct effect on immune cells, suppressing the function of some immune cells and overstimulating others. BPA, which is also used in baby bottles and in the resins that line food cans, has been discovered by the CDC in 95 percent of human urine samples tested and has been detected in newborn umbilical cord blood the world over.

In 1988, the EPA set a daily safe limit for humans of 0.05 milligrams of BPA per kilogram of body weight. Since then, investigative techniques for determining cell dysfunction in the lab have dramatically improved, allowing researchers to look at many chemicals' subtler effects. As it turns out, a number of studies show that BPA alters the activity in animal and human cell cultures at just one twenty-five-thousandth of the dose that the EPA deemed caused adverse health effects twenty years ago. Over the past two decades, BPA has meanwhile become an integral chemical in the packaging of millions of food products and other plastic goods; more than 6 billion pounds of BPA are used each year in resins lining metal cans, food packaging, hot beverage cups, and in blends with other types of plastic products. Lab research shows that the bond that secures BPA molecules to food and beverage packages changes over time, resulting in the release of free BPA into the food we eat and the beverages we consume, as well as into the environment. In 2006, researchers found that BPA—at concentrations lower than those already found in pregnant women, fetuses, and adults, and well within the range of our typical human exposure—causes estrogen receptors to initiate unnaturally rapid responses, changing our basic cellular function. Significant effects can be seen at extremely low levels of exposure—parts per billion and even per trillion—levels currently present in blood samples taken from people as well as animals.

Chemical manufacturers have worked hard to counter the mounting academic research showing that the negative health effects of endocrine disruptors can be seen at extremely low levels of exposure. In 2004, one researcher counted up all of the studies done to date on just BPA. Of 104 studies done by independent researchers, 94 found adverse effects. None of 11 studies conducted by the chemical industry's researchers on BPA identified adverse effects.

In the wake of the mounting data that endocrine disruptors wreak havoc on the human immune system, in 2005 the National Institutes of Health stated that investigations of exposures to pesticides and estrogenic compounds as triggers of autoimmune disease—about which we still know far too little—are now of "considerable research interest."

• • •

Another well-known endocrine disruptor comes in the form of a group of chemicals known as phthalates, which are added to cosmetics to make them creamier, to plastic bottles and plastics in general to make them more flexible and less brittle, to children's toys to make them more pliable, as well as to insecticides. As Becky heated up Zachary's baby bottle, and as she warmed up her soup in the microwave, she increased the likelihood that phthalates would leach from the plastic bottle and prepackaged plastic soup container into her lunch and Zachary's twice over: once from the bottle, and again through the trace phthalates mainlined to Zachary through her breast milk.

Whenever we heat plastics, we increase the likelihood of leaching out chemicals. Some drinking straws carry the warning on the label "not for hot beverages" for good reason: if you put that straw into a boiling cup of hot cocoa, you are creating something akin to a hot-water extraction technique—not unlike that used in labs to help isolate and draw out chemicals—causing the chemicals in the straw to be jettisoned directly into your yummy cup of cocoa. (As an aside, while urban myth holds that freezing water in plastic bottles draws out toxic chemicals and laces the water with them, in fact, freezing actually works against the release of chemicals, because chemicals do not diffuse as readily in colder temperatures.)

Phthalates are also key ingredients in Becky's newly purchased U.S. manufactured cosmetics (whereas in Europe and Japan phthalates have been banned because of their health risks). Every day when Becky puts on her face cream and body cream, she is lathering phthalates across the largest organ of her body. Like dioxin, bisphenol A, PBDEs, and pesticides, phthalates have been found in every American tested.

Becky Sandler might be especially disturbed to learn of data linking hair dye to a woman's likelihood of developing lupus, given that she has her roots dyed auburn to cover her premature gray every six weeks. Several studies have shown that women who use hair dye have three times the risk of developing lupus—that is, if they also carry specific genes that make them susceptible to autoimmune disease in the first place. This might not, however, reassure Becky all that much. She already has Raynaud's disease, an autoimmune disease that is certainly mild, but nonetheless shows her personal proclivity to autoimmunity. Most sufferers of any one autoimmune syndrome are three times more likely than others to develop additional autoimmune diseases down the road.

Of the many chemicals Becky is exposed to during her day, the one that is most directly linked to the exacerbation of autoimmune disease is the paint remover she uses to strip her daughter's chair and table. Although Becky is not a frequent user of solvents—and has little reason to fret over a one-time use in her garage—frequent use of paint thinners, removers, and mineral spirits by those who use them in occupations such as dry cleaning or airplane manufacturing (to degrease parts) or in the leather industry (to strip and tan hides) have been linked in occupational studies to a two- to three-fold risk of developing multiple sclerosis, connective tissue diseases, and the autoimmune disease scleroderma.

The problem is, Becky is breast-feeding. And that means that although her exposure to chemicals may be at one level, the exposure she passes on to Zachary exists at quite another. While it may seem counterintuitive, babies nurse at the top of our food chain. They feed one rung higher than we do, and in what is known as the law of biomagnification, that means that they receive a more concentrated level of all the contaminants that we have been exposed to over the course of our own lifetimes.

Noshing at the top of the food chain, we all receive a concentrated level of the environmental chemicals that persist in the air, water, and ground—because these contaminants have been ingested by all the animals that feed underneath us at each step, all the way down to the plants that grow in soil nourished by groundwater that has been steeped in industrial runoff before being eaten by the cow in the field. Or consider the mako shark that fed on the barracuda that fed on the fish that fed on the lugworms and tiny shrimplike crustaceans that dined on the tiny granular fragments of plastic that have been steadily accumulating in the environment over the past forty years. Fibrous bits of nine different synthetics—fragments from the gradual breakdown of larger plastic items like food packaging—are now routinely found in sediment in marine habitats from sandy beaches to the bottom of the open seas. When Becky eats a dinner of mako shark in a pepper crust at her favorite seafood eatery, she is ingesting those plastics as well as traceable levels of the highly active contraceptives—from the excretion of birth-control pills through our sewage system—that also now appear regularly in test samples of U.S. seawater. These industrial compounds—both of which are known endocrine disruptors—magnify in intensity as they are passed up the food chain from host to host, reaching their second to highest concentration in us—and their highest of all in human breast milk. And because babies eat far more for their size than do grown-ups, their dose of contaminants per meal is much greater than our own. Pound for pound, breast-feeding babies get more contaminants per meal, at more concentrated levels, from the healthiest known food source on the planet.

(One caveat here for nursing moms: no matter how contaminated breast milk may be, it is still the best food for babies. Not only does bottle feeding pose its own problems because of possible contaminants in the water used to make it, but for reasons we do not fully understand, breast-feeding provides protective measures against diarrhea and ear infections and even some childhood cancers.)

As if all that weren't enough for Zachary and his family to swallow, there is growing evidence that the sum of chemicals accumulating within us may be more toxic in combination than each chemical is alone. Think back to Becky's day. Now think of the multitude of trace chemicals such as chlorine, benzene, nitrate, and perchlorate documented to be in the tap water in many areas of the United

States (with which Becky makes her cup of tea), the chlorine bleach toilet cleanser, the dry-cleaning solvents in her newly cleaned clothes, the contact cement Becky uses to fix a broken toy, the benzene in the gasoline that she puts into her hybrid SUV, the new wooden pirate-ship climber that Selena clambers on, which has been treated with pesticides, and you can begin to get an idea of the chemical soup that researchers worry is circulating through our bodies.

Recently, scientists from the Environmental Protection Agency wondered whether contaminants that harm the endocrine system might produce a more toxic effect when they act in combination. As it turns out, blends of certain synthetic compounds do create a synergistic effect; two weakly estrogenic compounds create a more potent hit than one compound on its own. The harmful effects of endocrine disruptors are increased two- to threefold when these different chemicals act in unison to block endocrine receptors from normal functioning. Nevertheless, the Environmental Protection Agency is waiting to study the effects of low-dose exposure to endocrine-mimicking chemicals further, believing it "would be premature to require routine testing of substances for low-dose effect."

However, cautions Silverstone, "We know low levels of chemicals in the environment can cause many negative health consequences, including immune alterations, in animal studies. Funding for research to study these effects is still relatively small. As our knowledge of how the immune system works becomes ever more sophisticated, it seems reasonable to put more research dollars into how subtle alterations of the immune system can be caused by these simple and complex mixtures of environmental chemicals."

UNDERSTANDING HOW CHEMICALS TRIGGER AUTOIMMUNITY

At what level of contact do humans, versus lab rats, need to be concerned about such environmental hits? This is a question scientists in the field of autoimmune-disease research have attempted to answer only in the past five to ten years. In 2005, researchers from the National Institute of Environmental Health Sciences (NIEHS) and the Lupus Foundation of America cosponsored a meeting entitled Workshop on Lupus and the Environment: Disease Development, Progression, and Flares. This meeting followed on the heels of a 2003 meeting of nine such government agencies to address growing concerns about environmental factors in autoimmune disease. Likewise, a 1998 NIEHS conference also brought together immunologists, clinicians, epidemiologists, molecular biologists, and toxicologists to review current knowledge about links between chemicals in the environment and rising rates of autoimmune disease.

During these three conferences, investigators shared dozens of papers investigating links between industrial chemicals and autoimmunity, as well as data showing how damage is done to the tiniest immune cells by exposure to an array of environmental agents. Scientists linked exposure to compounds such as vinyl chloride—used in making plastic pipes (PVC), wire and cable coatings, and packaging materials—to a higher risk of developing mixed lupus, scleroderma, and rheumatoid arthritis in people. Silica dust, a by-product in ceramic factories, quarries, and construction sites, has also been linked to a higher risk of developing lupus and scleroderma.

One contaminant, trichloroethylene (TCE), a particularly troublesome chemical, received special attention at each of these gatherings. The most common contaminant in Superfund cleanup sites, TCE is a pervasive environmental pollutant that has leached into groundwater through industrial runoff in cities and suburbs across the United States. On military bases, TCE has frequently been used as a cleansing solvent to hose down planes, tanks, trucks, and other machinery, often draining off into streams or groundwater. Other common sources of TCE runoff range from dry-cleaning companies to airplane and machine manufacturers, where TCE is used in stripping metal parts, to leather production, as well as through household use of everything from paint thinners and strippers to many glues and adhesives. (Travel back again through Becky's day and think of her paint stripping and gluing projects, her dry cleaning hanging on her closet door, and the traces of TCE in the water in her afternoon tea and you get the gist of just how pervasive our exposure to TCE is.)

If you were to visit the National Library of Medicine's TOXMAP online and enter "trichloroethylene," a diagram of the United States would pop up showing 312 current sites where TCE has been improperly disposed of and where efforts are under way to clean it up—in addition to 360 TCE-contaminated Superfund sites. From Dallas, Texas, eastward, state lines on the U.S. TOXMAP are nearly obliterated by overlapping red and yellow dots and white squares, indicating TCE sites in every region. Military sites pose yet another source of contamination: today there are about 1,400 Department of Defense sites where the soil or water is contaminated by TCE. In many locations, especially those with porous ground that allows vapors to seep upward, TCE lingers in the air, particularly inside buildings. (Trichloroethylene is a highly volatile chemical, meaning that, like many chemical particles, it is easily released as a vapor into the atmosphere around us when used in industry or manufacturing.)

One of the most famous TCE hot spots of the past is that of Woburn, Massachusetts, where runoff from area tanneries ended up in the rivers, wells, and the general water supply. The story of the litigation surrounding the site became the basis of the book and movie *A Civil Action*. In other cities, including both Tucson and Phoenix, Arizona, as well as a small community in Georgia—three places where studies have been conducted to date—contamination of the water supply by trichloroethylene has been closely related to cluster epidemics of patients with lupus.

TCE is regularly detected in breast milk, and 10 percent of Americans now have detectable levels of TCE in their blood, from exposure through drinking water as well as breathing it in from the air around us. One of our most significant contacts, however, comes from taking showers. Exposure from breathing TCE released when shower water converts into shower steam is even higher, say experts, than what we get through drinking tap water or breathing TCE. (Exposure rate is so much higher because you are getting multiple types of exposure at once: direct contact with the water at the same time that you are breathing in vaporized TCE from the shower steam.) The National Academy of Sciences recently released a detailed study of how worrisome our daily exposure to TCE actually is, warning that evidence is growing stronger that the chemical is causing a range of disturbing human health problems. Nevertheless, the Department of Defense—which is responsible for cleaning up more than a thousand properties contaminated with TCE—has argued vigorously against the need to change regulations regarding TCE use and cleanup. Senators, including Hillary Rodham Clinton and Barbara Boxer, have appealed to the EPA, writing that TCE is not only a carcinogen but is also known to "damage the nervous and immune systems" and warning that "thousands of Americans may be exposed to unhealthful levels of TCE." As one epidemiologist put it, "It is a World Trade Center in slow motion. You would never notice it."

One immunotoxicologist has done much more than just take notice. Dr. Kathleen Gilbert, a forty-eight-year-old associate professor in the Department of Microbiology and Immunology at the Arkansas Children's Hospital Research Institute in Little Rock and coauthor of much of today's groundbreaking work on TCE and autoimmunity, has devoted the last decade to helping scientists understand how chemicals like TCE precipitate an autoimmune reaction at the cellular level in the body.

On any given Saturday afternoon, Gilbert's industrial white-walled and windowless lab on the fourth floor of the Children's Hospital is humming with activity like the inside of a well-run submarine. Manning the stations are seven scientists—six women and one man. Gilbert, along with her team of graduate students, postdoctoral fellows, and lab technicians—most of them young mothers—can be found here even on most weekends. Although the tools scientists like Gilbert and her team have to understand how autoimmunity is triggered by exposures at the cellular level have improved in recent years, they still remain fairly crude, explains Gilbert, a willowy woman whose sweeping red bangs frame piercing brown eyes. They are crude, she says, "because the field of immunotoxicology itself is still so new."

So new that ten years ago, when Gilbert first came to the Arkansas Children's Hospital, few researchers were experts in both immunology and toxicology; indeed, an experienced immunotoxicologist was hard to find. When Gilbert first arrived on the campus as an immunologist, she was immediately approached by a colleague in toxicology to see if she would be interested in collaborating on research on chemical triggers of autoimmunity. Dr. Neil Pumford was curious about whether TCE—one of the most common and pervasive toxicants in our air, water, and soil—might be implicated in autoimmune diseases such as lupus. Pumford's thought was that he could supply the expertise in toxicology, while Gilbert, who had made a name for herself in immunology while doing her postdoctoral research at Memorial Sloan-Kettering Cancer Center in New York, could supply the immunology know-how.

In 1997, Gilbert was fascinated by the prospect of opening one of the most tightly shut black boxes of modern medical science: she wanted to see in the lab how cellular processes break down when exposed to an environmental toxin. In particular, she wanted to pinpoint what happens when the body, unable to tolerate the toxic load, begins to destroy its own tissue in an autoimmune response.

And that was a tall order. Just to get a sense of how daunting a task that is, consider an imaginary scale of one to ten in which one represents a given environmental exposure and ten represents a person falling ill with an autoimmune disease. If we were to follow each number from one to ten to see how that exposure causes disease in our bodies, we would find that at steps four, five, and six, where we might hope to witness the precise activity of our innermost cells as they turn on self, researchers are still flying relatively blind. While we know from occupational studies that groups of people who are exposed to certain chemicals through their jobs, like those working with TCE-based solvents, have a much greater risk of developing autoimmune disease, we are still unable to see and document the cellular chain of events that causes that exposure to lead to disease. Nevertheless, the quest to make the invisible visible—and demonstrate, in lab animals, how exposure to a particular chemical causes autoimmunity—is the holy grail of autoimmune disease and immunotoxicology research.

The immune response involves one of the most complex systems in the body. Indeed, the number of cell interactions that go into one immune response—say, fighting off the microparticles that come out of a blast of diesel exhaust—would take up three consecutive chalkboards to show in its entirety. Kathleen Gilbert and Neil Pumford, however, have come about as close as anyone in giving us insight into what numbers four and five and six might look like in the human body. They began by working with young adult female mice in their Arkansas lab, to see whether TCE might stimulate an autoimmune reaction in their immune systems. Deliberately exposing human subjects to certain chemicals and waiting to see if they are more likely to develop disease would be clearly unethical, which is why rats and mice have had to stand in place of humans in autoimmune disease research, just as they do in cancer research.

First, they gave the mice drinking water that contained a fairly high dose of TCE. The dose was, in fact, about double what a worker in a dry cleaners or tannery might be "safely" exposed to under standards set by both EPA and Occupational Safety and Health Administration standards. For four weeks Gilbert and Pumford monitored the mice. "We had no idea what kind of immune-system alteration we might see," says Gilbert. So they did a whole battery of tests to look at what was happening with some of the cells in the mice that would tell them if there was, indeed, an autoimmune reaction.

To understand what they saw, it might be helpful to have one last tutorial on how the immune system functions when T cells—our front line of defense against foreign antigens—start to hunt for, and eradicate, harmful invaders. T cells work together in exquisite collaboration with a vast array of different types of immune cells to protect our bodies from bacterial, parasitic, fungal, and viral infections—as well as from other foreign invaders, including chemicals and toxins. The process starts when special markers—known as antigen receptors, which sit on the surface of T cells—detect pieces of foreign antigens entering the body. When they find an antigen that matches their antigen receptor, they make what you might think of as a bingo match.

To use another analogy, these antigen receptors are like homeland security police on high alert, scouring the body for anything they don't recognize as safe—anything that is "non-self." To give you some idea of what a challenging job this policing is, consider this: immune system helper cells, known as dendritic cells, present antigens from foreign invader cells to over a million of our T cells in a single day.

Once a T cell's antigen receptor finds an antigen has entered the body that it recognizes as foreign, the T cell forms what is known as an immunological synapse—think of it as a telephone call from the T cell to the dendritic cell—querying dendritic cells for additional information about the antigen and its source in the body. Is the antigen a deadly danger or simply, say, a harmless food protein? (In the case of food allergies, this might be a food protein that the body decides to mount an attack against as if it's a deadly foreign invader, as happens when a peanut is eaten by a person who has an allergic response to peanut protein.)

This interrogation may last hours. If, finally, the antigen is deemed a threat, the T cell starts multiplying, producing a posse in a rapid cellular population explosion. These T-cell police progeny are capable of killing invaders outright as well as marshaling other cells to destroy them.

In the case of autoimmune disease, however, T cells begin to function erratically. In a healthy immune system, regulatory T cells are able to make sure that other T cells never attack our own tissue. Part of their job is to ensure that T cells recognize our own body tissue as ourselves and never mistakenly attack "self." But in autoimmunity, T cells lose their "tolerance" to self. These self-reactive T cells stimulate other immune cells to produce autoantibodies that attach to the perfectly fine, healthy cells within our body—in any organ or tissue—and cause cells to die.

Environmental toxins appear to mess with normal internal signaling pathways, making it difficult for our immune cells to recognize what is foreign and what is self—a bit like a covert enemy force sending up smokescreens and spreading disinformation. Mouse studies show that even subtle signaling imbalances can predispose animals to produce antibodies against the self. In patients with lupus, for instance, certain signaling molecules that relay messages between cells and rally the production of antibodies have been shown to be present in abnormal amounts.

Gilbert and Pumford wanted to find out whether TCE might stimulate the production of an autoimmune response and, if so, see what cells might be involved. As is standard in this sort of research, they used a machine known as a flow cytometer to examine the surface of cells from the mouse, taken from immune-system organs such as the lymph nodes and the spleen. The flow cytometer uses a laser to light up cells if the cells express certain markers that should not, in normal circumstances, be present on the T cells. If, however, the cells light up, this could be considered as a "bingo" moment; a T cell that should recognize the mouse's tissue as self and tolerate it has, instead, become activated to possibly destroy the mouse's own tissue.

In Gilbert and Pumford's experiment, the T cells from mice exposed to TCE lit up all over the place. Yet no cells lit up in the group of control mice that had not been given TCE-laced water. Specifically, the flow cytometer told Gilbert that in the mice exposed to TCE, a T-cell activation molecule, CD44, was acting differently than it would have if there had been no autogen. CD44 molecules are usually activated when the body is fighting, say, a very bad viral infection. But in this case CD44 was signaling that, even in the absence of a viral infection, T cells had been activated—and they were most likely activated against self. Chances were that what Gilbert and Pumford were staring at was the mouse's own immune system, or T cells, being activated—and going on to destroy the mouse's own tissue and cells.

"It was a very robust effect," says Gilbert. "The more TCE we gave them, the more cell activation we got." Gilbert and Pumford were stunned. They were staring at not only an increase in the percentage of cells expressing CD44, but these CD44 cells were also producing a multitude of other inflammatory molecules known as cytokines, which are found in overabundance in patients with lupus and many other autoimmune diseases.

And so, they wondered, what would happen if they exposed mice to a lower dose of TCE over a longer period of time—a chronic exposure equal to exactly what a person might have in a tannery or airplane manufacturing company, an amount corresponding to limits already approved of as safe by the EPA for industrial workers?

This time around, even at these low doses, Gilbert and Pumford saw an increase in the percentage of cells that expressed CD44. But they also saw something else: after being exposed to TCE at lower doses over a longer period of time, the mice's T cells began to destroy their own liver tissue, causing a disease known as autoimmune hepatitis.

"It was a big moment," Gilbert recalls. In 2000, Gilbert and Pumford and colleagues published two back-to-back groundbreaking studies: they were among the first immunologists and toxicologists to show that low-dose exposure to environmental toxicants could be a potent stimulator of an autoimmune response.

While there have long been epidemiological studies telling us that people who work around certain chemicals are more likely to have autoimmune disease, those studies are complicated by the fact that people who might have been exposed to TCE are probably also exposed to other chemicals at the same time. This has made it simple for chemical manufacturers to cast such epidemiological studies as spurious; there is no way to tease out, much less prove, cause and effect based on occupational studies. Because the silent exposures that lead to disease are so often chronic, and happen slowly over time rather than in one fell swoop, it is difficult, if not impossible, to tie any single compound—or combination of contaminants—back to disease long after the fact.

"To suddenly see in the lab that occupational levels of TCE cause mice to come down with autoimmune disease was a huge jump," says Gilbert. In the world of autoimmune-disease research, what had been a mere hypothesis—that toxicants can promote autoimmune disease—had become proven fact in their Arkansas lab.

DIFFERENT AUTOGEN THRESHOLDS IN US ALL

Still, Gilbert and Pumford were admittedly working with mice known to already possess autoimmunity genes. They could only theorize as to how their findings might apply to the general population of humans.

Yet, like mice, many people possess a predisposing genetic susceptibility to autoimmune disease. The number of genes involved in each autoimmune disease are manifold; investigators are still uncovering new lupus genes every year. But the rough guesstimate is that about one in four—an estimated 20 to 25 percent of the general population—carry some combination of genes that make them more susceptible to one or more autoimmune diseases. For example, one in four people carries a gene variant that makes him or her more likely to develop rheumatoid arthritis, MS, and other autoimmune diseases.

For those who carry such subsets of genes, low doses of environmental toxicants are clearly a bigger deal than they might be for someone else. As the sixteenth-century Swiss-born physician and alchemist Paracelsus put it, the dose makes the poison. The quantity of a substance to which we're exposed is as important as the nature of the substance itself. Yet the dose at which a substance becomes dangerous differs for each individual, given his or her genetic makeup. For some, a minute exposure to a toxin may, for a period of time at least, be a manageable hit for the immune system—but at high or continuous enough doses, it will kill pretty much anyone. Even those who have no genetic susceptibility to autoimmunity will find that their immune systems flail in the face of a high enough dose of a toxic compound. They may not get autoimmune disease, but another disease—perhaps cancer, perhaps something else—will set in.

But for those with a genetic vulnerability to autoimmunity, even a small dose may trigger disease, creating a cellular mayhem in which the body begins to destroy its own blood, tissue, nerves, and organs. And this is what concerns researchers the most. For those 25 percent of people around the world who do have a genetic predisposition to autoimmunity, it may not take very much exposure to cause cells to miscommunicate.

For one in four people, the answer to the question of how much of a chemical has to exist in a person's body for it to wreak immune system havoc may indeed be very, very little. Twin studies show that autoimmune disease is roughly 30 percent genetic and 70 percent environmental. While two identical twins might hold the same genetic code for a certain autoimmune disease, either one of them will be struck with disease only if they meet up with the right environmental hit. As one researcher put it, while genetics may load the gun, it's environment that pulls the trigger. Or think of it this way: if genes are the icy mountain road, chemicals are the truck driving ninety miles an hour in a blizzard.

THE BARREL EFFECT

For patients who do possess the genetic variants predisposing them to autoimmune disease, reaching that threshold at which disease can more easily strike involves a number of factors. You might liken it to the "barrel effect." You can fill a barrel to the absolute rim, and even while water hovers about the edge, not a drop will spill. But add one more minuscule drop of liquid and the water will begin to cascade over the sides.

Think back, for a moment, to Jan Pankey. What factors might

have caused her immune cells to destroy the fatty proteins that her blood needs to clot? How did this happen so suddenly, seemingly overnight, and without warning? Jan's more obvious risk factors were clear enough. For starters, Jan was, like three-quarters of those afflicted with autoimmunity, female. Now, pour in Jan's personal genetic makeup: by the sheer fact that she has an autoimmune disease, Jan no doubt possesses a genetic vulnerability to autoimmunity. Add in the fact that Jan had recently increased her estrogen levels by going on birth-control pills, which may have toyed slightly with her endocrine system. A little more in the barrel. Mix in whatever industrial load of contaminants Jan might have stored up in her bloodstream and tissue over the course of her forty-nine years—which we can only guess at, based on the high amount of contaminants found in other women of her age—and which may already have been slightly, if unobtrusively, tinkering with the messages her cells are sending to one another. The water in the barrel rises just a tad farther. We might also wonder about whatever viruses Jan has been exposed to in her lifetime, which, as we will see in ensuing chapters, can also increase one's chances of developing autoimmune disease. Now imagine that the barrel is full to the brim with this mix of genes, hormones, and environmental and viral hits.

For some, the final drop that spills the barrel may be an infiltrating virus that taxes the immune system just one degree too much, setting an autoimmune response in motion (as has been the case in my own life); for others, it might be an unexpected environmental hit that pushes the immune system into overload and chaos. Given Jan's risk factors, Jan was hovering at that threshold. She was at that brim.

When Jan and David drove into those smoky Montana fires, they were steering into a chemical path of burning trees and nearly two dozen homes and other freestanding structures—a superintensified kind of air pollution made up of what are known in the scientific world as "microparticles." These air particles almost certainly carried not only forest debris but the chemical burn-off from possessions packed inside these homes—everything from flame retardants in the burning clothing, mattresses, and furniture to hundreds of additional toxins with which our household goods are laced during the manufacturing process. It certainly contained dioxin—since burning trash and trees are the largest source of dioxin in our atmosphere—as well as other known endocrine-mimicking chemicals.

Even though they themselves are physicians, Jan and David had no way of knowing, as they drove through those billowing smoke clouds, that in recent years environmental health researchers have documented the relationship between many such inhaled particles and the onset and exacerbation of autoimmune disease.

Indeed, in the same summer of Jan's ordeal, University of Montana chemistry professors and scientists were busy setting up sampling machines that sucked in that dense Missoula wildfire air and pumped it through tubing that collected the smallest particulates—the kind that are so tiny they find their way deep into people's lungs. In the process of looking at these particles, which are about one-thirtieth the diameter of a single strand of human hair, chemists found hundreds of chemical compounds in that smoke. These included a complex soup of pollutants including dioxin, mercury, and the same compounds found in diesel exhaust. Moreover, the sheer volume of particles was in and of itself shocking: the particulate matter in the air that wildfire season was ten times greater than the standard set as safe by the Environmental Protection Agency.

Five months after Jan's ordeal, three EPA researchers would publish a study on how twenty-four hours of breathing such densely polluted air particles can lead to dramatic, negative changes in our blood, including shifts in clotting factor. Eighteen months later, work would be published directly linking fatal blood clots with exposure to the airborne particulate matter in forest fires.

And in 2006, a shocking study based on hospital data from thirty-four cities over a fourteen-year span would show that people with autoimmune inflammatory diseases such as rheumatoid arthritis (RA) and lupus are at a substantially increased risk of death when they are exposed to particulate air pollution, or soot, for a substantial period of time. Individuals with rheumatoid arthritis or lupus who breathe in heavy particles of air pollution for a year or more face a 22-percent increase in their risk of dying from their autoimmune disease. An obvious question might be, Why don't we see headlines about those with autoimmunity being at such a heightened risk of dying in bigger, more polluted cities? The answer is very likely this: since, unlike cancer, there is no autoimmune-disease registry and no way to track these diseases or those who have them, no one—but a few researchers—has really been looking or taking any note.

Were Jan's blood clots exacerbated by the air pollution through which she and Dave drove and biked for three solid days? To say yes would be mere supposition. As we have seen, the steps connecting exposure (one on that scale of one to ten) to disease (ten), are still blurry at best. At numbers four, five, and six, we cannot go back in time and travel with Jan's cells to say definitively what prompted Jan's sudden and rapid onset of antiphospholipid antibody syndrome or prove whether those forest fires had a thing to do with it.

It is all supposition, yes, but it is a very good guess.

THE STORY IN THE NUMBERS

If you were to look today at a chart detailing incidence rates of autoimmune disease versus heart disease and cancer, you would see that while cancer and heart disease rates are, more or less, flatlining, autoimmune diseases are continuing in a steady upward climb. This raises some interesting questions. If an estimated 25 percent of people around the globe carry genes that make them susceptible to autoimmune disease, and if 8.5 percent of Americans already suffer from one or more autoimmune diseases—and if subtle, chronic exposures to the chemicals in our industrialized world are, as we know, playing a role in rising disease rates—how long will it take before an autoimmune disease breaks out in the remaining genetically susceptible Americans? Detectable levels of man-made chemical agents found in nursing mothers' breast milk have risen significantly over the past several decades—and they continue to rise dramatically. What is the threshold of chemical exposure at which an autoimmune reaction will be triggered in all who carry the genetic propensity?

Today, the National Institutes of Health spends only $591.2 million on autoimmune research annually—about one-sixth of the $3 billion spent on AIDS/HIV, which affects fewer than nine hundred thousand Americans. Cancer research claims ten times the annual research funding of autoimmune disease, although cancer affects less than half as many people. Despite the fact that autoimmune disease is the number-two cause of chronic illness and, on average, slices fifteen years off a patient's life, the level of autoimmune research funding is less than 2.2 percent of the National Institutes of Health budget. A report by the Institute of Medicine states that the United States still lags behind other countries in research into the processes and contaminants involved in autoimmunity.

Many of the contaminants discussed early in this chapter have been so little tested that we have no real idea as to what role they may be playing in rising autoimmunity rates. PFOA, for example, has barely been studied at all. Despite the fact that it is found in 96 percent of people and the chemical has a half-life of 4.4 years in the human body, and even though the one piece of research that we have on PFOA has shown it to be a potent immune suppressor, the Environmental Protection Agency does not require scientists to perform further study on this or any other chemical that has shown signs of toxicity in laboratory testing. While Japan recently spent $135 million on a research program identifying some seventy chemicals as endocrine disruptors, the total U.S. budget in 2003, 2004, and 2005 to study endocrine disruptors was less than $15 million for all three years combined.

According to Kathleen Gilbert, the current climate for funding federal research into how toxins affect the immune system has never been more dismal. The problem is twofold. First, the success rate for federal research grants for new investigators has decreased from 22.5 percent in 1998 to 16.8 percent in 2004. Second, as the result of recent restructuring, there are few toxicologists on the grant-review committees that evaluate these new grant applications. This makes it less likely that grants involving environmental toxicants will receive a high priority. These two factors combined make it very difficult to obtain and maintain funding for immunotoxicology research. "It would take an environmentally enlightened political climate to restore research funding and cleanup efforts at levels equal to the challenge," says Gilbert.

At the end of the 2005 conference Workshop on Lupus and the Environment: Disease Development, Progression and Flares, the National Institutes of Health asked scientists to provide suggestions for drafting what is known as a request for applications, or RFA. An RFA is a kind of clarion call from NIH that asks researchers to submit grant proposals in a specific area in need of more investigation—in this case the RFA is, should it ever get approval and difficult-to-find funding, to be used for researching autoimmune disease and environmental triggers more deeply. Yet to date, the National Institutes of Health has still not issued the request for researchers to submit applications for grants to investigate environmental triggers of autoimmunity.

Today, eighty thousand chemicals are registered for use in the United States and the U.S. Environmental Protection Agency approves an estimated seventeen hundred more a year with very little screening. We often assume that if no warning has appeared stating that a chemical is harmful, that must mean it's benign, when nothing could be further from the case. The 1976 Toxic Substances Control Act requires that new chemical compounds be tested for negative health effects before approval only if evidence of potential harm already exists—which is rarely the case for brand new chemicals. The FDA approves about 90 percent of these new compounds without restrictions.

And so, a great debate continues to rage in the scientific and political arena about what the growing number of studies linking environmental contaminants to autoimmunity collectively means, what the implications are, and—as we shall see in further chapters—what actions should be taken, if any.

Jumping ahead with the research that does exist in order to claim that the invisible chemicals around us are causing or exacerbating a rise in autoimmunity is the kind of connecting-of-dots and blame-the-environment speculation that makes many politicians crazy, and that chemical-industry publicists routinely deem as toothless.

In Arkansas, Gilbert is now deepening her research to see what the exact mechanisms are by which TCE activates T cells. "Industry interest seems to center on designing drugs to stop those T cells from activating after exposures," says Gilbert. "But what bothers me is that no one is talking about cleaning up the environment to help prevent these exposures in the first place."

Science, as a whole, does not make sudden leaps. Even when a body of research begins to form an arrow pointing in one clear direction, the standard scientific line remains predictably the same. At the end of almost every published paper appear the words "more data is needed to further our understanding."

Perhaps there is no better place to examine the ramifications of waiting too long for irrefutable proof of the role that environmental contaminants play in today's autoimmune epidemic than in the city of Buffalo, New York, where for far too long, residents, researchers, and society looked the other way.

CHAPTER THREE

DIRTY LITTLE SECRETS: CLUSTER EPIDEMICS FROM BUFFALO TO TEXAS

Try this exercise the next time you can spare a minute. Go to the web address http://www.epa.gov/enviro/emef and enter in zip code 14211 in the space provided. Now watch as your computer monitor morphs into a complex map of small green and black squares, each demarcating a hazardous-waste or toxic-release site within a few square blocks in Buffalo, New York. Take particular note of the number of black squares; each signifies a multihazard site—a combination of hazardous, toxic, and/or Superfund-classified substances and chemicals found at the locale. You might blink twice to think how foolhardy it would be for anyone to live smack in the heart of 14211 in the East Ferry neighborhood of Buffalo—it's just that toxic.

But in the mid-1980s the unusual number of residents in the East Ferry community who were falling ill with lupus and other debilitating autoimmune diseases had no clue about the toxic waste simmering within the soil, pavement, and streams around their homes and schools. The chemicals that had been seeping into the neighborhood from abandoned industrial-waste sites for decades hadn't yet been charted on any government website.

• • •

In 1980, Betty Jean Grant, a thirty-two-year-old African-American woman, and her husband, George, decided to open up a mom and pop store at 1055 East Ferry Street in Buffalo, N.Y. Serving the predominately African-American neighborhoods of East Ferry and next-door Delavan-Grider—zip code 14215—Grant's Variety Shop would meet local residents' needs, offering them milk, bread, and Afrocentric health-care products as well as items needed on the fly, like, say, a box of nails. Born and bred in Tennessee, and one of sixteen children, Betty Jean Grant possessed a general fondness for talking to people, and after having lived in Buffalo for ten years, she knew exactly what her neighbors' daily wants were and how far they had to walk or drive to purchase such everyday conveniences. Grant's Variety Shop quickly became, she says, "just like those neighborhood corner stores down South where people come in to see each other, talk, and socialize—and leave with a bit of food."

Amidst all that talking and listening, Grant got to know local residents—and know them well. In 1986, after having listened carefully to customers' woes for years, she began to divine a pattern in the stories they told that made her increasingly uneasy.

At first, it seemed no more than an isolated, tragic tale that could happen in any community. Karen Johnson,* a local teenager who often popped into Grant's store on her way home from school, stopped coming by. She lived only a block away at 428 Moselle Street, and Grant hadn't seen her in weeks. Grant heard one day that Karen had been diagnosed with the autoimmune disease lupus. A month later Karen died. She was eighteen years old.

She seemed to disappear overnight. And in a manner of speaking, Karen had. When lupus goes undiagnosed, the disease—which afflicts approximately 1.5 million Americans, or roughly one in

---

* This patient's name has been changed.

two hundred people—can shift from mild periods when chronic symptoms seem barely present to a suddenly life-threatening crisis overnight. In lupus, deranged immune fighter cells, triggered into acts of self-sabotage by a combination of genetic predisposition and environmental triggers, can turn against virtually any organ or tissue, including the joints, kidneys, heart, lungs, brain, blood, or skin, inflicting severe pain, inflammation, and cellular damage.

If the illness is caught before the body's rogue immune system significantly advances its attack, patients can work with their doctors toward a relatively decent outcome. To be diagnosed requires having an experienced physician who is also educated enough about the disease to detect lupus's complex, often intermittent symptoms and make the judgment call to run specific blood tests. The primary test, known as an ANA, looks for unusual antibodies detectable in the blood called antinuclear antibodies, which are able to bind with the nuclei of tissue and organ cells and inflict damage. A high ANA warns doctors that a patient's antibodies may indeed be turning against their own tissue, alerting physicians to the possibility of lupus as well as other connective-tissue diseases such as rheumatoid arthritis and scleroderma.

Although no new U.S. Food and Drug Administration–approved drugs have been developed for lupus in more than forty years, with the help of steroids and immune-suppressing drugs used to treat organ-transplant patients, those with lupus can control flares of their illness. Patients might always have to manage chronic pain and excessive fatigue, but life can often be reasonably good. However, left undiagnosed and untreated too long—as was the case with Karen Johnson—patients can experience sudden, serious organ damage and die. And nowhere was such a preventable and heartrending scenario more likely to occur than in the economically underprivileged African-American neighborhood of East Ferry in Buffalo, where few could afford regular preventative medical visits, quality medical care, and diagnostic tests for an emerging illness, much less the necessary interventions and medications for treatment.

Not long after Karen's death, her thirteen-year-old next-door neighbor, Devonne,* who lived at 426 Moselle, came into the store looking exhausted and depressed. Surmising that Devonne was low because of Karen's death, Grant asked her if she was doing okay. Devonne looked up and said, "Mrs. Grant, I just found out that I have lupus too."

Grant, a former nurse's aid, knew what a devastating disease lupus could be. "I just didn't know what to say to Devonne," she recalls. "It seemed to me a very odd and sad coincidence that two teenage girls living right next door to each other would be struck with lupus at nearly the same time."

Three months later a thirty-eight-year-old woman named Linda Winston,* who lived at 378 Moselle—almost across the street from Devonne—came into the store and told Grant that she was having a hard time because she couldn't go out in the sunshine anymore. Her doctor had just diagnosed her with lupus. Sunlight made the disease flare.

"Right then a warning bell went off in my head," says Grant. "Something just didn't sound right to me." Then, a few weeks later, Grant found out that one more woman living on Moselle Street was sick with the same autoimmune disease.

The next week there were five. A woman who lived three streets over from Moselle came in to say she'd been diagnosed with lupus as well.

That was it for Grant. "Five in a single block?" She called the City of Buffalo Department of Public Works and relayed her concerns to an official in the water department. Grant wanted to know, "Could our water be contaminated? Could something toxic in this area be causing multiple cases of lupus in a one-block radius?" A brusque answer shot back: absolutely not.

"I had no specifics," Grant says. "Just stories, like straws I was trying to pull together from out of the air." Twice she called

---

* These patients names have been changed.

different department heads at the Erie County Department of Health, only to be met with a more vehement response. "They told me, 'Look, lady, you're being paranoid, you're creating a fantasy, looking for something that just isn't there,' " she says. After making a few more phone calls, Grant was told point-blank to "stop creating a conspiracy theory."

In the ensuing years, more and more cases of lupus would quietly emerge among people living in the East Ferry and Delavan-Grider neighborhoods, as would incidences of other autoimmune diseases such as rheumatoid arthritis, scleroderma, multiple sclerosis, Hashimoto's thyroiditis, Sjögren's syndrome, antiphospholipid antibody syndrome, Graves' disease, type 1 diabetes, and myasthenia gravis. Most of those afflicted, however, would remain unaware of how many others were falling ill with similar autoimmune diseases—much less why.

Fifteen-year-old LaShekia Chatman* was one of these young women. In 1992 she was about to go through a kind of hell no teenager should ever have to experience. LaShekia had grown up pretty much like any American city kid, in a white two-story with sky blue trim on the corner of Mapleridge and Deerfield. She worked hard for A's and B's in school and in fifth grade was tapped for Buffalo's gifted and talented program, City Honors School. By her freshman year of high school she performed on the cheerleading squad, starred in *Godspell*, and began an African step dancing group. She was well loved up and down her block by grown-ups and kids alike—including by her friend Kayla Jordan,* with whom she played from the time she was a toddler.

At the age of fifteen, however, she began to experience muscle pain, joint aches, and a constant fatigue that she likens, looking back, to "that feeling you have during those first few hours when

---

* This patient's name has been changed.

you're getting the flu but you don't know yet what's wrong with you." LaShekia's flulike malaise lasted for weeks. As one month passed and then two, LaShekia's mother worried that her daughter's problems stemmed from something more serious than the normal wear and tear that comes with being an overachieving teen. Their pediatrician ran a battery of blood tests and discovered that LaShekia had Epstein-Barr virus, or EBV, a fairly common viral infection. Also known as mononucleosis, EBV could hit teenagers especially hard. At last, her family assumed, they'd discovered what was dragging LaShekia down.

Several months after mono ought to have run its natural course, however, LaShekia was no better. Her bone-deep lethargy was worsening. She noticed other small, worrisome signs. LaShekia would get a minuscule cut on her hand and the wound wouldn't heal for weeks. She came down with one cold after another, until it seemed as if she'd been born with a raw throat and flooded sinuses. It hurt just to walk; LaShekia felt as if small ash fires smoldered in every joint. The pediatric practice reassured LaShekia's mother that it could take a good amount of time for a fifteen-year-old to get back on her feet after mononucleosis.

LaShekia spent several days a week unable to go to school, struggling to keep up with homework from bed. Half a year slipped by this way in illness, as time often will when an undetected autoimmune disease mounts its attack, and LaShekia was not improving. The pediatrician agreed that they needed to run more tests and sent the Chatmans to a local rheumatologist to investigate LaShekia's joint pain. This time, a new diagnosis emerged. LaShekia's blood work revealed what is known as a "high sed rate." Blood sedimentation rates, or sed rates, are lab tests that gauge how fast red blood cells fall to the bottom of a glass test tube. How fast they fall tells doctors, as a crude sort of measure, whether there might be inflammation going on in the body. The higher the rate at which the red blood cells fall, the more inflammation there is.

LaShekia's sed rate was sky high. Bone X-rays confirmed that LaShekia's joints were badly inflamed. The two findings together pointed to the diagnosis of juvenile rheumatoid arthritis, known for short as JRA. In JRA, as in all autoimmune diseases, fighter cells in the arsenal of the body's exquisitely synchronized immune system, what we might think of as the body's central intelligence agency—which normally safeguard us against dangerous infiltrators such as viruses, bacteria, or environmental toxins—skew off kilter. Instead of defending the body, a faction of fighter cells become akin to rogue agents, activating other cells to destroy healthy cells and tissue. In this case, fighter cells, or T cells, were activating autoantibodies, antibodies directed against self, to destroy the lining of LaShekia's joints. The result, for LaShekia, was the kind of burning pain, swelling, and inflammation from which JRA patients so often suffer.

Upsetting as a diagnosis of JRA was, however, the Chatmans—LaShekia, her mom, dad, and grandmother—were happy finally to have something to work with. LaShekia started taking Tylenol for joint pain, with the hope that she would begin to feel better. For a while she did, although her physical improvement, if any, was slight.

In 1995, at the age of eighteen, LaShekia set off for Pace University in New York City, hoping to be the first college graduate in her family. Despite her physical setbacks, she had managed to graduate from high school with the rest of her class. She got as far as Halloween during her freshman year at Pace, when it became clear that her physical torpor was worsening. She had lost significant weight. Twice since she had left for university, LaShekia had blacked out and ended up in New York Downtown Hospital's emergency room. Her mother worried that the stresses of college life were too much for her daughter and insisted that she return home to Buffalo.

LaShekia, who stands five foot six, had dropped to an emaciated ninety-five pounds by the time she returned home. Her long ebony hair had noticeably thinned, and her once-glowing brown complexion was lackluster and sallow. LaShekia recalls that when her mother saw her she was so upset that "she locked herself in the bathroom for nearly an hour. She said she had to finish her shower, but I could hear her in there crying, trying to hide from me how scared she was."

LaShekia's rheumatologist, whom she saw a few days later, couldn't fathom what was happening; he sent LaShekia to Buffalo's Roswell Park Cancer Institute to rule out any sort of cancer. In between stays in Roswell for tests, LaShekia would come home for a week or so. She was so weak and in such acute pain she couldn't walk to the bathroom, turn a doorknob, or bear the pressure of her body's weight against the mattress. When she did manage to sleep it was for a few fitful hours, only to awake in a pool of sweat. Her hair was falling out on her pillow, and the bright light of the outdoors made her wince. LaShekia's mother, Renita, recalls feeling as though she were watching her daughter "die before my eyes."

LaShekia sometimes overheard her mother speaking in hushed, worried tones with her friend Kayla's mom over coffee at the Chatmans' kitchen table. The two moms were close friends and had more in common than they might have liked: like LaShekia, Kayla had been growing increasingly unwell. For months, Kayla had been experiencing severe lethargy and debilitating headaches. Then she woke one morning and had trouble seeing out of her right eye. Kayla had seen several local doctors who, despite the severity of her symptoms, had been unable to discern what was wrong with her.

Kayla's mother, Marion Jordan,* happened to be friends with Betty Jean Grant, who had shared her concern that something toxic in the area was causing young women to fall sick with autoimmune disease, lupus in particular. As Marion and Renita talked, the same terrible and terrifying suspicion washed over them. Could it—whatever *it* was—be making their daughters sick, too?

Marion and Renita started keeping track, informally, of all the people who had become sick with lupus in their own square-block area in the Delavan-Grider neighborhood. There was the young mom down the street who had just been diagnosed with lupus and who hobbled with a cane to ease the pain of her thick, swollen legs. Then there was LaShekia's sixty-year-old adoptive grandpa who lived around the corner from her and who had already lost a leg to

---

* This patient's name and the names of her family members have been changed.

lupus because the disease had been caught too late. He made sure to let Renita and Marion know whenever he got wind of yet another neighbor who should be added to their lupus tally.

Then Kayla joined the list. She began to have terrible joint pain along with her other symptoms. At first, given her vision problems, doctors diagnosed her with MS. They did a brain biopsy and found, however, that Kayla had central-nervous-system vasculitis, an autoimmune disease of the blood vessels of the brain. Then, after more testing, they added the diagnosis of lupus.

The majority of those struck with lupus were young women of childbearing years. If they lived in East Ferry they tended to be poor, while those in Delavan-Grider, LaShekia's neighborhood, tended to be mildly-making-it middle class. All of them were African American.

For neighbors in the small urban communities of East Ferry and Delavan-Grider, terms like "lupus" and "scleroderma" were on the verge of becoming household words. In these two neighborhoods it was beginning to seem almost a natural course of events to be diagnosed with lupus or rheumatoid arthritis or type 1 diabetes by the time you were twenty or thirty years old. Still, other than Grant, few ventured questions. When locals did get an uneasy feeling about how many were falling sick with autoimmune diseases on their block or street they usually shared their worries with one another over the fence or on the front porch or after church. No one was officially counting heads, keeping charts; no one was connecting the dots.

By Christmas of 1995, LaShekia still did not have a diagnosis. Roswell oncologists had performed lung, lymph node, bronchial, and bone-marrow biopsies on LaShekia Chatman and had come up empty-handed. They asked Alan Baer, a well-known local rheumatologist, to consult in her case, and gave the Chatmans a referral. Before the Chatmans could call Baer's office to request an appointment, Alan Baer phoned Renita to say that he had heard of LaShekia's struggle and was hoping that he might be able to help her.

Would they like to come in and see him? It was extraordinary for a doctor to reach out into this economically sidelined community. The Chatmans were awed and gratified. They had already seen six physicians during LaShekia's three-year downward spiral. Not one had been able to shed light on why LaShekia seemed to be silently slipping away.

The first time Alan Baer met his new patient, he knew nothing of the other patients with lupus in the area. But he did know that many of LaShekia's symptoms—hair falling out, night sweats, excessive weight loss, fatigue, photosensitivity, and severe pain in every joint and muscle—suggested lupus. LaShekia already had one autoimmune disease, which made her statistically much more likely to have others. Lupus was a better than good hunch. Alan Baer tested LaShekia for antinuclear antibodies, and her ANA and other lupus biomarker tests proved positive. There was no time to lose. Baer immediately put LaShekia on a trial course of the steroid prednisone.

Within weeks of starting prednisone, LaShekia's pain and inflammation began to diminish. Her appetite started to return. Dr. Baer added the drug Imuran, an immunosuppressant developed to help prevent the bodies of transplant patients from rejecting their new organs, to help tamp down her overenthusiastic immune system.

In subsequent visits, it became clear to Baer that LaShekia was also developing the features of scleroderma. A progressive autoimmune disease in which the immune cells attack the connective tissue in the body—the collagen within human skin and tissue as well as the elastin in the ligaments that connect bones—scleroderma can leave damaging scar tissue in the skin as well as organs. Baer diagnosed LaShekia with what is sometimes called "overlap syndrome," a connective-tissue disease with features of both lupus and scleroderma. Between 1995 and 2003, Dr. Baer would go on to see LaShekia through several additional diagnoses of Raynaud's disease, a condition that causes the fingers and/or toes to turn white as a result of diminished blood supply after even slight changes in temperature; and vasculitis, an inflammation of the blood vessels.

By 2003, scar tissue from scleroderma had developed in all eight of LaShekia's fingers, making it difficult to move them, and had immobilized both sides of her mouth so that she couldn't open it very wide. Taking a bite out of an apple, for instance, had become a joy of the past.

THE PERSONAL BECOMES POLITICAL

During the same years that LaShekia was bearing the burden of additional autoimmune diagnoses, Grant was growing increasingly disturbed by how many people were growing ill in her area. She realized that if she wanted to help the community and get to the bottom of this troubling issue, she first needed to have more clout. For that, she would need to be on the inside track—meaning inside city hall.

In 1997 Betty Jean Grant ran for a seat on the city council but lost the election. She lived not far from the East Ferry neighborhood in an area known as the University District, so called because it was home to the University at Buffalo. Because of her long hours at the store she rarely spent much time on her home turf, however, and wasn't known in the wider University District community nearly as well as she was in East Ferry. Still, her loss just made her more determined to gear up and run again.

In November 1999, Betty Jean Grant made her second bid for election to the city council, and this time she won. On January 1, 2000, she was sworn in as city councilwoman representing the University District of Buffalo, New York. She began to juggle her work on the city council with running Grant's Variety Shop, where she continued to hear far too many stories of residents who were far too sick.

Shortly after Grant was elected, a neighborhood resident named Rhonda Dixon Lee, who had once rented a house from Grant at 851 East Ferry Street and who later lived on Moselle Street—yes, that Moselle Street—came into the store. Lee, a former nursing student, ran a nearby day-care center. Many of the young women whose babies she took care of were single teens who often ran into hard times. Lee regularly took foster kids into her home and was well known for the indefatigable vigor with which she, as she terms it figuratively, "beat up on teen moms so they would get their lives together and take care of their kids." Often, she succeeded. But once in a while there would be a mom who couldn't overcome her drug habit, and Lee would adopt that baby into her own family. Lee's family eventually expanded to eight boys and two girls.

One day, she went into Grant's Variety Shop to pick up a few staples. She was moving with difficulty and clearly in pain. Grant asked if she was okay and mentioned to her that everyone in the area seemed to be getting sick. A lot of them had lupus. Lee stopped in her slow-moving tracks. Lupus? She had lived in the area all her life and had been diagnosed with lupus in 1990. Lee's father had lupus, and her best friend had recently died from lupus. Lee had been taking numerous medications to help control her lupus for the past ten years, and despite her illness she had managed to keep giving, helping out young teens, fostering needy children. Until, one day in 2000, Rhonda became a bit like Shel Silverstein's *The Giving Tree*, with almost nothing left to give away. That was the year she was diagnosed with breast cancer for the second time on top of having lupus, and her indefatigable vigor began to wane.

Grant and Lee couldn't stop talking that day in the store. They were both health professionals trained in nursing. They couldn't fathom it: why were so many in their neighborhood sick with a relatively rare autoimmune disease? Grant shared with Lee her suspicion that one of the causes might be some kind of contamination that was silently and invisibly percolating in the area. It was just a hunch, yes, but it was a hunch that had only intensified over the past fourteen years.

As it would turn out, after waiting a decade and a half for a single clue as to whether or not she was right, practically overnight synchronicity would step in and answers would begin to materialize.

THE STRANGE HISTORY OF 858 EAST FERRY STREET

Three months into working at city hall, Grant was going through a stack of papers to prepare for the next city council meeting when she came across a startling memo from the Buffalo Environmental Management Commission, or BEMC. Attached to the memo was a record of decision, also known as an ROD, detailing plans to address a highly toxic waste site situated on the east side of Buffalo. The memo, dated April 27, 2000, was sent from the BEMC to the city's common council. It noted that the New York State Department of Environmental Conservation, or DEC, had designated a nearly three-and-a-half-acre undeveloped property situated at 858 East Ferry Street—smack in the center of the East Ferry neighborhood—as a class-two toxic waste site due to the high concentration of polychlorinated biphenyls (PCBs) and lead found there. A class-two designation meant that the site, according to the DEC, posed "a significant threat to the public health or environment" and that "action was required" to remediate the site. The odd thing about it was that the investigation that had found the property to be highly hazardous had taken place three years earlier—yet this memo was just now coming to the city council.

Grant was both upset and baffled. She knew that property well. The lot was a deceptively lush piece of land two blocks from her store. No one in the community really knew who owned 858 East Ferry Street or why it had sat unused for as long as anyone could remember. Everyone referred to the property simply by its street address, 858 East Ferry. Neighborhood children played hide and seek among the weeds, bushes, and trees on the empty lot, and people frequently dug in the dirt to uncover the unusual antique bottles that could be found there. Some neighbors who lived in the public housing project nestled behind 858 East Ferry tended a pumpkin patch there. Grant also owned a rental house at 851 East Ferry, directly across the street—about nine yards—from the lot. Rhonda Dixon Lee had lived in that house for six years between 1982 and 1988.

Grant read and reread the memo and the document. She was dismayed by the details of what she learned. In 1996, an environmental restoration program known as the Clean Water/Clean Air Bond Act had provided the state of New York with money to clean up its municipalities' brownfields, or vacant properties that might be contaminated. The purpose was to see whether such brownfields—if they were indeed contaminated—could be cleaned up enough to prove to be prime development lots. In 1997 the city of Buffalo, which was hoping to develop such brownfields within the city to further economic expansion, had asked the New York State Department of Environmental Conservation to investigate the site. The lot claimed a strange history. Although the property had never housed any type of building, a Michael Heyman Company had operated a zinc and lead smelting and refining facility on the adjacent lot for sixty-one years, between 1917 and 1978. The factory had routinely transported highly contaminated waste and dumped it next door at 858 East Ferry. The factory itself had since been demolished. Today, a used car lot, TNT Auto, stood in its place.

In 1997 the DEC took soil and water samples from the site, at the city's request, to see what the status of the lot might be. If it was contaminated, the goal would be to clean it up enough to make it attractive to commercial developers. Under state regulations, a brownfield has to fit a specific definition to be considered a hazardous waste site. First, a toxic agent found on location has to fall on a predetermined list of chemicals or be a by-product of industrial processes known to produce toxic waste and/or the material must meet a chemical test characteristic of hazardous waste. Soil and groundwater testing at 858 East Ferry quickly revealed that the property more than met the criteria for a hazardous waste site, on many levels. PCBs were found in both soil and groundwater in a high-enough concentration to qualify by state definition as a hazardous waste site. But that was the lesser menace. A heavy concentration of lead ash intermingled with the soil sat several inches thick across the 3.32-acre site. The lead existed at a shockingly high concentration. The majority of soil samples showed lead levels ranging from 19,900 to 46,700 parts per million—far exceeding the Environmental Protection Agency's safety level of 400 parts per million in areas where children play, or 1,200 parts per million in other areas of a property. The site at 858 East Ferry exceeded New York State's criteria for a hazardous waste site nearly forty times over.

In March 1999 the Division of Environmental Remediation of the DEC issued a record of decision, or ROD—the document that Grant now held in her hands—which outlined plans to remove soil from the site by truck and dump it elsewhere, at a cost of $1.3 million. Although the city had asked for the investigation to take place, the remediation, the document read, would now be "carried out under the State Superfund Act." The city owned the land, but once the state had placed the 858 East Ferry site on the state Superfund cleanup list, remediation became the state's responsibility overnight.

However, the memo attached to the top of this record of decision spelled out a very different course of action; it informed city council members that, in fact, 858 East Ferry would not be remediated as planned. The toxic PCB and lead-laced soil would not be trucked out of the neighborhood. In fact, nothing was going to be done about the site for the foreseeable future: the state Superfund had just gone belly up, and there was simply no money left to remove the hazardous waste that permeated the 858 East Ferry property. Case closed.

Grant was dumbfounded by the senselessness of what she was reading. There was no money to remediate a toxic waste site that had been sitting there unbeknownst to residents for decades—and that the city had known about for the past three years? How could that be?

Several other facts concerned her. A line in the record of decision said that the New York State Department of Environmental Conservation had sent a bulletin to surrounding residents and business owners in February 1999 alerting them that a toxic waste site sat in their midst. Grant, who checked her mail carefully every day at her store, was certain she had never received a letter there. Nor had any letter ever arrived at the home she owned at 851 East Ferry, where her own daughter had been living for the last few years, practically smack on top of the 858 East Ferry site itself.

Over the next few days Betty Jean asked the dozens of customers who came in and out of Grant's Variety Shop if they'd ever gotten a letter in the past about East Ferry being classified as a class-two toxic waste site. Had anyone heard a single word about the problem? Not one had. She asked the next Sunday at True Bethel Baptist Church—which sat directly across the street from 858 East Ferry—if any clergy or members had received such a memo in their mailboxes. No one at church had ever heard a word about it, either.

"No one ever got those letters," Betty Jean says emphatically. "That is not the kind of thing you get and throw away. People have been wondering for fourteen years why everyone is getting so sick—and you think they'd get a letter telling them that they're living next to all those toxic chemicals and just toss it in the trash can?"

But perhaps the thing that disturbed Grant the most about the memo she received as councilwoman was that it was already slated—by the city's common council—to be "received and filed." That, says Grant, was code for "fait accompli. It was designated as received and filed, because the city felt there was nothing more to be done; that we should consider ourselves informed and file the issue away, no discussion necessary." But, she fumed, if no remediation was going to be done, how could they possibly be expected to accept that and file the papers away? What about the residents they had been elected to protect?

At the next full council meeting in May when the issue was raised and about to be checked off with a cursory nod with the understanding that it was out of their hands, a done deal, Betty Jean was ready. She held up her hand in a pause motion. "Not so fast," she told her fellow councillors. "This is really serious. This is a class-two site, and I happen to think our neighbors are getting sick from this."

Grant found support from the councilman who represented the East Ferry area where the site was located. While the majority of the council wanted to drop the issue, arguing that the Superfund had no money, so why press a hopeless case, the two council members persevered. They called the New York State Department of Environmental Conservation to suggest firmly that, at the very least, a fence be erected around the property with signs posted stating No Trespassing—Toxic Waste Site. The DEC responded by saying that since the city owned the lot, only the city had the legal right to erect a fence on it. The DEC added that they had written several letters to the city requesting that they erect a fence, but the city was not willing to do so. Calls made to the city were no more fruitful. The city claimed that since the state had already listed the site for cleanup, the city no longer bore any responsibility to remediate the area in any way—including putting up a fence to keep people off the property. It was now strictly the state's responsibility to find the money to clean it up because it had investigated the contamination, determined a course of action, and placed the East Ferry site on the Superfund list. The city was not to blame, they said, for the fact that the Superfund went bankrupt. It quickly became evident to Grant that the city and the DEC were engaged in a dead-end blame game.

As for the letter that the DEC said it had sent out to the community to warn them about the site, it was unclear what had actually occurred—and it may always remain so. The DEC held that they had sent residents a bulletin informing them about the site and alerting them to a meeting to discuss it, but no one had come forward except for a single developer interested in building on the lot. Grant and others in the community were adamant that they had never received any such letter. Today, no one at the Albany, New York, office of the DEC, from which the East Ferry project was overseen, is willing to talk about what might have happened back then to result in so many residents remaining uninformed for so long.

Yet ironically, those missing letters and the lack of willingness on the part of the city to erect a simple fence would end up being the two catalysts that would galvanize residents to stand up and say they were mad as hell and weren't going to take it anymore.

Grant was so infuriated that she wrote a letter to the local African-American community newspaper, the *Challenger,* and to the local *Buffalo Criterion,* letting residents know about the toxic waste site. In her letter she pointed out the possible correlation between autoimmune disease in the area and proximity to the East Ferry locale. She asked anyone in the area who had an autoimmune disease to give her a call. She went to the local True Bethel Baptist Church and asked the pastor there, the Reverend Darius G. Pridgen, to get the word out as well. Within a week, her list of who was afflicted with lupus and other autoimmune diseases within a few blocks of East Ferry grew to nineteen.

Rhonda Dixon Lee, up until that point, had been getting involved with helping those with lupus through an entirely different avenue. Having trained as a nurse, Lee felt that much more could be done to enhance local residents' understanding of the disease so that those who were sick received proper treatment before irreversible tissue or organ damage occurred. She had been putting her efforts into assisting another local resident, Judith Anderson, a fifty-five-year-old African-American woman and founder of a local advocacy and support group, sponsored by the Lupus Alliance of America's Western New York affiliate, called Sisters with Lupus. Anderson had established the group to help low-income African-American women who were suffering from the disease. Anderson knew all too well what these women were facing; she was a lupus sufferer herself.

Anderson, a petite woman whose demure demeanor belies her resolve for her mission, had also come of age in the East Ferry/Delavan-Grider area of Buffalo. She had been ill since the age of nineteen. As a young child in the 1950s and 60s, Anderson had grown up about a mile from 858 East Ferry. Later, she lived on Carl Street, a third of a mile from the site, for three years. And between 1973 and 1987, her parents had owned and operated a family business called Anderson Lanes, a bowling alley with a bar and restaurant on Northland Avenue, which ran along the north side of the 858 East Ferry lot. For fourteen years, as a young wife and mother, Anderson had worked part-time at Anderson Lanes, which was located a little more than half a mile from the East Ferry site.

Anderson, like most of the women in the area, had spent long, difficult years unable to secure a medical diagnosis for her disease. By her early twenties, as a divorced single mother working for the local telephone company, she would set the alarm at four a.m. in order to get to work by nine. Her muscles and joints and connective tissue ached so much it took an hour to get in and out of the shower and another hour just to coax on her pants and shirt, with breaks in between to rest from the exertion.

Doctors, of whom Anderson saw dozens during office visits and intermittent hospital stays, were perpetually stumped. At times, she thought she must simply be insane. Not one doctor ever thought to test her for lupus. In 1989, her disability progressed to the point that when she did arrive at work, where her company enforced strict employee sick-day rules, coworkers would have to meet her at the door, put her in a rolling chair, and wheel her to her desk so she could start the day. She had to write with a felt tip pen, because she lacked the strength to bear down hard enough with a pencil or ballpoint to mark the page.

In 1990 she was finally tested for and diagnosed with lupus. By then she was forty-four years old and had lived with lupus, without the right treatment, for twenty-five years. All that time, she had somehow managed to avoid going into kidney failure. She was lucky to be alive, and she knew it.

After being diagnosed she would sometimes scan the obituaries in the local paper and read that another twenty- or thirty-year-old woman had died of lupus or of "unknown causes" that seemed clearly lupus-like in nature. It made her angry to think of women suffering as she had, without ever knowing why—without getting treatment and support or knowing that there were steps doctors could take to help them manage their disease. Judith Anderson wanted to change things for the women of Buffalo. In 1991 she began to volunteer for the Lupus Alliance of Western New York. What started as a part-time volunteer job soon turned into a full-time paying position as program director. By 1993 she had started the Sisters with Lupus support group in hopes of helping women in Buffalo get the diagnosis and medical therapy they so desperately needed.

• • •

In the spring of 2000, when Betty Jean alerted the community about the contamination at 858 East Ferry Street and shared her strong concern that the toxic waste site might be connected to higher than average rates of autoimmunity in the neighborhood, Rhonda and Judith were as alarmed as Betty Jean that the state and city were doing nothing. "We know that our dirty earth is related to disease," Anderson says. "So is that what we're going to leave for our children? Once you know of a problem, you need to fix it, so future generations won't face the same ordeal. If you don't do anything about it, that's plain wrong." The state and city weren't willing to fix it? Then Betty Jean, Rhonda, Judith, and fellow citizens would make it happen.

A GATHERING STORM OF PROTEST

Where to start? Betty Jean sought help from a well-respected community activist and friend, Ausur Afrika, because of his diligence in assisting with work against discrimination and unfair conditions in the community. Afrika regularly held meetings for the area's Black Chamber of Commerce, which he had helped to found, at a local bookstore, Harambe—its name an eastern African word referring to the tribal custom of all pulling together to help one another in times of need. Afrika was ready to help. He had seen Betty Jean's letter in the newspaper before she came to him to share her suspicions about how the toxicity at 858 East Ferry had played a role in why so many people in the area had lupus.

After that letter appeared, a piece ran in the larger Buffalo paper, the *Buffalo News*, arguing that it was "unlikely" that there was any relationship between 858 East Ferry and the area's lupus cluster. The counterargument being made, Afrika recalls, "pointed out that the direct cause of lupus was not known so therefore you couldn't say that lead and PCBs could be part of what was triggering people's disease." But that seemed illogical to Afrika. "If you don't know what is triggering lupus, how can you say that a particular source isn't triggering it?" he asks.

In the summer of 2000 Betty Jean Grant, Ausur Afrika, Rhonda Dixon Lee, and several others came to a Black Chamber of Commerce meeting in what would be the first of many such gatherings. They agreed that they had to compel the city and state to take action. They continued to hold weekly meetings at Harambe over that summer, fall, and winter, naming themselves the Toxic Waste/Lupus Coalition, with the specific goals of alerting residents to the hazardous site at 858 East Ferry as well as forcing the city and state to do something to better protect the people who lived in the neighborhood.

Around that time a new city council member, Antoine Thompson, was elected to represent the nearby East Ferry area. Thompson was concerned about what was happening in East Ferry and joined the cause wholeheartedly. Antoine Thompson, Ausur Afrika, and Betty Jean Grant, in conjunction with the rest of the Toxic Waste/Lupus Coalition, kept meeting and sending suggestions to the Department of Environmental Conservation about how it could temporarily address the site for a small amount of money until more could be done.

"We came up with a million ideas as to what they might do that wouldn't cost nearly as much money," recalls Afrika. "We suggested they put a tarplike ground cover over the area so the lead ash wouldn't drift off the site. We asked again for a fence and that they put up a sign stating that the site was a hazardous waste site." But again no action was taken. The Toxic Waste/Lupus Coalition feared that the DEC and the city wanted to sweep the issue away, which simply goaded them on more. On Sundays they went to the public housing development next to the property and flooded the area with flyers. They put flyers in doorways and on car windshields, warning people not to go into the field at 858 East Ferry and telling them why. They asked Pastor Pridgen at True Bethel to alert his congregation to the site's toxicity.

Betty Jean, who as councilwoman had a weekly radio show, informed listeners that there was a toxic waste site in their area and that the coalition was concerned that if someone lived in the area that person might be more likely to have lupus. She asked them to call in. "Every week we heard from more and more who were afflicted," she says.

The coalition decided to go door to door and try to find out who else was ill. Rhonda, along with others, started going from house to house, handing out pamphlets, encouraging residents to come to their meetings to talk about the excessive number of neighbors suffering from autoimmune diseases and whether or not the toxic site at 858 East Ferry might have anything to do with their debility.

"On just the two streets that I canvased we found seventeen people with lupus—eight on Bissell and nine on Moselle," Rhonda recalls. "Some had already died by the time we started knocking on doors." Bissell and Moselle were each only three blocks long. By the end of that process the group had found thirty-seven residents in the immediate vicinity with lupus.

Headlines announcing "East Side Residents Fear Site May Be Causing Lupus" and "Decision to Shelve Cleanup Draws Fire" began to appear in the local *Buffalo News*. The number of concerned citizens who wanted to learn more about the toxic waste site multiplied. Darius Pridgen of True Bethel offered his church as a meeting site to allow the Toxic Waste/Lupus Coalition to accommodate its increasing membership. Still, while the coalition's numbers were growing, their clout remained nil—despite two city council members spearheading their cause. They were a group of African Americans in a downtrodden neighborhood. No one cared. No one was paying attention.

They needed reinforcements. And they had a hunch as to where they might get just that. At the coalition's request, Dr. John Vena, then a professor in the Department of Social and Preventive Medicine and director of the Environment and Society Institute (ESI) at the University at Buffalo, joined their cause and agreed to organize a university-community partnership. The institute occasionally provided funding to examine environmental problems relevant to the regional community; helping the residents of East Ferry with their environmental health crisis was exactly in keeping with the institute's mission statement.

Having secured Vena's involvement, the Toxic Waste/Lupus Coalition decided to call a community-wide meeting at True Bethel Baptist Church, the windows of which looked directly out upon the toxic waste site at 858 East Ferry. The coalition invited local residents, Vena, and David Locey, a midcareer environmental engineer who had been working for New York's Department of Environmental Conservation for more than a decade and who had overseen the initial evaluation of 858 East Ferry Street.

As the date of the meeting approached, Afrika held an unusual press conference. He stood alone in the toxic field of 858 East Ferry and told reporters about the dangerous levels of lead and PCBs the DEC had found there. He related how for more than a year the Toxic Waste/Lupus Coalition had been asking the city and state to deal with the problem, but still nothing was being done to remediate the site or to fence off the area. It was an effective strategy. On April 22, 2001, the *Buffalo News* came out with a photo of Afrika standing alone in the open, contaminated lot. The caption announced that the next day there would be a community awareness forum at True Bethel open to all residents of the City of Buffalo.

Twenty-four hours later, after having known about the property for four years, the city suddenly located the funds to pay for a fence and erected one around the entire site. A sign went up stating No Trespassing, but the words "hazardous waste" were not mentioned.

On April 23, 2001, Betty Jean Grant, Ausur Afrika, Antoine Thompson, John Vena, Rhonda Dixon Lee, Marion Jordan, and Judith Anderson as well as nearly fifty others from the community gathered at the True Bethel Baptist Church. They wanted answers from the Department of Environmental Conservation.

That night, they would learn not only about the unexpected extent of the problem at 858 East Ferry Street, but about two other

toxic waste sites in their midst that had also been leaching contaminants into the area for decades without residents' knowledge.

"THE SITUATION IS WORSE THAN YOU THINK"

That night was the first time the community heard about the full
extent of the pollution on the East Ferry site from the DEC's representative, David Locey. Many sat there in utter disbelief and horror
as they listened to the report: the lead ash, which in some areas
existed at a concentration nearly forty times higher than the EPA's
safety limit, sat two inches to as much as two feet thick on the surface of the property. Not only was the soil full of lead, but PCB-
contaminated sediment had been found on and near the lot from
industrial debris—tires, televisions, and construction rubble—ille-
gally dumped at the locale. The lead contamination, the DEC suspected, probably extended to the ground under the used-car lot
west of the site, which was as large as the lot at 858 East Ferry itself. Usually, the DEC would run more soil and water tests to determine if the surrounding area was affected, but the Superfund, as
everyone knew, was bone dry. The property at 858 East Ferry could
not be cleaned up until the state put more money in the Superfund,
Locey informed residents. The DEC had no way of knowing if or
when that might happen.

Afrika was incensed. "Now you're talking about doing more
surveys," he said. "Why are you wasting time with more surveys
when you've already issued a recommendation for remediation?"

The meeting was fraught with conflict, which only intensified
when the State University of New York at Buffalo environmentalists working with Vena presented a map to residents that night
charting two other major waste sites that had, for years prior
to being cleaned up, lingered unaddressed in the East Ferry and
Delavan-Grider neighborhoods. The history of the sites and their
rampant contamination—and how long it had taken for them to be
addressed—left residents doubly infuriated.

The first of these other sites, located at 537 East Delavan Avenue, sat two blocks south of both Marion Jordan and LaShekia Chatman's homes and two blocks north of East Ferry Street. The lot had been owned by a company named Vibratech Inc., which had for years manufactured trucking and railroad parts. The industrial facility, in operation since 1927, had also been used as a paint coating operation, a tire warehouse, and, most recently, an automobile operation that dismantled cars for their recyclable materials.

The DEC had investigated the site in the mid 1980s and found the 6,250-square-foot locale to be heavily contaminated with degreasing solvents such as trichloroethylene (TCE), vinyl chloride, and other particularly dangerous toxic agents commonly used in the manufacturing of metal items to clean off oils, greases, and other petroleum products, as well as a large number of other volatile organic compounds, known as VOCs. VOCs vaporize easily at room temperature and enter the surrounding atmosphere, where, studies show, vapors can linger as pollution for long periods of time.

The VOC contamination was the result of repeated and frequent industrial spillage over the past fifty years. In addition, ten ten-thousand-gallon tanks full of degreasing solvents as well as other chemicals—four below ground and six above—that had never been disposed of were leaching chemicals onto the site. PCB spills from transformers also soaked some areas. The local Scajaquada Creek, which accepted the majority of stormwater overflow in this area of Buffalo, was located about eleven hundred feet south of the property. The DEC survey in the mid 1980s reported that TCE-contaminated runoff from the site was found in high concentrations in nearby groundwater along the creek as well as down along a railroad spur area in the rear of the Vibratech facility. Rains caused TCE-laden runoff to course into the stream and railroad spur area, and TCE and other VOCs were continuing to leach slowly into the area groundwater from the facility's chemical spillage. Full remediation of the soil would be a huge and costly challenge.

Little was done in the 1980s to address the problem. At that time, only the four below-ground tanks of degreasing solvents, fuels, and unknown chemicals were emptied. Despite the fact that the soil and groundwater were contaminated at what were termed "high concentrations," the state classified the site as an inactive hazardous waste site—the area was not deemed as "presently constituting a significant threat to human health or the environment." The reasoning was thus: the area was restricted from public use, and the localized contaminated groundwater did not affect public drinking-water supplies since drinking water in the area came from public water storage sources. Cleaning it up was not a priority.

A decade later, in 1995, the same year that LaShekia Chatman, who lived amid this constellation of contaminated locales, was diagnosed with lupus, the DEC finally began full remediation at the East Delavan site two blocks away from her home. Much of the TCE- and PCB-contaminated soil was turned up and excavated from the facility. The six remaining full tanks of chemical waste were emptied, and the basement hazardous waste storage area was closed off. Even so, in May 1996, follow-up testing showed that volatile organic compound contamination still existed in the groundwater, albeit at lower levels—slightly half of what it had been prior to remediation in 1994. However, in one monitored area, the contamination level of VOCs had actually risen after the cleanup.

In March 1997, the DEC filed its final report, the record of decision, indicating that the site at 537 East Delavan was taken care of. The VOC-polluted soil, runoff, and groundwater that still exist there flowed down to the nearby sewer and were pumped away, with the sewer surge acting as a kind of natural barrier preventing any outward migration of contaminated soil and water from the spot.

The cleanup process had taken ten years. Aside from the question of whether the cleanup was fully complete, the fact would always remain that TCE—a highly volatile organic chemical that quickly and invisibly vaporizes into the surrounding air, including when the toxic vapors are unearthed as the soil is excavated during cleanup—had seeped into the environs for decades.

• • •

That night was also the first time residents learned of a third toxic hotspot—a PCB "inactive hazardous waste site" located at 318 Urban Street—a few blocks south of East Ferry Street and little more than a stone's throw from Rhonda Dixon Lee's home. The site had been investigated in 1990 but was not remediated until 1999. The New York Department of Environmental Conservation investigated the site, which was owned by General Electric and the Pyramid Steel Corporation, as part of its routine oversight into industrial manufacturing plants. They found it to be heavily contaminated with PCBs, which had been seeping into the ground for decades. Although the manufacture of PCB had been outlawed in the United States in 1976, it was used for decades prior to that as an industrial adhesive—a kind of toxic glue—in manufactured heat and ventilation systems, appliances, and electrical parts. The building had been used to store such electrical equipment. Both the surface and subsurface soils were discovered to be heavily contaminated by PCBs escaping from the equipment.

Starting in 1999, the area soil was removed and the PCB-laced drains leading from the facility into the sewer system were cleaned. But such environmental cleanup can never return an area to its former unblemished state. Residents learned that night that traces of the chemical remained in nearby sewers and that the sewer system ran through a heavily populated part of the East Ferry area, where, local advocates worried, PCB levels might still pose some health risk.

Together, this string of waste sites formed a kind of toxic Orion's belt that stretched across the East Ferry and Delavan-Grider neighborhoods—only this Orion's belt remained dangerously invisible to the naked eye. All three of these sites, all within less than a mile of Grant's Variety Shop, contained contaminants that were known to be implicated in immune dysfunction and, in many cases, were tied directly to autoimmune disease.

Lead, a well-documented neurotoxin, is not a substance that scientists have studied a great deal as a trigger of autoimmune disease, or autogen. But that isn't because researchers don't believe it is one. By the time scientists fully recognized autoimmunity and its umbrella of diseases in the 1970s, lead was already on its way to being understood as one of the most noxious substances on earth. Asking the question of whether it could also promote autoimmune disease was pushed aside by the pressing scientific effort to understand lead's role in impairing neural development in children. Nevertheless, in 2005, in research unrelated to the Buffalo lupus cluster, researchers set out to discover whether one of the additional legacies of lead hidden in our environment might be that it also tampers with the human immune system. Indeed, exposure to lead in lab animals disrupts immune-system cells that normally control runaway immune responses and prevent the autoimmune response from happening.

In the years between 1985 and 1995, as the site at East Delavan Street was going through various stages of DEC investigation and remediation, scientists in labs across the globe—including California, England, Italy, and France—were becoming extremely concerned about the emerging connection between TCE exposure and autoimmune disease, be it through vapor inhalation, skin contact, or ingestion. Occupational studies of workers exposed to the chemical through their jobs had already begun to show that those workers had a higher risk of developing lupus, scleroderma, and other autoimmune diseases. Indeed, in 1997, when the DEC filed its record of decision on East Delavan Street and deemed it remediated, Arkansas scientists Kathleen Gilbert and Neil Pumford were already immersed in research that would lead to their series of groundbreaking studies proving TCE to be a highly potent autoimmune-disease and lupus trigger.

During those same years, residents had been exposed to leaching PCBs at 318 Urban Street. PCBs, like plastic additives such as bisphenol A (BPA) and common pesticides, are endocrine-disrupting chemicals that have been shown in numerous lab studies to stimulate increased production of autoantibodies—antibodies against self—which are the hallmark of autoimmunity in action. Indeed, as we have seen in the previous chapter, the science demonstrating the way in which estrogen disruptors such as PCBs promote autoimmune disease is emerging with profoundly disturbing conclusions.

That April night at the Toxic Waste/Lupus Coalition community awareness meeting at True Bethel Baptist Church, Rhonda Dixon Lee, sitting with members of her community whom she had known all her life, was stunned by what she was hearing. She turned to Judith Anderson and asked her, "Did I just hear what I think I heard? The city and state knew about these sites all these years? And all three of those sites sit within a mile of my home?" She had been sick, her whole family had been sick—for ten years. "All those years of people being sick and dying and people are only now telling us the truth about what's really going on?" she asked. Lee burst into tears.

John Vena informed residents that he wanted the Environment and Society Institute to partner with them to seek a grant from the National Institute of Environmental Health Sciences to bring together University at Buffalo scientists and community members for a five-year study on the health impact of 858 East Ferry, focusing on the prevalence of autoimmune disease. Vena called it "the community's project."

Judith Anderson stood up to say that her lupus organization would assist residents in any way it could.

Residents headed home, reeling from what they had learned. Kayla's mom, Marion Jordan, was one of them. Her daughter had been terribly ill lately and was now living in Atlanta with her older sister, who was helping to care for her. After the meeting Marion called Renita, who had been unable to attend, to tell her that their worries had been justified: their neighborhood lupus/autoimmune cluster seemed to be related to contaminated industrial waste that had sat unaddressed in the community for decades.

"Oh my goodness, I was angry," recalls Renita Chatman. "All I could think about was how when I was pregnant with LaShekia I did everything right. I didn't smoke, I didn't drink, I exercised, I slept, I ate the healthiest foods. When she was born, I nursed her, I fed her the right things. I was so careful. I worked hard to give her a good start and to protect her. But I couldn't protect her from the fumes and the particles in the air and the water full of stuff that I couldn't even see. I couldn't stop thinking about it. When I was pregnant I used to love to eat ice chips all day. Was that what made LaShekia sick? Was it all those ice chips full of all the runoff from those waste sites that sullied our water system? I didn't know. And I knew that I would never know."

THE NEAR IMPOSSIBILITY OF PROVING A CLUSTER

In 2001 John Vena received a grant from the National Institute of Environmental Health Sciences to bring together University at Buffalo scientists and community members to study the health impact of 858 East Ferry Street on area residents. Although he would serve as the principal investigator, the Lupus Coalition would work as co-investigator. Part of the funding allowed for the creation of the Buffalo Lupus Project, to help experts reach into the community, find out who was suffering from autoimmunity, and aid them in getting the help they needed.

Although the university team was interested in whether or not a lupus cluster existed in East Ferry, proving that a cluster did exist was not their primary goal. Their main mission was to help the community deal with their immediate and critical environmental health crisis. It would be a mistake to focus their efforts on trying to demonstrate that there was a cluster because proving a scientific cluster is a nearly impossible epidemiological task, and nowhere is that more true than in the field of autoimmune disease. Technically, a cluster can be defined as a greater than expected occurrence of disease cases in a geographically defined region that is unlikely to have occurred by chance alone. Several elements are necessary in determining any cluster: the underlying disease prevalence should be known with some reliability, and the boundaries of the geographic area need to conform to natural population patterns. In other words, the area cannot be artificially constructed to include the maximum number of cases. Researchers also look for "biological plausibility": is it already well established that the chemical or agent present in the community can lead to this particular disease? There is also the question of proximity: are you more likely to suffer from the disease the closer you live to the contaminated site?

In considering whether East Ferry would fit such criteria for a cluster, the university team had to ask some fundamental questions. Could it be sure that the link between the environment and the group of people with disease was causal? People living in communities where industrial toxic waste sites tend to be situated are, frequently, at the lower end of the socioeconomic ladder. If they weren't, they might well have moved from such an economically depressed neighborhood long before. Life in such rundown neighborhoods is inherently more stressful. Dealing with poor housing conditions—broken heating systems, busted windows and doors, potholes in the sidewalks, high levels of industrial or traffic noise—can all make it more difficult to get through each day. Moreover, if you don't have enough money for the rent, the car has broken down again, and you live with a continual shortfall in groceries, your days are more stressful than if you have no such worries. Stress in and of itself is known to play a strong role in disease manifestation. Stress also leads to more "health risk behaviors"—poor diet, alcohol abuse, and so on, which can in turn lead to poorer health outcomes.

Could the researchers prove that the number of people with autoimmune disease in the East Ferry area of Buffalo was statistically significant enough to be a cluster? Or was it merely a statistical aberration resulting from the difficult life circumstances of people in the area? These are the questions that the University at Buffalo team would ask in trying to judge whether East Ferry qualified as a cluster site. A number that looked high, compared to another area of the country, still might not prove the cause and effect relationship between toxic waste sites and autoimmune disease that they were looking for.

Researchers were further limited by the nature of autoimmune disease itself. It often takes years for autoimmune diseases like lupus to be diagnosed, and even longer for those living in underprivileged populations who lack access to good care or who might be more easily dismissed by doctors because of their difficulty in covering hefty medical bills. Moreover, during the decades that these toxic waste sites had been quietly left active like forgotten landmines in the neighborhood, residents had moved, and many had died. More people might have been sick, yes, but some were no longer around to be part of any head count.

Even for those who had stayed put and who had been accurately diagnosed, there remained the issue of how to find them. Lupus and other autoimmune diseases, unlike cancer, are not reportable diseases, meaning health departments do not collect information on who has an autoimmune disease, much less how many are afflicted with each of the nearly one hundred different diseases that fall under the autoimmunity umbrella.

On the other hand, if your great aunt were to be diagnosed with lung cancer tomorrow, she would be added automatically by the physician or hospital treating her to statistics systematically gathered on the 9 million Americans who have ever been diagnosed with any sort of cancer in the United States. The National Cancer Institute, the Centers for Disease Control and Prevention, and the North American Association of Central Cancer Registries all fund surveillance research on who has which cancer by age, sex, race, and locale. So we know, at any given juncture, how many Hispanic women at age forty have breast cancer in New York City. Or how many sixty-five-year-old African-American men have survived prostate cancer in Florida. The National Cancer Institute's Surveillance, Epidemiology, and End Results (SEER) Program's data program is so specific that patient information includes the stage of each patient's cancer tumor at diagnosis, the first course of treatment, and follow-up status. This information is available to all through the National Cancer Institute's Web portal, through its SEER Cancer Statistics Review.

By comparison, the 23.5 million patients who suffer from autoimmune diseases do not claim megabytes in cyberspace in any national database. Physicians are not required to report who has autoimmune disease to any national registry, because no national registry exists. The data we do have is based on small epidemiological studies from which experts have extrapolated as best they can. No true numbers are available on where these patients live or when they fell ill, or even what autoimmune disease they might have. Search for details about them and what emerges is a dark screen.

Finally, researchers faced one more substantial hurdle in proving the biological plausibility of an autoimmune-disease cluster. Since the very concept of autogenicity—that chemical and toxic agents can prod the immune system to overreact, resulting in autoimmunity—is in and of itself new, how can we go about proving there is a cluster of people who have autoimmunity as a result of exposures to toxic waste in their area?

The State University of New York at Buffalo environmental scientists were unsure if they would be able to meet all the criteria for an ironclad cluster. However, they felt that they had more than enough information to warrant investigating the question further. Moreover, as scientists concerned with public health, they needed to reach those who were ill and help them get the treatment and care they needed. With the aid of Vena's grant money, Judith Anderson was asked to be the lupus educator for the project and chair of the Research and Survey Committee. Since federal law does not allow access to patients through doctors' offices or health records, Judith had to be creative. She examined old tax records to find those who had lived in the area and moved, then, if she was able to track them down, she asked about their health status. She arranged for billboards to be raised alongside the highways in the vicinity. The signs showed three African-American women standing side by side and big bold letters saying "We live near 858 E. Ferry St. We all have Lupus. Are you sick too? Take 5 minutes and call Judith to join the registry." The Buffalo Lupus Project, working together with the community's Toxic Waste/Lupus Coalition, held a massive two-month radio campaign asking those with lupus and other autoimmune diseases to join its lupus registry. It distributed pamphlets titled "Are Toxic Waste Sites Affecting Your Health?" In 2003, Anderson took over as community health coordinator for the Buffalo Lupus Project. She distributed flyers that mapped out for residents the locations of the three toxic waste blocks in East Ferry and Delavan-Grider, which included detailed explanations about the connection between chemicals and autoimmune disease.

Around that time, Vena left the University at Buffalo and turned the project over to Carlos Crespo, an associate professor in the Department of Social and Preventive Medicine at the university, who had worked in minority health epidemiology both at the National Institutes of Health and at the Centers for Disease Control and Prevention. Crespo had a personal interest in studying autoimmunity. At the age of sixteen, his hair had begun to fall out in large chunks—a traumatic experience at any age and especially so for a teenage boy. Crespo was diagnosed with alopecia areata, an autoimmune disease in which, for reasons unknown, the body's own immune system attacks the hair follicles and disrupts normal hair formation. Doctors gave him nearly fifty steroid shots directly into the scalp to try to stop the autoimmune response, but his hair didn't grow back until he was twenty-two. At the age of thirty, it fell out again. He went with it and shaved his head. A hipster blue-jeaned professor who looks a bit like a Latino cross between Yul Brynner and Kojak, Crespo took on Vena's cause with great interest.

The university environmental scientists involved in the project were disturbed that even by 2003—two years after the meeting at True Bethel—there were still no plans to remediate East Ferry. The Toxic Waste/Lupus Coalition approached Joseph Gardella, professor of chemistry at the University at Buffalo's Environment and Society Institute, who is well known in western New York for taking on tough environmental causes, such as helping homeowners in Buffalo's Hickory Woods development whose houses had been built on contaminated soil from a Superfund site. Gardella, a wry, shorts-sporting, suntanned, and bulldogish fifty-one-year-old, volunteered to use his expertise in environmental chemistry and the effects of exposure to toxins to help residents pressure the DEC to find funds to clean up East Ferry. Gardella didn't care that the Superfund was dry, and he didn't see any point in waiting around to find out whether East Ferry met all the statistical criteria for being an official cluster or not. As an environmental chemist he cared about the pure facts staring them in the face: a known toxic agent was contaminating the residential area and not a darn thing was being done about it. He took on the project, he says, "with a conservative approach: if a toxin is there and you know it's bad you need to do something to remove it. I see it as my job to push walls to make that happen."

CLEANING UP THE MESS, FINALLY

In August 2003, Gardella, along with community members and a group of chemistry, geology, and geography students, did just that. He and his team took thirty soil samples outside the East Ferry lot itself—throughout the surrounding East Ferry streets and neighborhood. They tested the samples for lead and ferried the disturbing results to the DEC. Meanwhile, Toxic Waste/Lupus Coalition community members continued to demand meetings with DEC representatives, calling for action. In 2006, relentlessly badgered by an outraged community and faced with Gardella's lab findings, which showed that high levels of lead had migrated offsite and across East Ferry Street to the exposed soil on the easement beyond the curb, the state finally promised to take action to clean up the site. They agreed to extend the area of remediation significantly to include four adjacent contaminated lots west of 858 East Ferry Street, an area approximately four times as large as the original Superfund site.

As for whether East Ferry presents a disease cluster that will meet the stringent and statistical guidelines for determining an environmentally triggered cluster, it will be some time before the emerging data can be fully quantified, much less published. Either way, the question of whether the Buffalo lupus cluster is officially the direct result of toxicity in the area seems increasingly moot. Between 2002 and 2006, through the Buffalo Lupus Project and the Toxic Waste/Lupus Coalition's combined efforts, the number of people discovered to have lupus and other autoimmune diseases in the community quadrupled. On Carl Street alone, where Judith Anderson had lived for several years as a young wife and mother, she found four young women who had already been diagnosed with lupus.

According to the Lupus Foundation of America, which conducted several nationwide telephone surveys, approximately 1.5 million Americans have lupus—which translates to roughly 1 in 200 people. Based on the latest census, the East Ferry area studied in the Buffalo Lupus Project has a population of 11,000. By 2006, the Buffalo Lupus Project had identified 143 individuals—110 with lupus and 33 with other autoimmune diseases—in that same East Ferry population, which translates to approximately 1 in 100 individuals suffering from lupus in the East Ferry neighborhood. Those who live in this district of Buffalo have twice the likelihood of developing lupus as individuals living elsewhere.

Although the University at Buffalo has not yet wrapped up the Buffalo Lupus Project, Carlos Crespo's "personal bias," he says, is that "epidemiologically, there is a lupus cluster in this area. The distribution of lupus cases in the East Ferry area is outside of the average that you would see in a similar community to this one."

In 2005, Crespo moved on to be the director of the School of Community Health at Portland State University in Oregon. In his stead, Laurene Tumiel-Berhalter, PhD, the vice chair of research and development in the Department of Family Medicine at the University at Buffalo, has taken over the Buffalo Lupus Project. Tumiel-Berhalter agrees with Crespo that "these numbers raise eyebrows. One in one hundred Americans do not normally have lupus." She points out that although African Americans in general have higher rates of lupus than do Caucasians—and East Ferry is largely, though not entirely, an African-American community—even so, "it still doesn't account for this lupus cluster." Moreover, one can never know how many patients researchers missed since limited funds did not allow them to knock on every one of those eleven thousand doors. How many patients never saw a billboard or a flyer and so never reported to the registry; how many were ill but had no idea as to what it was they were suffering from; how many had died from lupus complications before the Buffalo Lupus Project even began? And then there were no doubt others who had moved away and left no trace. The numbers were, in fact, likely to be higher than what the researchers could tabulate.

Of more importance to residents, as well as to activists like Crespo, Gardella, Grant, and Anderson, is this: by 2006 they had succeeded in presenting enough of a case—and exerting enough relentless community pressure—to force the cleanup of 858 East Ferry despite the Superfund being empty. Today, the Department of Environmental Conservation admits that the problem at East Ferry involves "more volume of material than we initially thought." To fully clean up the area will cost not the $1.3 million originally projected in the DEC's record of decision in 1999, but nearly six times that—$7.7 million. In late 2006, remediation commenced, and contractors began to dig up the area and truck the contaminated soil to a landfill.

Not surprisingly, the DEC remains dubious that the toxic waste about to be remediated is linked to the plethora of illness in the area. "To this day we still cannot say that there is any connection between this site and the disease of autoimmunity in this area," says David Locey. "I think anyone working on this project has to admit that they can't know that with any certainty." Nevertheless, when asked if he would allow his kids to play on the East Ferry site, he pauses and says, "No, I wouldn't let my kids play on that lot."

Although cleanup had finally begun—after five years of fighting for it and nine years after the problem was first discovered—few feel victorious. Most feel it's far too little too late. "I've raised all ten of my babies here," says Rhonda Dixon Lee. "I just found out that now one of my daughters has lupus, too. All of these neighborhood kids have grown up, just like she did, walking up and down these blocks past all these chemicals every day, without ever knowing they were there."

Residents like Lee ask themselves the following questions: Although the two nearby sites on Delavan and Urban have already recently undergone remediation, and 858 East Ferry is now beginning to be addressed, what about the effects these fugitive leakages have already had on the parents and children who have lived in this area all their lives? Might someone appear healthy now only to get autoimmune disease in the future as a result of their earlier exposures? Aren't chances high that their immune systems have already been taxed by this slow, invisible, and continuous exposure to autogenic chemicals—whether they have yet seen any physical signs of disease or not?

It's particularly troublesome to Crespo that, like so many disease clusters, this happened in a minority community that is economically depressed. Indeed, one 2004 study conducted in the city of Buffalo reports that neighborhoods with predominantly minority populations have more than thirty-two times the number of air-polluting facilities as nonminority neighborhoods. Had East Ferry been a more affluent, nonminority area this probably wouldn't have occurred, Crespo believes. Industry in the area has certainly not been motivated to clean up its toxic waste. Cleanup and remediation are time-consuming and enormously expensive. Validation, much less help, didn't arrive until the number of people sick and dying with lupus in the area had already reached such critical mass that the cluster could no longer be ignored. For the many years that PCBs, lead, and TCE sat smoldering on those three sites, Buffalo was a disaster just waiting to be revealed.

CLUSTERS AROUND THE GLOBE

As population explosions and urban sprawl intersect with our increasingly chemical-laden landscape, other neighborhoods face similar concerns to those in Buffalo. Elsewhere in the United States and around the world, autoimmune studies include reports of a high number of lupus patients and those with biomarkers for lupus (a higher than average prevalence of antinuclear antibodies, which indicates an increased likelihood that a person will develop lupus in the future) near toxic sites, including a waste site harboring TCE and heavy metals in Tucson, Arizona. In another case, in El Paso, Texas, a forty-two-year-old former resident with multiple sclerosis contacted the Texas Department of Health in 1994 to report an apparent cluster of MS cases among people who had spent their childhood in the Kern Place–Mission Hills area of El Paso. Fifteen adults, aged forty-two to fifty-three, who had lived in that neighborhood as children—most of whom had attended the nearby Mesita Elementary School—had multiple sclerosis. The Texas Department of Health investigated and concluded that those who attended Mesita during the same years as those in the MS cluster had double the expected rate of MS. This was, they said, a conservative estimate; numbers might actually be higher. Investigators linked the cluster to the fact that children growing up in the area were exposed to a high level of heavy metals. Mesita Elementary School was located about one mile east from what had been, during these patients' childhood years, the American Smelting and Refining Company, which processed primarily lead, copper, cadmium, and zinc, along with emitting high levels of sulfuric acid. Many residents had, in fact, grown up referring to their neighborhood as "Smeltertown." Further investigation found that these MS patients' hair samples showed that they had been exposed to a number of heavy metals.

Seven other heavy-metal-based clusters of MS have been investigated and established, in addition to others linked to varied types of toxic waste. One MS cluster now under investigation is in Morrison, Illinois, and its environs. There, researchers from the Agency for Toxic Substances and Disease Registry of the Department of Health and Human Services are looking into what may be one of the highest rates of MS in the world—related, residents believe, to chemical pesticides and toxins from manufacturing and hazardous waste sites. Investigators looking into high rates of MS in Morrison are also studying four neighboring towns: Lewiston, DePue, Savanna, and Paw Paw. DePue and Savanna are both Superfund sites. A combination of chemical exposures in the five-town area includes those from pesticides, fertilizers, zinc smelting, heavy industrial manufacturing, unexploded weapons stored at a now defunct army depot, and toxic waste sites housing city sludge transported to the area from Chicago.

Likewise, a heightened incidence of lupus in a small African-American community in Georgia has been attributed to environmental pollutants from industrial sources. In a four-year study of Choctaw Native Americans in southeastern Oklahoma, researchers found a higher than average occurrence of scleroderma. Although genetics in the closely related Choctaw population was likely a contributing factor, relatives who moved away did not have as high a rate of scleroderma. Other high rates of scleroderma include those being investigated in Woodstock, in southwestern Ontario, and that of a small rural area in the province of Rome, Italy. In the south of Boston, there has been a four times higher than normal incidence of scleroderma (PBS and *Nightline* have both aired segments about the Massachusetts Department of Health's investigation into this emergent cluster), just one of several inquiries under way in the United States today. In Anniston, Alabama, investigators funded by the Agency for Toxic Substances and Disease Registry are conducting studies to determine whether high rates of autoimmune disease in the area are linked to an industrial manufacturing site where most of the PCBs in the United States were once manufactured and dumped. Blood serum levels of PCBs have been measured in a number of local residents in excess of 100 parts per billion. The CDC considers a blood PCB level in excess of 20 parts per billion to be significantly elevated. In 2003, two lawsuits against the PCB manufacturer and its spinoff companies resulted in a close to three-quarter-million-dollar settlement that was split, after lawyers' fees, among twenty thousand residents. Many of these residents were from socioeconomically underprivileged families who formerly sharecropped near the plant when it was dumping factory waste from PCB production. And in Libby, Montana, a town polluted by asbestos, recent studies conducted by the University of Montana's Center for Environmental Health Sciences show that local residents are 28.6 percent more likely to have antinuclear antibodies in their blood than a control group from a nearby town without asbestos pollution.

From Buffalo to Arizona, from Boston to Oklahoma, we live in an increasingly complex sea of autogenic agents. Added to that is the chemical load that we import into our own homes through the products, foods, and home goods we buy and consume. You can green your home as best you can, eat organic, avoid dry cleaning the clothes, throw out the solvents, and buy bedding *sans* flame retardants, but can you find that hallowed ground far from the chemical-driven American industrial machine? It is difficult to locate that halcyon land where toxic waste sites, nasty landfills, dry-cleaner TCE spills, and PCB-laced soil don't linger nearby—which is part of the reason why it is so hard to prove cause and effect between toxic waste and any disease cluster. So much toxic waste exists everywhere, how can we definitively compare what autoimmune-disease rates might be in a pristine area with those in a highly contaminated area when such clear-cut lines rarely exist in the cities and suburbs where we live?

To see how true this is, go to the Environmental Protection Agency's EnviroMapper yourself and plug in your own zip code. You can search any reported spots in your neighborhood that discharge toxins into the air or water, as well as hazardous waste and Superfund sites, though you may not be thrilled with what you find. Just take a peek at one small community (zip code 37055) along Eno Road in Dickson County, Tennessee. The largely African-American community that lives on Eno Road is surrounded by garbage dumps, landfills, and three toxic waste sites. Residents were recently informed that for the last decade they've been drinking tap water with levels of TCE that are twenty-four times higher than the maximum level deemed safe by the Environmental Protection Agency. For ten years water laced with TCE has been leaching into the groundwater from those nearby landfills and ending up in Eno Road residents' coffee cups and water glasses.

There are many, many other Eno Roads. In 2002, the Agency for Toxic Substances and Disease Registry (ATSDR) and its partners prepared public-health assessment documents for 122 toxic waste sites. Of those sites, 28.5 percent were found to be leaching contaminants into the community, posing a public health hazard. In another 2002 assessment, ATSDR estimated that more than 1.7 million people live within one mile of 371 sites under assessment—the majority of which are contaminated with a range of volatile organic compounds including TCE, arsenic, and other toxic chemicals.

Today, 1,200 designated Superfund sites around the country still await cleanup. At about 10 percent of these sites, toxic chemicals are known to be seeping out into communities or people are still freely entering sites and being exposed to the hazardous waste there. The Environmental Protection Agency does not release projections for what it plans to spend to remediate these 1,200 sites, when these areas will be cleaned up, or how long it will take.

All of which begs the question: Are there 1,200—or more—silent, hidden Buffalos spread across America, where residents simply haven't yet thought to ask why they're being struck by these debilitating diseases at disturbingly high rates? Since the majority of patients take years to be diagnosed, we have no records of who has autoimmune diseases in America, and studies linking specific autogens to the triggering of autoimmune diseases are relatively new and all too easily dismissed by industry, chances are that in most communities where such clusters surreptitiously exist no one is even asking the question.

SEARCHING FOR A FRESH START

Today, LaShekia Chatman and her mom, Renita, live in the more economically prosperous community of Cheektowaga, not far from downtown Buffalo, in a brick house with wrought iron fencing—identical to every other house on their street. The Chatmans moved out of East Ferry four years ago, hoping for a fresh, chemical-free start—only to find that they had relocated to the vicinity of yet another autoimmune-disease cluster in the making. Soon after the Chatmans moved in, the local Cheektowaga Homeowners Association released a report citing high incidences of autoimmune diseases in their community. Residents and environmental scientists from the University at Buffalo believe that several chemical-laden landfill dumps and the Buffalo Crushed Stone Quarry, which surround the neighborhood in what some refer to as a "toxic triangle," are predisposing Cheektowaga residents to autoimmune illnesses. Mine blasting at the quarry throws large amounts of crystalline silica, one of the most documented triggers of lupus, rheumatoid arthritis, and scleroderma, into the atmosphere. Hydrogen sulfide, a toxic ingredient in mining wastewater, races through the area creeks.

When the Cheektowaga cluster became public through the work of local activists, LaShekia said it hit her like "an anvil striking someone in the head in a cartoon with the balloon: 'Are you KIDDING me? Not AGAIN.'" Having jumped from one frying pan into the next, the Chatmans understandably feel it might do little good to move elsewhere in Buffalo. Who knows what hidden toxic waste they might end up living near next time?

Today, LaShekia, who has since graduated from college and begun work on a novel, has spent nearly a decade and a half battling a total of five different devastating autoimmune diseases, two of which—lupus and scleroderma—can bring normal existence to a halt, or even end a life. Still under Alan Baer's care, she manages her illnesses on a finely tuned combo cocktail of prednisone, Imuran, Plaquenil, Prilosec, and aspirin. At the age of twenty-nine, she confesses she sometimes feels lonely and "envious" watching other young people enjoy the normal things that twenty-somethings with their whole lives ahead of them do. She longs to be like them, to "be able to think about having a career, getting married, and having children," she says. "Or even just to get to be irresponsible and stay out late with friends and eat junk food and go dancing all night, because you don't have to do the super-responsible things that someone with a chronic illness has to do, like get plenty of rest, go to bed early, eat right, and watch your every move."

After speaking many times by phone, LaShekia and I finally meet for the first time on a beautiful, crisp August day in Buffalo. The sky is a photogenic blue with bottlebrush marks of white—an optimistic backdrop for a city where the streetscape exudes a gray and downcast feel that, by comparison, would make a Hopper painting seem cheerful. Judith Anderson is driving LaShekia and me on a whirlwind tour through LaShekia's past—starting with LaShekia's old jump-roping ground, on the street where she first lived. The small colonial in which LaShekia once lived in the community of Delavan-Grider lies a ten-minute stroll from 858 East Ferry and a three-minute walk from the TCE site on Delavan. As we drive slowly through her old neighborhood, LaShekia, a stately young woman sporting a chic chignon and hip black cat glasses, points through the car window to the car manufacturing plants and abandoned brick smokestacks of factories rising along the landscape in every direction—a kind of industrial ghost town.

For a moment we linger in the car outside her old house, and I can imagine LaShekia racing on lanky legs up and down these front steps as a child, full of vigor and promise. "How does it feel, looking back at growing up here?" I ask.

"I feel this rush of shock and anger that this cluster could develop without any of us knowing what was happening to us, or why," she says. "The fact is, if I had grown up, say, in Colorado, this wouldn't have happened. I hate to think of other teenagers living in industrial towns who might have to forfeit everything because other people have decided that cleaning up chemical waste isn't important."

The stew of environmental contaminants in which Buffalo residents and their children have marinated for years clearly has tipped many of their immune systems toward disease. Each individual's unique combination of genes, gender, hormones, exposure to environmental chemicals and heavy metals, and viral hits determines his or her future. In many patients like LaShekia, it may well be that environmental chemicals first torque the immune system so that it sits just

a hair trigger shy of becoming deranged. Suddenly, one last hit occurs; a virus enters the system and an autoimmune reaction is
spurred into motion.

LaShekia lived in an area with waste sites containing TCE,
PCBs, and lead—all known or suspected autogens—her entire life.
After fifteen years of her immune system's being taxed in a slow
and continuous manner by the toxic agents that surrounded her, a
seemingly harmless, common virus, Epstein-Barr, attacked. The
point at which LaShekia's immune system could continue to maintain balance was suddenly breached, and her immune cells raced
out of control. The role that viruses play in reaching this final point
is, as we are about to see, also emerging as a critical factor in today's
autoimmune-disease crisis.

CHAPTER FOUR

A POTENT PACKAGE: VIRUSES, VACCINES, AND HEAVY METALS

There may be no better example of how a common virus can trigger the body to sabotage itself than my own story. In the past seven years, a slew of viral attacks have changed my body permanently. The first incident occurred in 2000, when I was sidelined by a flu with the usual fever and muscle aches and pains, the kind of virus from which most people quickly recover to get on with their lives. A few weeks after the flu had come and gone, however, the skin on my forearms, hands, calves, and feet became curiously numb—as if the surface of my skin had fallen asleep and only half awakened. The strange deadened feeling was accompanied by odd shooting pains in my fingers and wrists, like sparks of fire spreading from one hot nerve to the next.

The first doctor I saw, a local internist, suggested my symptoms might be related to the fact that I have a pacemaker. He thought there might be a connection between my heart problems and the tingling and numbness in my extremities. My cardiologist, however, scoffed at the idea. He referred me to Dr. Ahmet Hoke, a well-known neurologist at Johns Hopkins, who ordered biopsies in which pencil-eraser-deep tissue samples were taken from my thighs. Hoke, a Middle Eastern–born physician who serves as the director of the Division of Neuromuscular Diseases at Johns Hopkins, discussed my test results with me a few days later. My biopsies showed that I had suffered damage to my small-fiber sensory nerves, the tiny nerves that tell us whether what we touch is soft or rough, hot or cold. The disease, known as small-fiber sensory neuropathy, was, he elaborated, "probably the result of a recent virus."

"How does a virus attack my nerves?" I wanted to know.

"An autoimmune reaction," he said. "Most likely a protein on the surface of a molecule of the virus you had looks like a protein on the surface of the molecules of your nerve tissue. The body gets tricked by their similarity and attacks the small-fiber sensory nerves as it fights the virus. We call it molecular mimicry."

It was the first time—in that summer of 2000—that I fully grasped precisely what "autoimmune" meant. Our immune cells could mistake our body's own tissue for a virus or bacteria or other foreign invader, or antigen, and the mechanisms by which the immune system should prevent such cases of mistaken identity from happening could fail abysmally. I had always known, theoretically, that hypothyroidism, which I also had, was autoimmune in nature, but I had never fully understood before how autoimmunity actually occurred within the human body.

Hoke reassured me that, in my case, my biopsies showed that something quite hopeful had occurred. In some patients with small-fiber sensory neuropathy, the nerves, after degenerating, regenerate to some degree. My sense that my skin had fallen asleep and only partially reawakened was more accurate than I could have known.

Small-fiber sensory neuropathy would turn out to be the least distressing of the three autoimmune reactions I would experience over the next six years—each of which Ahmet Hoke would tie back to infections I'd had a month or so prior to the episode. In 2001, and again in 2005, after having had a seemingly innocuous bout of vomiting, I developed Guillain-Barré syndrome, or GBS, and became paralyzed as my immune system systematically damaged the myelin sheaths that coated my nerves, the same sheaths that are injured in multiple sclerosis.

Once again my immune fighter cells were flubbing up, making similar molecular mistakes—each time with more disturbing consequences.

Yet something puzzled me. Although a virus had triggered each of my autoimmune episodes, I knew that viruses had to be only part of the story. I had had many feverish flus prior to the one in 2000 that led to small-fiber sensory neuropathy. And I had had many stomach flus in my life prior to 2001. While I clearly possessed the genetic predisposition to autoimmunity, and, yes, a virus had attacked, these two factors had been true for me many, many times before, yet I had never demyelinated and undergone the "flaccid paralysis" of Guillain-Barré syndrome after having had the stomach bug. Clearly, like most people who develop autoimmune disease after a virus, something else in my environment had to have been slowly pushing my immune system to this precipice—a precarious edge from which one viral hit could send me tumbling, like Jill, all the way down the hill. Nevertheless, in my case—as well as for the majority of patients with autoimmunity—keen attention had to be paid to the catalytic role of viruses in my disease and the astonishing manner in which viruses are somehow able to pull that final switch that tricks the immune system into attacking the cells of the body it is meant to safeguard.

THE LUPUS HUNTERS

For decades, researchers investigating Guillain-Barré syndrome have held the suspicion that GBS might be linked to infectious pathogens—not only because patients so often report having been ill in the six weeks prior to getting the disease, but also because clusters of cases have been linked in timing and locale to large, national vaccination programs with vaccines containing viral antigens. Yet the idea that autoimmune diseases as a broader group might be triggered in part by viruses has been anathema to most researchers.

Ironically, the first scientists to emerge with startling lab evidence that lupus might be triggered by a ubiquitous virus almost all of us are exposed to by adulthood was a professor and grad student team that wasn't even looking to make that connection.

Dr. John Harley, a transplanted West Virginian whose dry, quick humor and deep smile wrinkles soften his exacting edge, today manages a research staff of two hundred as chief of the Arthritis and Immunology Research Program at the Oklahoma Medical Research Foundation (OMRF). Most days he can be found more or less racewalking through the halls of his research institute as he moves between his research lab, teaching classroom, and the hospital, often shadowed by a handful of students and an assistant towing a cart full of files. Harley also serves as a professor and chief of the Rheumatology, Allergy and Immunology Division at the University of Oklahoma Health Sciences Center and as a staff physician at the Oklahoma City VA Medical Center, where he cares for patients with lupus and other autoimmune diseases.

For the past thirty-two years, Harley has committed himself to pinpointing the first step that goes awry in the pathway that leads patients to develop lupus. He has deep personal reasons for pursuing the triggers for the disease. When Harley was working toward his MD/PhD at the University of Pennsylvania three decades ago, his best friend at Penn died of lupus. They were working together as senior lab partners when his friend's kidneys began to shut down. Harley, who often stopped by to visit his friend at the hospital in the evenings, found him lapsing in and out of consciousness one night, suffering from kidney failure. Although treatment for lupus has not progressed much in the intervening decades, there were even fewer options for lupus patients in 1974, even at Penn, considered one of the best hospitals in the world. That night, Harley held his friend to comfort him. Not long after, his friend died in Harley's arms.

Nearly twenty years down the pike, by the early 1990s, Harley—after a residency at Yale and postdoc training at the National Institutes of Health—was in charge of the large-scale lab operation at the Oklahoma Medical Research Foundation, where he had been working for eight years. Judi James, meanwhile, was a fourth-generation Oklahoman from Pond Creek, a small northern Oklahoma town of fewer than nine hundred people, who'd come to OMRF as an undergraduate and never left. The first student of the newly established MD-PhD program at the University of Oklahoma Health Sciences Center, James wanted to pursue research in asthma. Unable to find a lab dedicated to asthma research, she headed to Harley's lab to get experience "so that I could move on to asthma research" later on. Then she had an encounter that shifted her career focus forever. One morning she accompanied Harley on rounds at University Hospital and "met a woman with lupus in the intensive care unit who was exactly my age—twenty—who was extremely sick. She had two small children. I was struck that we still lacked anything but broad immunosuppressants to help her and that we knew so little about the disease, or what triggers it." In an instant James was caught, she says, "by the lupus research bug."

Harley and his lupus team were already engaged in exceedingly meticulous work trying to isolate potential triggers for lupus. All cells have many proteins contained within them. Such protein molecules are, in turn, made up of sequences of amino acids. These amino acids make up specific, codelike patterns and are present in—or sometimes on the surface of—our body's cells, as well as in the foreign invaders that enter our bodies, be they viral or bacterial. Each sequence of amino acids forms a unique pattern, something like the bar codes on supermarket items that the scanner in the grocery store recognizes as you go through the checkout line. Let's say a flu virus enters your body. Immune cells that are programmed to recognize the proteins from the flu virus set out to find it and attack it. They are able to recognize these proteins as dangerous because they recognize the unique code of amino acids on the surface of the virus.

Once these immune fighter cells recognize the flu virus based on its similar "identification bar code," they send out a posse of antibodies that begin to bind with the intruders, often engulfing and destroying them.

But in a less than healthy body—one compromised by genetic

predisposition, a heavy burden of chemicals, stress, a processed-food diet, or some combination thereof—the immune fighter cells and the antibodies they send forth begin to make costly mistakes. They may see a set of amino acids, or a bar code, in healthy body tissue that is very like those in the flu virus, and instead of recognizing that pattern as being similar yet distinctly different, they goof, mistaking the sequence of amino acids in the healthy body cells for those belonging to the infiltrating germ. They set out to obliterate all the cells and viruses that share the same sequences, just to be sure they are getting the job done.

Such was the case in my own episodes of neurological auto-immunity. The fighter cells of my immune system mistook the amino acid sequence in the proteins of my own healthy myelin sheaths for a similar amino acid sequence in a foreign stomach virus and attacked both in the process of trying to scourge the flu from my body. When such a scenario occurs, autoimmune disease strikes.

Broadly speaking, this drama of mistaken identity is what Harley and James suspected was happening inside the bodies of lupus patients. They knew that some antigen out there had a sequence of amino acids—or bar code—very similar to that found in lupus patients' healthy cells. They knew this because they could identify a key sequence of eight amino acids in the actual structure of lupus patients' autoantibodies. "Autoantibody," the word scientists use to designate antibodies that have attacked and bound with healthy tissue in error, literally means "antibody against self."

This particular string of eight amino acids, taken by researchers from what is known as the "Sm B amino acid sequence" was bound by the autoantibodies of lupus patients. It existed as a kind of smoking-gun evidence after a crime. Harley suggested James look at the sequence more closely. By looking at its structure, Harley hoped he and James might be able to peer into the past and see what pattern of amino acids on a foreign antigen so closely imitated the pattern of eight amino acids in the Sm B sequence that it could cause lupus patients' immune systems to err, triggering the whole cascade of events leading to lupus.

Still, he wasn't overly hopeful. There were literally thousands of potential antigens out there.

Yet what Judi James found was startling. James searched a database of similar amino acid sequences in hopes of finding a clue as to what might be a potential lupus antigen. She showed Harley that this Sm B sequence bore a striking resemblance to an amino acid sequence that researchers had previously identified in the Epstein-Barr virus.

Epstein-Barr virus, or EBV, is a common viral infection that ordinarily causes anything from low-grade fever and sore throat symptoms in children to mononucleosis in teenagers and adults. When Harley saw that the sequence of a part of EBV was so similar to the Sm B amino acid sequence, "bells went off in my mind," he recalls. "I thought that if that's really right, that would be really tremendous." If they knew the virus did trigger the disease, could they intervene to stop it? At that point the connection remained just a virtual experiment—portrayed only on a computer screen—and Harley knew the match might have occurred as a coincidence and not show causation.

Besides, the question of whether EBV might play a role in lupus was, for any researcher of Harley's ilk, a scientific hot potato, one best left untouched. Years earlier, researchers had wondered if there was a link between Epstein-Barr and autoimmune disease. Scientists had studied the Epstein-Barr–autoimmune connection in the early 1970s—in the news headline heyday of Epstein-Barr—and found, by and large, nothing there. That seemed to make sense—after all, by age forty 96 percent of people have been infected with Epstein-Barr, a member of the herpes family, while only a fraction develop autoimmune disease. In the world of autoimmune-disease research, the question of whether Epstein-Barr could cause lupus had been asked and answered and the answer was no.

But resuscitate it they did. Harley and James were applying much more sophisticated lab techniques than had been available to the scientists in the 1970s. They had actual amino acid sequences in hand to study and compare. Still, Harley was cautious. One doesn't overthrow a supposedly watertight conclusion of modern science overnight. He asked Judi to replicate her results. Each time, the answer came up the same: it appeared that EBV might indeed play a direct hand in triggering autoimmunity by being a hauntingly close match to the Sm B sequence.

Harley ruefully recalls the day they decided to push ahead with their research. "Judi came to me with what she'd found and said, 'We should study EBV further.' I said, 'Judi, you had better hope and pray EBV is not involved here, because it has been claimed to cause everything and been proven to cause very little. No one in the entire medical community will believe us, we will be treated like scientific pariahs, and it will take us the rest of our careers to prove we're right.' " The suggestion that Epstein-Barr virus might have a hand in autoimmunity, would, Harley knew, "be irritating to our colleagues because our predecessors had looked at it and found very little there. Resuscitating it before the medical community was going to be even worse than if it had never been looked at before."

The next step was to test their prediction that Epstein-Barr played a role in lupus. Harley told James that they would immunize some of the animals in the lab with EBV peptides that looked like the Sm B self-protein, and that if these Epstein-Barr protein pieces produced lupus in them he would shut down several other projects in order to test whether that association could also be found in humans. Sure enough, the lab animals got a lupuslike disease. James was astounded to find that she could "take one piece of the structure of EBV and cause lupus by immunizing the animals with it."

Harley and James quickly published their findings and applied for a grant from the National Institutes of Health seeking research funding. They were so gung ho, in fact, that, in a story well known to colleagues, Harley was once racing a grant application to Federal Express when his old Ford Pinto burst into flames. Firefighters were still extinguishing the fire when Harley bummed a ride to FedEx to send the grant proposal. The front of the car, meanwhile, "melted like icing."

As he'd predicted, fellow scientists were not supportive. He and James were, Harley says, "body-slammed." Nevertheless, true to his word, Harley closed down some other areas of research and he and James went to work. In order to see if the same association was found in humans, they decided to study children and teens—an easier population to study than adults because children have a lower rate of EBV infection, which makes testing for association with lupus easier and more straightforward. The research team took blood samples from healthy children and teens and found that roughly 70 percent of these children had EBV DNA present in their bloodstreams. But when they examined lupus patients from the same age group, they saw that virtually every one of them tested positive for Epstein-Barr exposure. Ninety-nine percent of the same children who had lupus were also positive for Epstein-Barr—a statistically significant higher percentage than in their control group.

Harley and James's results, published in 1997, provided striking evidence that Epstein-Barr plays a role in triggering lupus—and that the same relationship that exists between Epstein-Barr and autoimmune disease in lab animals also exists in humans. "For most patients with lupus, Epstein-Barr is a necessary condition for autoimmune disease," submits Harley. Although EBV works in connection with many, many other factors, says Harley, "without the Epstein-Barr connection I think most patients would not be affected with lupus."

In lupus research, Harley is what social psychologists might refer to as a "change agent"—someone so far out on the cutting edge of a new line of thought that by the time early adopters of that new concept sign on to it as well, they nevertheless lope far behind. Since 1997, Harley and James have published numerous other studies in top medical journals that continue to affirm their conclusions about Epstein-Barr. And in the fall of 2006, Harley was given the first ever Excellence in Scientific Mentoring Award by the American College of Rheumatology for his achievements in helping young researchers, like Judi James, to make their mark resolving cutting-edge research questions such as this one.

Meanwhile, the wider scientific community has come on board

as multiple studies at other institutions around the world have supported Harley and James's original findings. One recent study supporting the link between Epstein-Barr and lupus shows that African Americans who test positive for Epstein-Barr are five to six times more likely to have lupus. Not surprisingly, genes play a specific role in the connection between Epstein-Barr and lupus as well. African-American and white patients who have lupus and Epstein-Barr are more likely to possess a genetic variation in the way their T cells control the immune response. Having this genetic variation significantly increases the risk of developing lupus if one has been exposed to Epstein-Barr.

Still, few diagnosing physicians think to ask about recent viruses when struggling to detect whether or not a patient has autoimmunity. In a sense, this is hardly surprising, because there is often a significant time lag between viral exposure and the onset of autoimmune illness. It can take days, weeks, months, and even years to develop autoantibodies against one's own body tissue after having been exposed to a virus. In a clinical setting, cause and effect are difficult, if not impossible, to ascertain.

Just think of LaShekia Chatman. For years after coming down with and being diagnosed with Epstein-Barr, LaShekia suffered from the symptoms of—and nearly died from—undiagnosed lupus. For decades, scientists had dismissed not only the chemical-autoimmune link but the viral-autoimmune connection as well. As it would turn out, both featured in LaShekia's autoimmune story. And that scientific blindness played a subtle part in why, for seven years, no physician suspected that LaShekia had lupus—even though her history so clearly pointed to both a viral and chemical overload.

What Harley and James were able to do by first isolating that "smoking gun"—that Sm B protein sequence targeted by lupus patients' antibodies—was to demonstrate, on the smallest cellular level, that the body can be tricked into attacking itself. Their research was a dramatic example of molecular mimicry at work between a protein in a virus and a protein in the body. They had, in a manner of speaking, been able to travel back in time and show that the autoimmune reaction in lupus patients was a slow-brew reaction to an Epstein-Barr exposure that had occurred months, years, or even decades before. As Harley puts it, "I do not know of a human model of molecular mimicry as convincing as this."

Today, a bevy of other researchers is on the hunt for similar links between viruses and autoimmune disease in the hopes of better understanding the mystery of how an infectious agent might interact with other factors to induce autoimmunity. One 2006 study reported in the *Archives of Neurology*, published by the American Medical Association, shows that young adults who have high levels of antibodies against the Epstein-Barr virus are significantly more likely to develop multiple sclerosis fifteen to twenty years down the road. Harvard School of Public Health and Kaiser Permanente researchers were able to determine this correlation by examining records of more than 100,000 patients who joined health plans between 1965 and 1974, when they were in their early thirties. All participants had undergone multiple examinations and all of them had had their blood samples stored. In the late 1990s, Kaiser researchers went back and scoured the medical lab records of forty-two of these women and men whose earlier blood samples had been kept and who later went on to develop MS. A control group of patients who did not develop MS—three times the size of the group with the disease—was also studied. Scientists looked at all the participants' preserved blood samples to determine what their levels of antibodies against the Epstein-Barr virus had been fifteen years earlier.

Measuring those antibodies yielded marked results. Those with the highest levels of antibodies against Epstein-Barr were twice as likely to develop multiple sclerosis fifteen to twenty years later. Researchers concluded that mounting evidence relating "Epstein-Barr virus infection to other autoimmune diseases, particularly lupus, suggests that Epstein-Barr virus may have a broad role in predisposing to autoimmunity." Likewise, National Institutes of Health researchers recently found that patients with multiple sclerosis carry a larger than normal number of antibodies against Epstein-Barr. One particularly provocative study out of the Hospital for Sick Children in Toronto shows an association between pediatric multiple sclerosis and the Epstein-Barr virus, indicating that exposure to the virus in childhood may be an important environmental trigger for developing MS early on.

Epstein-Barr is hardly the only viral infection that has been under the microscope in recent years in autoimmune-disease research labs. Scientists can now show the precise process by which proteins in streptococcal bacteria mimic cells in the heart, resulting in the autoimmune reaction known commonly as rheumatic heart disease. Other scientists are examining the relationship between the measles virus and multiple sclerosis, suggesting that viral outbreaks of measles might contribute to some localized epidemics of multiple sclerosis. And for many years, one of the more unsettling questions in the field of viral autoimmune-disease research has been whether individuals exposed to common viruses while in their mothers' wombs, or as newborns, are more likely to develop type 1 juvenile-onset diabetes.

In type 1 diabetes, an autoimmune disease also known as insulin-dependent diabetes mellitus, or IDDM, the pancreas undergoes an attack by the body's own immune system and becomes incapable of making insulin. Investigations into whether viruses might be implicated in type 1 diabetes go back decades. But it has only been with the help of more recent and sophisticated lab techniques that scientists have been capable of pinpointing how certain viruses, called enteroviruses, second only to the common cold as the most common cause of viral infections, incite some cases of type 1 diabetes. Enteroviruses, those ordinary viral infections that keep young children home from day care or school with cold and flulike symptoms and sometimes fever and muscle aches, cause an estimated 10 to 15 million infections a year in the United States. The most serious of these, the family of polio enteroviruses, have been eradicated in the United States as a result of aggressive vaccine campaigns. But researchers today are concerned about a more common and seemingly innocuous type of virus within the family of sixty-one nonpolio enteroviruses known as the coxsackie B viruses.

In the mid 1990s, researchers in Sweden examined stored blood samples from mothers who had delivered babies in Swedish hospitals, in hopes of better pinning down the relationship between coxsackie B viruses and childhood diabetes. They compared blood samples of 57 mothers of diabetic children with those of 203 mothers of nondiabetic children. Coxsackie B antigens turned out to be significantly more prevalent in mothers whose children later developed diabetes. The researchers concluded that enteroviral infection during pregnancy put the baby at risk for developing childhood-onset diabetes, particularly for developing the disease before the age of three.

Other studies tie mumps infection to the onset of diabetes. Although childhood immunization programs begun in the late 1950s have all but eradicated mumps, a recent resurgence of mumps outbreaks in the United States coupled with today's skyrocketing rates of childhood diabetes seems likely to resurrect this inquiry again in the near future.

It all sounds quite grim. One viral infection and you end up with a lifelong, debilitating autoimmune disease? Well, not exactly. Remember the barrel effect? While researchers and physicians are concerned by rising rates of children with autoimmunity—especially type 1 diabetes—most researchers agree that the causes of autoimmune disease in children, as in adults, are exceedingly multifaceted. The disease erupts in a given person at a given time due to a barrel effect, and viruses play just one part in filling that barrel. In the past, our understanding of what factors coalesce over a patient's lifetime and cause the barrel to suddenly spill over has been sorely lacking. Today, as more and more lab evidence pours in, clues, if not answers, are beginning to emerge.

Still, the profound link between viruses and autoimmune disease has not yet trickled down to the majority of medical practitioners. Few doctors know to address the potential role that a recent viral attack may play in developing autoimmunity when they are struggling to diagnose a patient who may have autoimmune disease.

It may also help to think of our growing understanding of the association between common viruses and autoimmune disease in the context of what is happening today in medical research in general. For centuries, scientists failed to recognize that pathogens played a role in a whole range of what were deemed to be noninfectious diseases. Up until the late twentieth century, health professionals believed that cancers and such chronic diseases as peptic ulcers were probably caused by a combination of genetics, diet, stress, and other lifestyle factors. But researchers now know that most peptic ulcers are caused by an infection with the bacterium *Helicobacter pylori* and can be treated with antibiotics. Treating patients surgically, it turns out, has been completely unnecessary. Infection with human papillomavirus, the cause of genital warts, is now known to be the major cause of cervical cancer. Epstein-Barr virus, in addition to being a culprit in lupus and multiple sclerosis, is now fingered in certain cancers such as Burkitt's lymphoma and nasopharyngeal carcinoma. Hepatitis B is thought to be associated with an increased risk of some liver cancers. Even some psychiatric conditions, such as schizophrenia and certain types of obsessive-compulsive disorder, are believed to be directly or indirectly the result of infections. And scientists are now finding tentative links between viral infections and obesity as well.

A recent report from the American Society of Microbiology highlights how widely this "new germ theory" applies to some thirty viral and bacterial microorganisms for which there exists strong evidence of an association to chronic disease.

In a sense, then, today's emerging relationship between common viruses and autoimmune disease merely mirrors what is coming to be better understood in all areas of health research: infectious pathogens play a far greater role than scientists once surmised in the onset of diseases, including cancer, heart disease, psychiatric illness, and autoimmune diseases, from Guillain-Barré syndrome to type 1 diabetes to lupus.

A WALK ON THE WILD SIDE: CHANGING VIRUSES AND GLOBAL WARMING

One can hardly talk about viruses in the twenty-first century without grappling with the emergence of a number of virulent new pathogens such as the H5N1 virus (avian or bird flu), West Nile virus, Ebola virus, and severe acute respiratory syndrome, or SARS.

These new potential plagues tend to result, in part, from the global spread of industrialization, which pushes humans toward ever-closer contact with wildlife as we encroach into what were once solely wildlife habitats. Ebola virus outbreaks are linked to mining development in previously untouched areas as well as hunters looking for exotic bush meat; the AIDS pandemic is believed to have originated from human encroachment into African forests where wild chimpanzees were a reservoir for the virus; and fruit bats in remote areas are thought to be the original source of several high profile zoonotic pathogens which have spread to humans, the most recent of which is SARS.

Similarly, H5N1 virus, or avian flu, is often the result of farmers and infected fowl crowding together in prime living space. Andrew Cunningham, a zoologist with the Zoological Society of London, recently raised a red flag about new viruses emerging from global encroachment into wildlife in an essay in the British medical journal *BMJ*, arguing that while this has probably happened many times in the past, such viruses failed to spread because those infected lived in remote enough areas that they either died or got well before they interacted with larger human populations. In today's world, however, the increases in international trade and travel make any kind of virulent new flu outbreak an overnight global emergency. The international trade in wildlife is now enormous, with hundreds of millions of wild animals and their products being transported around the world every year. The emergence of West Nile virus in North America, and AIDS and SARS globally, Cunningham points out, arose from such travel and trade in an age when "travelers can be in the middle of a tropical jungle one day and commuting to their desk in London the next." With world air travel expected to grow at about 5 percent a year for at least the next twenty years, the global crisis of newly emerging infectious diseases is unlikely to disappear anytime soon.

Others argue for the impact of global warming and hotter weather on growing rates of infectious diseases. In Al Gore's 2006 movie *An Inconvenient Truth,* a disturbing chart cites rising rates of illnesses, among them SARS, malaria, Ebola virus, and avian flu. The documentary's accompanying Web site states that with continued warming, deaths from climate-related illness are expected to rise sharply over the next two decades, according to projections by the World Health Organization. The question emerges: As the planet warms from pollution and infection-bearing mosquitoes and ticks proliferate in more temperate climates, how much will illness rates rise? Mosquitoes that transmit diseases such as West Nile virus thrive in warm weather. Simply lengthening the warm season will allow mosquitoes more time to reproduce, which means more generations of mosquitoes each year. Warmer climates may also allow mosquitoes to expand into areas that were too cold for them before. To make matters worse, the heat could also speed up the reproduction of the viruses the mosquitoes transmit.

Some viruses thrive in colder climates, others in warmer ones. In fact "colds" were first given that name because researchers were trying to grow a common cold virus in the lab and no one could manage it. One day, a researcher accidentally left the door ajar on the incubator and the temperature dropped. When the scientist came back the next day he discovered to his astonishment that the virus was now growing. That's how researchers came to understand that "cold" viruses grow better at cooler temperatures.

Other viruses, like coxsackievirus, however, favor warmer conditions. These viruses don't replicate over the winter, but neither do they die. They lie in wait until temperatures are warmer and suitable for their growth. If temperatures are consistently warmer, that allows viruses that grow in warmer temperatures to abound. Common viruses such as RSV, or respiratory syncytial virus, a major cause of respiratory illness in young children, also thrive in warmer weather. If both viral and chemical triggers of autoimmunity are mounting simultaneously, what exactly will that mean for today's already disturbing increase in autoimmune disease?

AVIAN FLU: AN AUTOIMMUNE-INDUCING VIRUS

The most feared of these new pathogens is no doubt the H5N1 virus, headlined, at this writing, to be the cause of the next flu pandemic. Because of the unusual way in which the virus can cause the body's immune system to rapidly turn from friend to foe, the avian flu is particularly troublesome for the quarter of the population that possesses the genetic predisposition to autoimmunity. Avian flu is feared because it could provoke a repeat of the influenza pandemic of 1918. The 1918 flu, or H1N1 virus, was—like the avian flu—an influenza A virus. Like that earlier flu, avian flu unleashes an unusual hurricanelike storm of immune-system signaling proteins called cytokines, which signal the immune system to combat microbial invaders. Cytokines signaling to the immune system to fight disease is a good thing, but when cytokine levels are elevated for too long and their signaling becomes uncontrolled, they can hijack the body's immune system to turn against the body itself. In avian flu, just as in autoimmune disease, too many cytokines are released, stimulating the immune system troops to run amok, killing not just avian flu–infected cells but healthy cells throughout virtually every organ of the body. In avian flu the result is fast, furious, and all too often deadly.

Moreover, one doesn't need to possess a genetic predisposition to autoimmunity for the avian flu to unleash its autoimmune-like cytokine fire. The H5N1 virus is so virulent that it bypasses the need for any genetic predisposition; anyone can suffer avian flu's severe friendly-fire effect. In 1918, those most likely to die were people with strong immune systems rather than the elderly and very young. Whether those with a predisposition to autoimmunity—who by the very nature of the disease have overly strong immune system responses—are in some way more at risk is a question researchers and patients alike can hope they only have to answer hypothetically.

VACCINATION STATION: AUTOIMMUNITY GETS A SHOT IN THE ARM?

As anyone who watches the six o'clock news well knows, the emergence of pathogens with the potential to become global pandemics is driving a frenzied search for new vaccines for avian flu and viruses such as SARS. For those with autoimmune disease, however, these vaccines might prove just as worrisome as they are reassuring. Although individuals with an unrecognized genetic predisposition to autoimmunity or who have an autoimmune disease may be more in need of protection against flu pandemics and infectious-disease outbreaks than others with less overexcitable immune systems, vaccines may in and of themselves prove to be dangerous for them.

Just over thirty years ago, in 1976, the Centers for Disease Control investigated and confirmed that a severe influenza outbreak at Fort Dix, New Jersey, had been caused by the "swine flu"—an influenza A–type virus. The Department of Health, Education, and Welfare grew concerned that the United States might be about to see another large national flu pandemic, involving numbers of influenza deaths reminiscent of the flu pandemic of 1918. The federal government deemed it prudent to vaccinate all Americans. In October 1976, the National Influenza Immunization Program officially began. Initially, nearly 1 million Americans were vaccinated each week, with the number growing to more than 4 million a week by the end of that first month. By the middle of November, 6 million Americans were being vaccinated each week. From the very start of the campaign, the National Influenza Immunization Program ran a well-organized surveillance system, monitoring for adverse side effects. Within the first two months, concerns from that early warning system began to emerge. More than ten states reported cases of Guillain-Barré syndrome in individuals who had been vaccinated recently. The relationship was so profound that the vaccination program stopped cold on December 16, 1976. By January 1977, more than five hundred cases of Guillain-Barré syndrome had been reported as a direct result of the vaccine. People were being vaccinated to protect against the influenza A swine flu, but literally hundreds of them were ending up with an uncommon neurological disorder leading to acute paralysis, from which some recovered wholly, others partially, and twenty-five died. Later calculations showed that the relative risk of acquiring GBS during the six weeks after the vaccination was ten times higher if you had been vaccinated than if you had never received the swine flu vaccine.

The cases of GBS that resulted from the swine flu vaccine were no different, in terms of the severity of paralysis and weakness, from those that had emerged in nonvaccinated individuals, except for the fact that those who developed GBS without having been vaccinated were, as in my own case, far more likely to have had an acute illness in the month preceding GBS.

When we catch a disease naturally, we usually produce antibodies to the organism that causes it. These antibodies, or proteins in the blood, remember the organism that caused the disease and can recognize and inactivate it when we come into contact with it again. Vaccines—made up of bits of virus that have either been crippled so that they can't trigger serious illness or have been killed before being injected—teach our body's immune system to produce antibodies and identify the virus so that when the immune system encounters it again it will recognize it and inactivate it without our ever having to suffer the disease itself.

Epidemiologists wondered if the cause of so many people developing GBS after getting the swine flu vaccine might have been a residual protein taken from the myelin of embryonic chicks that existed in the vaccine through all its manufacturing stages, though the idea that this myelin protein had caused a case of molecular mimicry was a guess at best. Back then, investigators could not imagine that the virus in the vaccine itself was the cause. Still, it seemed a freak occurrence having to do with something unique to the swine flu vaccine.

Then, in 1992, 1993, and 1994, it all happened again. People developed Guillain-Barré after widescale influenza vaccination programs, cementing the epidemiologic evidence that influenza strains other than the swine flu could also induce GBS. This isn't all that surprising, given Harley and James's discovery that molecular mimicry between a protein in a virus and a protein in the body could lead to autoimmune disease. But it was a startling realization at the time.

Sadly, those most in need of protection—people susceptible to demyelination and paralysis should they come down with an acute infection—are also those most likely to be at risk of severe adverse effects from the very vaccines meant to help them. For that reason, most physicians advise those who have had Guillain-Barré syndrome not to receive flu vaccines.

While concerns over the ill effects of vaccines make up as many headlines as do our efforts to invent new ones, it nevertheless seems prudent to underscore how much society as a whole has benefited from wide-scale vaccinations before launching into a deeper examination of the growing data finding a causal link between vaccines and autoimmune disease. If you were born about a hundred years ago and came down with a case of diphtheria, your life would have been at stake. At that time, thousands of people died routinely during disease outbreaks of mumps, rubella, and diphtheria. Enough generations have passed in the interim that few of us are viscerally cognizant of how lethal these diseases once were. As a public health tool, vaccines are an astonishingly beneficial and cost-effective life-saving intervention against infectious disease.

But they have their downsides, and autoimmune disease is emerging as a potentially dark one. In 1994, the *Journal of the American Medical Association* reported a dangerous relationship between diphtheria, tetanus, and oral polio vaccines and a number of autoimmune disorders, including Guillian-Barré syndrome. Similarly, a correlation has been reported and debated in scientific journals for years between the hepatitis B vaccine and multiple sclerosis as well as rheumatoid arthritis. Other evidence links the measles vaccine to multiple sclerosis and the measles, mumps, rubella (MMR) and hepatitis B vaccines to rheumatoid arthritis. Many scientists also believe strong anecdotal evidence exists between receiving the hepatitis B vaccine and developing lupus. Yet another noted connection between vaccine and illness is evidence relating the *Haemophilus influenzae* type b vaccine, known as Hib, to type 1 diabetes. Like Epstein-Barr, however, the Hib vaccine may take time to wreak its damage and spark disease: a statistically significant association between receiving the *Haemophilus* vaccine and developing type 1 diabetes in children exists as much as three years after receiving the vaccine. More recently, reports have emerged linking the new human papillomavirus, or HPV, vaccine to a statistically significant increased risk of Guillain Barré syndrome, especially when the vaccine is co-administered with the meningococcal vaccine.

As one top researcher who prefers to speak off the record puts it, "If you are looking for what the big 'ahas' in autoimmune research are going to be in the next few years, you have to look at vaccines." Since our understanding of autoimmunity in general is still relatively young compared to national research campaigns into so many other diseases, and our epidemiological data linking autoimmune disease to standard vaccination programs is even newer, it's easy enough to dismiss most of what we do know as speculative. The frequently long time frame between getting a vaccine and developing autoantibodies as a result can make it hard to cast such associations as cause and effect. Still, the data we do have clearly shows that certain autoimmune diseases such as Guillain-Barré syndrome and type 1 diabetes can be triggered by vaccines. Is it so surprising then to consider that others can be as well?

How vaccines spark autoimmune disease and how large a role they may play in setting the disease in motion in combination with other triggers is still an open question, however. Yet as researchers begin to delve more into this troubling correlation with newer lab techniques that allow them to trace antibodies back to the very thing that made them overproliferate in the first place, the answers they come up with may prove increasingly tricky for individual physicians, parents, and patients to grapple with.

Meanwhile, in a larger societal sense, whether vaccines pose a significant enough risk to question their widespread use remains, at best, a philosophical quandry, since nationalized immunization programs protect the masses against a number of devastating diseases and do it quite efficiently, whereas autoimmune disease due to vaccination has not been shown to afflict overwhelming numbers of children and adults. In any risk-benefit analysis, the numbers of lives saved from vaccines far outweigh the numbers of people who react by developing autoimmunity. Still, this is little comfort for the parent whose child goes in for his Haemophilus influenzae type b vaccine and ends up with a disease as devastating as childhood diabetes before the age of seven.

All this points to a more important mystery that has yet to be solved. Why don't more people who experience common infections or who receive vaccines get sick? Why aren't all 25 percent of people who have a genetic predisposition to autoimmunity falling ill as a result of molecular mimicry? Why does a viral hit cause the immune system to make such a monumental gaffe in some people and not others?

THE ROLE OF HEAVY METALS

It's important to remember that there are multiple factors involved in the onset of autoimmune disease. Each of us has a different genetic susceptibility to autoimmunity, and we each also carry very different degrees of genetic ability to withstand the onslaughts of chronic toxic autogenic hits from the day-to-day environment in which we live. And that individual difference directly impacts how compromised our immune system becomes over time. The more compromised our system becomes, the more likely our immune cells are to become confused and overwhelmed, so that when we do meet infectious viruses or bacteria, mistakes can all the more easily happen.

To grasp how genetics, toxic agents, viruses, and vaccines become interlocking forces that can kick-start autoimmunity, we have to remember how environmental hits and chemicals can tax the immune system through long, slow, and continual environmental exposures—priming the pump, so to speak, so that the now proverbial barrel sloshes dangerously close to its brim and viruses can all the more easily "spill" the immune system over the brink.

Recent studies into how differently individuals process one particular autogen, the heavy metal mercury, bear this out all too perfectly. In the past decade, scientists in the field of autoimmune-disease research have become particularly concerned about mercury for two reasons—first, its increased ubiquity in our environment, and second, a stack of recent data proving that even low-level exposure to mercury, especially in people who are more genetically prone to develop autoimmunity, directly impairs the delicate balance of the immune system, playing a kingpin role in predisposing them to autoimmune disease.

Mercury, in one of its forms, thimerosal, is still used in some flu vaccines and some over-the-counter pharmaceuticals. Present until recently in virtually every vaccine children received throughout the 1990s, including hepatitis B, bacterial meningitis, diphtheria, whooping cough, and tetanus, thimerosal is now the subject of a well-known heated controversy questioning whether cumulative doses in childhood vaccines may play a role in autism and other developmental delays. While the thimerosal debate is best covered by authors focusing solely on investigating those claims, mercury in general, and mercury in vaccines in the form of thimerosal, are nevertheless pertinent to our discussion as to how an autogen can influence how fast or furiously an individual's barrel fills to reach the onset of disease.

Our most significant exposure to mercury comes, as adults, from the air we breathe and the food we eat—especially from larger fish. Like all environmental toxins, mercury accumulates up the food chain. (The tiniest fish are consumed by bigger fish, which are eaten by large swordfish and tuna, so that by the time the tuna consumes his dinner, he's packing in all the mercury ingested by the smaller creatures.)

How did so much mercury get into the oceans and lakes to be consumed by fish in the first place? Since the advent of the industrial age, the atmospheric burden of mercury in our environment—meaning the amount falling from the sky from waste from coal combustion, incineration, mining, coal-fired utilities, and industrial boilers—has tripled. In the United States, coal-fired power plants alone spew about fifty tons of mercury into the air each year. Dry particles of mercury travel effortlessly in effluent clouds across the American landscape—migrating from coal-burning power plants in the Midwest to points often thousands of miles away, where they literally rain out of the sky in what environmentalists commonly refer to as "mercury polluted rainstorms." Once mercury particles shower to earth, they lace every acre, from forest floors to neighborhood parks to rippling ocean waves.

To measure how much mercury exists in our day-to-day environment, researchers tested mercury levels in fish, birds, and mammals across remote areas of New England and found that even animals far from industrialized cities carry disturbingly high amounts of mercury in their bodies, mercury that could be specifically traced back to power plants thousands of miles away in the Midwest. That's telling to scientists, because it means even supposedly pristine air, water, and food sources—including those on seemingly distant mountaintops of New England—are already highly contaminated from mercury fallout.

Mercury finds its way into our bodies from other, more direct sources, of course, such as industrial waste releases and toxic spills. Today, the National Library of Medicine's TOXMAP site lists a combination of 1,432 known current sites and 431 Superfund locales nationwide where mercury or mercury compounds have been released or leaked. All these external sources add to the burden of heavy metals we already carry in our bodies. According to the Centers for Disease Control, 12 percent of women of childbearing age now have mercury levels that exceed the Environmental Protection Agency's safety standard. The 10 percent of women with the highest mercury levels tend to live in coastal areas, especially along the Atlantic coast, and carry body burdens of mercury at 5.9 parts per billion, way over the 3.5 parts per billion limit the EPA cites as a known health threat. Meanwhile, a 2007 New York City Health and Nutrition Examination Survey recently reported that a quarter of adult New Yorkers have elevated blood mercury levels. Similarly, in 2004, a study conducted jointly by the Environmental Quality Institute at the University of North Carolina at Asheville and Greenpeace analyzed women's hair samples (one of several scientific means of testing for heavy metal exposure) and found that 21 percent of women of childbearing age have mercury levels higher than the EPA's safety limit of 1 microgram of mercury per gram of hair.

This is no small thing: researchers know that mercury can cross the placenta and affect the developing brain of the fetus. Mercury, like lead, is a potent neurotoxin. EPA scientists estimate that one in six infants born in the United States is now at risk for developmental disorders because of exposure to mercury while in the mother's womb. Mercury can accumulate in the umbilical-cord blood of pregnant women at a level that's 1.7 times as great as the concentration in the mother's blood itself. That means that a newborn's mercury level might reach 5.8 parts per billion in a mother whose mercury concentration is just 3.5 parts per billion— at a particularly dangerous time in fetal brain development. Recently, researchers found that low levels of mercury can target critical stem cells in the brain that are essential to the growth and development of the central nervous system and cause them to prematurely shut down, especially when exposures happen during critical development periods like fetal growth and early childhood.

THE GENES-MERCURY DANCE

One of the major players in today's cutting-edge research on how low-level exposures to mercury can directly stimulate autoimmunity or accelerate the disease is Kenneth Michael Pollard, PhD, associate professor in the Department of Molecular and Experimental Medicine at the Scripps Research Institute in La Jolla, California. For the past twenty years, Mike Pollard and his colleagues both at Scripps and at Linköping University in Linköping, Sweden, have been exploring how the interplay between genetics and mercury influences whether one will develop autoimmune disease—as well as how mercury stimulates autoimmune disease in some genetic groups more than others.

Pollard, a fifty-five-year-old native of Australia, is the author of sixty scientific papers, an international conference presenter, and has participated on six National Institutes of Health committees. He has made a career both in Australia and in California, investigating the way mercury influences the function of different sets of proteins in human body tissue and leads to autoimmune disease. Inside Pollard's molecular laboratory at Scripps, the California sun beating down outside seems as remote as that on a tourist postcard; all one can hear is the hum of freezers that hold tissue samples and occasionally the sound of mice running through the sawdust of their cages. Pollard's quest is to understand the effects of mercury on human biology, and on the autoimmune process in particular. As the average body burden of mercury that Americans carry increases by the year, Pollard's mission "to prevent mercury exposure from leading to disease in the first place" has become all the more pressing.

Various types of mercury—elemental mercury, inorganic mercury, methyl mercury, and ethyl mercury (a by-product of thimerosal)—all affect people differently because they are metabolized by the body differently. Elemental mercury is the type that you find in dental amalgam. People who have fillings with dental amalgam can build up body burdens of mercury because, over time, mercury from their teeth leaches into the body and accumulates in the kidneys. Although a recent 2006 Food and Drug Administration report concluded that mercury dental fillings are safe, an expert panel for the FDA rejected that agency report only a week later. Panel members complained that the report excluded some important studies, making it impossible to reach a clear answer as to whether fillings are safe, especially for pregnant women and children. They concluded that far more study was required. Meanwhile, in the field of autoimmune-disease research, studies tie abnormal amounts of heavy metals such as mercury to scleroderma, with other research relating having a high number of dental fillings to one's likelihood of developing scleroderma. One recent case-control study reported that severely affected scleorderma patients were more likely to have higher levels of mercury in their urine.

Methyl mercury, an organic mercury, is the form that's commonly found in fish. Methyl mercury passes readily from the human gut to the bloodstream and into all organs and tissues. For reasons not yet completely understood, methyl mercury exposure does particular damage to the central nervous system. Once inside the body, some of that methyl mercury is converted into an inorganic form that can fasten on to and disable many of the cellular proteins and enzymes essential to cellular function. This inorganic form of mercury is the same type of mercury that Pollard is using in his experiments. Inorganic mercury is the major form of mercury that accumulates in the kidneys—and has been found to induce autoimmune disease in many different inbred strains of laboratory mice. Even low-dose mercury exposure increases the severity and prevalence of autoimmune myocarditis in mice.

"When you ingest fish that has mercury in it, that mercury is more highly reactive in the body than many people realize," says Pollard, who is also the editor of a new book for scientists, *Autoantibodies and Autoimmunity,* a comprehensive look at the latest research on autoantibodies in autoimmune disease. Investigations by a number of researchers show that mercury reacts with proteins in the body by combining directly with body tissue. This interaction of mercury with the protein sequences that make up our body tissue changes the actual structure of these proteins. The result is a heavy-metal plus body-cell amalgam—an utterly new complex hybrid that is astonishingly part heavy metal, part body tissue. Not surprisingly, this half-human, half-heavy-metal complex, which sounds a bit like something out of a sci-fi movie, is wholly foreign to our bodies.

You might logically assume that the immune system now reacts against this new hybrid protein and, in the process of trying to destroy it, also destroys the organs and tissue of the body itself. But what Pollard has found in lab animals exposed to mercury is that the actual autoantibodies produced against the mouse's own body tissue form not against these new hybrid proteins but directly against the mouse's pure, unadulterated body tissue. Somehow, mercury produces such a potent response in the body that it not only creates these surprising hybrid proteins, it also forces the immune system, in a process not fully understood, to react against pure body tissue. But this damage does not necessarily happen in the same part of the body where mercury exposure first occurred. Pollard points out that "although we are exposing mice via injection under the skin, and getting inflammation there, the autoimmune response occurs in more distant tissues such as the kidney." It's almost as if the immune system is so traumatized by trying to figure out what to do with these different protein sequences—those from the mercury–body tissue hybrid and those that exist in the body's own pure tissue—that immune cells moving through the body can no longer determine which is safe and which is harmful. They can attack the wrong target in the body anywhere.

But Pollard, who has been a faculty member at Scripps since 1992 and has since added a great deal of scientific understanding to the way mercury stimulates this two-step autoimmune response, is perhaps best known for showing how a slight difference in genetic code can dramatically change mercury's impact on the immune system, causing it to induce an autoimmune response swiftly, more moderately—or even not at all.

Because researchers would never expose human beings with differing genetic profiles to mercury on purpose in order to see exactly what genes might help some people avoid disease, mice are used instead. As it turns out, mice provide a clear lens through which scientists can view how different degrees of genetic susceptibility contribute to mercury-induced autoimmunity. Over the course of several studies Pollard and his Swedish collaborators have exposed strains of mice with different genetic susceptibility to autoimmune disease to inorganic mercury. The mice in their experiments displayed varied degrees of autoimmune responses to mercury depending upon their genetic backgrounds. A few strains that were not genetically susceptible to lupus were resistant to developing mercury-induced autoimmunity, while a number of other strains that were genetically susceptible to lupus developed a disease closely resembling lupus in humans.

But the salient question was: How did these exposures in mice relate to the amount of mercury that average Americans are exposed to in their day-to-day lives?

In order to replicate in lab mice what everyday contact with mercury in our environment might translate to for humans, Pollard and his colleagues had to figure out the average level of mercury—the mercury body burden—that most Americans are carrying in their tissues and bloodstreams. His team looked at data showing the standard amount of mercury that has accumulated, over time, in the kidneys of healthy people who did not have a history of occupational exposure to mercury and who died in accidents or from other non-disease-related causes. It turns out that the average level of inorganic mercury in healthy people's kidneys is about 0.5 micrograms for every gram of kidney tissue. Pollard's lab set that level as a guideline for dosing lab mice with mercury so they could build up a load in their kidneys analogous to that which most humans are unknowingly walking around with. They then exposed groups of lupus-prone female mice, known as BXSB mice, to doses of mercury that they thought might produce a similar burden of mercury in their kidneys.

Just as the investigators had found with the other lupus strains of mice, not only did mercury exposure make the disease occur earlier in these BXSB mice, but the greater the dose of mercury the earlier the disease appeared. After thirty-eight weeks of slow, continuous exposure, one group of female BXSB mice developed a level of mercury in their kidneys equivalent to that of a typical human exposure. This group of mice, and groups with higher levels of exposure, showed accelerated development of autoimmunity, while mice given a lower dose of mercury developed disease at a rate similar to the control mice, which were exposed merely to a saline solution. Pollard and his colleagues concluded that "environmentally relevant tissue levels of mercury"—meaning levels analogous to that which many Americans have in their bodies—"could be associated with exacerbations of autoimmune disease in genetically susceptible individuals."

Genetics is therefore key to understanding how mercury influences autoimmunity. To see how this works, let's imagine that we have in front of us a group of ten mice, each with a different genetic susceptibility to lupus, and a train with ten boxcars that each mouse must race through. Before attempting to make it through the train, each mouse is first exposed to a dose of mercury that's analogous to what many of us carry in our bodies right now from a combination of mercury amalgam dental fillings, fish consumption, and the amount of mercury we absorb from other foods, water, and the atmosphere around us. When a mouse possessing a high genetic susceptibility to autoimmunity gets exposed to a low dose of mercury, it develops the autoimmune disease lupus quite quickly. We might visualize this mouse as falling ill before it even gets through the very first boxcar of the train. Other mouse strains, however, which possess more genetic resistance to lupus, might only get sick after they've made it as far as the third or fifth boxcar—they've lasted that much longer before succumbing because they possess a bit more genetic resistance. And then there is that one lucky mouse strain that packs so much genetic resistance to autoimmune disease that it flies through to boxcar ten and still feels quite plucky—even though it has been exposed to the same amount of mercury in the same doses as all the other mice who developed autoimmune disease.

In this sense, different strains of mice are a good substitute for researchers to work with when considering the myriad possible different genetic subsets that make people who have been exposed to heavy metals vary in their susceptibility to autoimmune disease.

Others, possessing fewer susceptible variants of genes, are less prone. Some people, like the mouse who gets to the tenth box, are remarkably resistant regardless of what you throw at them.

"The mice in our experiment are sort of like humans going through life, building up mercury exposure," says Pollard. "This long-term chronic exposure to mercury can set autoimmune disease in motion—and certainly, for those who already suffer from autoimmunity, make disease more severe over one person's lifetime."

LOOPING BACK TO VACCINES

Even as the evidence pointing to the harmful effects of mercury mount, the Institute of Medicine announced in May 2004 that it had reviewed earlier studies asking whether thimerosal in vaccines could be linked to the tenfold increase in childhood autism spanning from the early 1980s through the late 1990s—and concluded that there was no link. Nevertheless, in the United States, thousands of parents of autistic children and those with certain learning disabilities are going to the mat to demand a deeper investigation into whether thimerosal has had any role in their children's disabilities. They cite alleged evidence that the CDC covered up critical information that, throughout the 1990s, federal health officials had inadvertently nearly tripled the amount of ethyl mercury being injected into some babies during a critical period of brain development. This was at a time when new thimerosal-containing vaccines were added to the list of a child's required shots in unprecedented numbers. By 1999, a baby who received all recommended vaccines at her two-month checkup might well have been injected with up to 118 times the EPA's safety limit for daily exposure to mercury.

Recent research from the University of California, Davis shows that extremely small levels of thimerosal can alter the normal activity and function of critical immune cells by stimulating the production of cytokines—the body's signaling proteins that can whip up the immune cells to trigger a full-blown immune response.

By inciting immune cells at the wrong time, the cytokines lead the immune system to turn on the body itself. Researchers believe that the genetic background of some individuals may render them especially susceptible to the effects of thimerosal.

Meanwhile, in Sweden, where researchers may feel freer to write the inciting word "thimerosal" on a grant application, Mike Pollard's close collaborators in the Division of Molecular and Immunological Pathology at Linköping University are looking closely at whether mercury in the form of thimerosal (an organic mercury) might induce the same autoimmune conditions observed in mice after exposure to inorganic mercury (inorganic mercury being the type Pollard used in his studies). Their findings, published in 2006, indicate that thimerosal does induce a systemic autoimmune response similar to that seen with inorganic mercury itself. Another recent study caused a stir within the scientific community by finding that even the low level of mercury used in vaccines preserved with thimerosal can trigger irregularities in immune-system cells in test-tube experiments. Even so, if there is an interplay with mercury, top scientists in the autoimmune-mercury field caution that there is probably no one single environmental trigger that is causing autism, just as there is no one single gene that is causing it. Any environmental role that mercury plays in autism may well be due to cumulative effects of mercury—including heightened exposure in the womb because of the way in which mercury concentrates in fetal cord blood—combined with specific viral hits, which also may occur in utero. And, just as in mice, each child's unique genetic makeup will make it easier or harder for mercury, in combination with many other factors, to wreak its damage.

THE AUTISM-AUTOIMMUNE CONNECTION

Although we are a long way from understanding the interplay of these triggers in the rapidly rising rates of autism across the industrialized world—including the United States, Japan, England, Sweden, Denmark, and France—one of the more stunning recent findings about the syndrome is that autism may in fact have an autoimmune component. In what researchers believe is a major new discovery about the origins of autism, scientists recently detected aberrant antibodies in the blood of kids in families with a pattern of autism and in mothers with more than one autistic child. The working hypothesis is that these antibodies are actually raised against proteins in the fetal brain; indeed, researchers have found that autistic brains have chronic inflammation, a sign of immune activity. A number of scientists are now investigating whether autism might conceivably be attributed to the formation of autoantibodies against the central nervous system in genetically susceptible individuals. All of which begs the question: Are researchers about to determine that autism is also—at least in some cases—autoimmune in nature? If so, are the triggers similar to those with other autoimmune diseases? Would it then seem at all surprising if mercury were one of them, given what we know about mercury as a trigger for autoimmunity in general?

As for the role of thimerosal in autoimmunity, when I ask one researcher, who prefers to go unnamed, whether thimerosal exposure from vaccines might bear any responsibility in today's rising rates of autoimmune disease, she is decidedly candid. She reminds me that at the same time that we are "pricking up" the immune cells to be reactive by administering a vaccine, we are also introducing that foreign antigen in a bath of mercury. For some patients, this is a potential double whammy. Think of it: in the old days, only a certain percentage of kids got mumps. Some of them suffered life-altering consequences or died, which underscores the need for the mumps vaccine. Now, however, every child gets exposed to the foreign antigen of the mumps virus (and the many other diseases we vaccinate against) via vaccines, with many of them exposed to that foreign viral protein sequence at the same moment in time that they are exposed to foreign ethyl mercury. Now, says this expert, "you have a child patient who doesn't get measles or mumps—but they do get an autoimmune disease. Only we may not see that relationship in broad epidemiological terms, because we haven't been look-ing for it." In correcting one problem, we may have been creating another.

Some worry that our exposure to mercury from fallout from the atmosphere, intake from foods, and exposure from vaccines and dental amalgam has reached such a level that it may be contrib-uting across the board to today's international rise in autoimmune-disease rates—creating one widespread, global cluster, if you will. A cluster so widespread that we are all but blind to the connection.

THE HYGIENE HYPOTHESIS

The idea that our immune systems are so barraged by an onslaught of viral hits and vaccines, so vulnerable to an environment dirty with mercury, TCE, dioxin, and a hundred other known autogens that it's sparking an autoimmune crisis, doesn't pass muster with everyone. In fact, according to scientific proponents of what's termed "the hygiene hypothesis," the root cause of rising rates of autoimmunity stems not from the fact that we are living in too dirty a world, but, rather, from the fact that we are living too clean.

The too-clean theory is based on the argument that in the same century that we've seen a considerable rise in the prevalence of allergies and autoimmune disease, we've seen a dramatic decline in many previously common childhood infections such as rubella, mumps, measles, and diphtheria. That leads many scientists to argue that a lack of exposure to viruses and the swill of bacteria that most of our ancestors were exposed to living *sans* vaccines or modern hygiene means children's immune systems are no longer forced to build up the necessary immune defenses they need. In a world of well-vacuumed homes, scrubbed bathrooms and kitchens, and more time spent in minivans than mucking about through woods, forests, and farmland, coupled with massive vaccination campaigns that prevent full-fledged infection from many childhood diseases, children's immune systems are, in a sense, overprotected.

If a child's immune system were a military academy, you might think of invading pathogens (be they bacteria or viruses) as sergeants providing a comprehensive set of military drills. Academy trainees need a certain number of drills to learn how to perform against a wide array of attacks. Each time they experience a practice exercise, their ability to respond with accuracy and precision is enhanced. But an underdrilled immune system may result in too few key immune cells becoming educated enough to know how to recognize and fight back against different attacks in an effective manner.

Hence, believe the too-clean theorists, the true culprit behind rising rates of autoimmune disease may be the fact that we simply don't have enough disease and germ-laden dirt challenging our immune systems as children. Because we've been so well vaccinated, our homes are kept largely free of dust, dirt, and disease, and we lather up with antibacterial soaps, our immune systems haven't had to do enough battle to become seasoned fighters. And that makes our immune cells a bit like dangerously underchallenged teenagers who are loose on the street just looking for something, anything, to occupy themselves. So when a foreign virus invades, our immune system overreacts, kick-starting a hyper-driven response, provoking everything from allergies to allergy-induced asthma to autoimmunity.

Indeed, researchers increasingly believe that triggers behind today's rising rates of autoimmune disease may be similar to those behind skyrocketing rates of childhood allergies and allergy-induced asthma. Many investigators worry that such increases are further testament to the fact that the human immune system—especially a child's more vulnerable immune system—is becoming unable to differentiate properly between what is safe and what is foreign. Consider the rise in food-related and inhalant allergies. More than half of Americans test positive to one or more allergens, more than double the percentage who did thirty years ago. Go into any elementary school these days and the basket of inhalers and EpiPens—a device for delivering a shot of epinephrine in the event of a severe allergic response—sitting on the teacher's desk makes this all too evident. Ditto asthma, which is often allergy induced. Twenty million Americans now suffer from asthma, and 7 million of these are children. The number of people suffering from asthma in the U.S. increased 74 percent between 1980 and 1996.

The fact that autoimmunity and allergies are rising in tandem makes complete sense, since the mechanisms behind allergies and autoimmune disease are so similar: both are the result of an inappropriate overresponse, or hypersensitivity, of the immune system to something that the body doesn't recognize as safe. An allergic reaction to food occurs when the immune system incorrectly identifies a food protein as a threat to the body. This immune response elevates the level of a blood antibody known as IgE. When IgE levels increase and a person is exposed to the food again, the body releases histamines and other chemicals to protect the body. This results in symptoms of an allergic reaction. The similarity between an allergic response and an autoimmune response is clearest in the autoimmune disease known as celiac disease—what some term a gluten allergy—in which the body perceives gluten as a foreign invader. In order to protect the body from the foreign substance in the digestive tract, the immune system produces antibodies that mistakenly attack the lining of the gut as well, resulting in autoimmune disease. Eliminate the allergen—gluten in wheat and other grains—and the autoimmune disease subsides.

Both allergies and autoimmune disease are the result of the immune system's efforts to hold a potentially harmful foreign substance at bay. In allergies, the immune system reacts to an external substance that would normally be harmless. With autoimmune disorders, the immune system reacts to normal tissue in the body that would normally be seen as harmless. The difference is that in the case of allergies, the trigger is a known, quantifiable external stimulus (peanut butter, eggs, pollen, dust mites, trees, grass, mold), whereas in most cases of autoimmunity (other than celiac disease) the causes can often only be ascertained (or only guessed at) after disease strikes. When the immune system is pushed to turn haywire in one area, it's more likely to go haywire in many areas.

• • •

Some studies support the theory that rising rates of immune-system-mediated illnesses are attributable to our living in too pristine a world. For example, some studies show that adults who were around infant siblings during their first six years of life have a reduced risk of multiple sclerosis. The theory is that having younger siblings increases one's likelihood of having had infections early in life, and a lack of contact with siblings may mean one's immune system is understimulated during those crucial years when the immune system is being educated for the future.

One new study found that gutter rats and field mice exhibit far fewer allergies and autoimmune diseases than their superhygienic laboratory counterparts. Researchers found that the immune systems of flea-ridden wild rats are busy fighting off everything from germs to parasites, whereas the immune systems of lab rats had nothing major to occupy them. With no real dangers to fight off, lab rats were more likely to make antibodies that attacked substances like pollen, or the body's own tissue. In other words, the lab rats' immune systems became hypersensitive to substances that would not bother their wild counterparts. One might compare this to an old person who lives alone in an apartment and has few true concerns, and so they get upset by the least little thing, like the mailman not coming on time. By contrast, someone who is experiencing a true trauma, say the loss of a loved one, is going to see small things like the late mail as entirely inconsequential.

But blaming hygiene as the sole source of today's autoimmune epidemic doesn't wash with all scientists, and this basic conflict of ideas is at the heart of a growing controversy. One well-known researcher who feels the too-clean theory can't possibly fully explain today's rising rates of autoimmune disease is DeLisa Fairweather, PhD, a young assistant professor at the Bloomberg School of Public Health's Department of Environmental Health Sciences Division of

Toxicology and a protégé and co-author with Noel Rose of many scientific papers on viral-induced autoimmune disease.

In the doorway of her office, Fairweather apologizes for the state of disarray. "Always looking for more time to read," she says, gesturing to a picnic-sized worktable to our left, laden with dozens of research-paper stacks, some so high they're near to toppling. To our right hangs a large whiteboard with hundreds of Fairweather's small jotted notations, arrows flying in varied directions stressing connections between scribbled thoughts and lists punctuated with question marks.

I ask her what she thinks about the hygiene hypothesis as the primary explanation for rising rates of autoimmunity, at a time in our evolution when we're living in the most chemically polluted environment ever. To elucidate her answer, Fairweather, her warm blue eyes animated behind tortoiseshell glasses, lines up three eight-and-a-half by eleven sheets of paper, turns them horizontally, and lays them side by side in one thirty-three-inch stretch. As she talks she diagrams for me why, in her estimation, the too-clean theory is too flimsy to explain today's autoimmune epidemic.

Although it is true, she agrees, that allergies, asthma, and auto-immunity may be higher in countries where there are more vaccines and fewer infections in early childhood, it is also true that immi-grants from other countries (who may be exposed to more infections and fewer vaccines as young children) develop allergies and auto-immune disease at rates similar to those of Americans soon after they immigrate to this country. Likewise, countries that adopt a Western diet and become more industrialized, but don't have the same vac-cination program as we have in the United States, tend to develop allergies and autoimmune disease at the same high rates of illness that we do. Moreover, she asserts, "The hygiene hypothesis cannot explain all the babies who are born today with allergies."

But what diminishes the too-clean theory most in her mind is that although certain childhood illnesses have lessened due to vac-cination programs against well-known childhood viruses, other childhood infections haven't let up in the least. Most respiratory and stomach-flu bugs children get are moving-target infections scientists can't easily develop vaccines against because they mutate so quickly that by the time a vaccine is developed to fight them, the germ has already changed its structure so significantly that the vaccine is rendered ineffective. These bugs challenge the immune systems of children with unfettered constancy, as you can witness should you enter any preschool classroom or daycare center in America. Inquire of any veteran preschool teacher of thirty years and they will tell you that kids today certainly don't seem to be out less with colds and viruses and stomach bugs than they were decades ago. Rather, it seems whole grades of preschoolers will get hit with a stomach bug one week and another virus the next, leading to half-empty classrooms several times a year. Meanwhile, new viruses such as West Nile and the spread of such infections as Lyme disease pose additional challenges to the immune system that children a generation ago never had to face. "Not all infections have lessened," believes Fairweather. "There has to be something bigger at play."

As someone who has dealt with numerous autoimmune disorders since puberty, I look back over my own childhood and wonder if it could have been too clean. My three siblings and I were all a year apart, and illnesses flew through our house with such vengeance that my mother says there was once a stretch of forty days during which there was always someone vomiting or feverish. Most of the time we were pretty hearty and spent every day in the summer or on weekends mucking about in the swamp to one side of our house, the woods behind us, or swimming or sailing or waterskiing like river rats in the less-than-pristine Chesapeake Bay. We were deeply in the swill, as it were, and in our younger years carried about dead mice and birds and turtles and fish skeletons, seldom washing our hands. It was life on the bay, and we'd only return after hours of getting caked in the dirt of the great outdoors when we heard our parents blowing the foghorn to let us know it was time to traipse homeward over the fields or swamps. I cannot imagine a dirtier childhood. I also had mumps and measles both. But somehow, I ended up with numerous autoimmune diseases.

The biggest point of controversy with the hygiene hypothesis, says Fairweather, is that "it does not take into account the increase in pollution and chemicals in our environment in the past fifty years, which stimulate our immune system in a similar way that infections do. We are certainly not cleaner in a chemical sense than we used to be. In autoimmune disease, the immune response looks as if it has seen an infection. Why would the lack of disease—or a too-clean environment—produce a response in the body that looks as if it has seen an infectious agent?" We know that autogens can stimulate an autoimmune response in a similar way that infectious agents do, and we know that our exposure to autogens has sky-rocketed in the last half century. If our immune systems could talk, chances are they would tell us not that they are feeling challenged too little, but that they are feeling challenged too much.

BLASTING OUR CELLS

To grasp fully how our twenty-first-century immune systems may be overtaxed by constant hits, it's critical that we understand what occurs in that very first moment when the immune system mounts its defense against either a virus or autogen. In fighting off danger-ous pathogenic hits, our bodies are equipped with two basic types of immune responses. The initial immune response, known as the innate immune response, occurs when the body first detects a for-eign antigen working its way past the body's barriers. Scientists, Fairweather says, used to assume this innate immune response was not terribly sophisticated, because it only recognizes foreign invad-ers in generalized groups, rather than with any detailed specificity. For example, it might recognize an infiltrating germ as belonging to a broad group of viruses, but it does not register what kind of virus it's looking at exactly. You might imagine the innate immune re-sponse's means of dealing with an antigen kind of like the way you deal with a garden pest you've just noticed on your rosebush. You might spray the bush with a generic garden spray you've had sitting around on a garage shelf and hope for the best; it may not be a product that's specifically meant to conquer the exact insect that's destroying your bush, but it will probably help nonetheless because it defends pretty well against garden pests in general.

The other kind of immune response is the adaptive immune response, which takes place long past the moment when a foreign invader first infiltrates the body. It has always been assumed that all the real defensive action took place during the adaptive immune response—when the immune system sets out to detect exactly what specific type of antigen has infiltrated the body and to mount a response that targets it for destruction. Scientists believed that it was here that the immune system made the grave mistakes that would lead to autoimmune disease. Yet in her Hopkins lab, Fairweather has been able to prove that assumption to be incorrect. The innate immune system, which no one bothered to look at very closely, is a whole lot smarter and more influential in the autoimmune process than scientists have assumed it to be. Fairweather's most recently published papers contend that the adaptive immune response is, in fact, "completely controlled by what happens at that critical initial meeting when the innate immune system reacts for the very first time to an invader." It's that initial moment when, say, a virus enters your body because you put your fingers—which have just touched a doorknob just touched by someone who is sick and contagious—to your lips. The innate immune response—influenced, of course, by one's genetic susceptibility and exposure to chemicals—sets the stage for what the adaptive immune response will then decide to do.

After painstakingly uncovering the workings of the innate immune system in mice, Fairweather has concluded that the human immune system can become so besieged by unrelenting contact with a toxic barrage of viruses, chemicals, and heavy metals that it's practically forced to run amok. The synergistic combination of chemicals in our daily food and air coupled with common viral hits, she contends, puts our immune systems through so many drills that they are on constant high alert and simply can't handle it. According to Fairweather, when the innate immune system meets a constant onslaught of potentially dangerous challenges, be they infectious or toxic substances, it behaves like a car whose accelerator is stuck at eighty miles an hour and whose brakes aren't working.

To understand how the brakes fail on a cellular level in the human body requires a short course in one more group of immune cells, known as mast cells. Mast cells are part of the innate immune system's initial response team, and they work by recognizing patterns on the surface of foreign invaders through what are called "toll-like receptors." These toll-like receptors sit on the surface of mast cells and identify all invading antigens, announcing to the body, much like an alarm system might, "Alert! Alert! Trespasser!" In response, mast cells release cytokines to signal the immune system to attack the antigen. Infectious agents aren't the only things that can cause mast cells to react; chemicals can as well. Should mast cells be bombarded with one questionable environmental interloper after another, they signal the immune system to hit the gas pedal over and over again, until it's as if the engine is being gunned full throttle, 24/7. The master control switch that tells the immune system to fight with all its heart gets stuck in the on position and can't be turned back off.

To see how this process occurs in real time, Fairweather works in her lab with mice that have been exposed to a common virus such as coxsackievirus B3, known for short as CVB3, which can cause low-grade abdominal distress and diarrhea. When coxsackievirus B3 first enters the immune system, it enters the mast cells, where it gets broken down and chopped up. Toll-like receptors on the surface of the mast cells take a bit of that chopped-up virus and communicate the information they've gathered by presenting a piece of the virus to the T cells as if to say, "Hey, look, we've got a virus here!" The immune system must now decide whether to fight the coxsackievirus B3.

What happens next is critical. Should the mast cells signal the immune system to stay turned on just long enough to fight that virus, all is well. But should the mast cells stay turned on for too long and continue to release cytokines that further stimulate the immune system to attack the invading virus—and then seconds later send that same message alerting the immune system to respond to a chemical in a processed, food-colored cheese sandwich, and a second later do it again when it senses that the body has been exposed to flame retardants—the innate immune system never gets to rest from its state of high alert. The cellular interaction that puts on the brakes fails.

What ought to be putting the brakes on these cellular high jinks? At the crux of Fairweather's research is the discovery of an entirely new gene, called *Tim-3*. The job of *Tim-3* is to tell the immune cells to stop firing off fighter cytokines. *Tim-3*, when able to do its job correctly, is the master brake in the system.

THE ALLERGY CONNECTION—AND WHY EVEN THOSE WITHOUT A GENETIC PREDISPOSITION TO AUTOIMMUNITY ARE NOW AT RISK

Ironically the *Tim-3* gene turns out to sit in a location where no scientist would ever have dreamed to look: smack on the chromosome that determines certain types of allergic reactions. Finding the *Tim-3* gene on this spot completely shocked researchers, says Fairweather. "At first they were confused; what was the *Tim-3* gene, involved in autoimmunity, doing on the allergy gene?"

As it turns out, this makes complete sense. The way in which mast cells ignite a rapid blast of cytokines that leads to autoimmune disease is very "reminiscent of the hypersensitivity of mast cells during allergic responses," says Fairweather. When mast cells respond to allergic stimuli or infections they release cytokines and start an inflammatory response, which is the same process that initiates autoimmune disease.

As she talks about her research, Fairweather charts out these cellular interactions on the papers she's spread before us: a rough Rube Goldberg diagram. It's not easy to follow, and it's incredible to consider that in the time it's taken to read these last few paragraphs, our mast cells have made such split-second decisions about whether to launch an attack on each and every substance we've come into contact with thousands, if not millions, of times.

Like Fairweather's Rube Goldberg drawing, the immune system seems booby-trapped with control mechanisms that, when breached, cause the body to go haywire. When that point is reached—because, as in the case of Fairweather's mice, the immune cells never get the message to put on the brakes—her lab animals develop myocarditis, an autoimmune disease in which the body's immune fighter cells attack the tissue of the heart. "It's a matter of balance," says Fairweather. If the body is constantly fighting new autogens, that balance goes out of whack. Mast cells begin to proliferate even more, causing more cytokines to be produced—when the exact opposite ought to be happening and the immune system ought to be damping down. All gas, no brakes.

Fairweather believes that this overwhelming response of our mast cells, and not the hygiene hypothesis, is what's driving today's autoimmune and allergy epidemic. Indeed, Fairweather contends, the synergistic effect of shifts in our lifestyles over the past fifty years is so profound that even people who do not possess a genetic predisposition to autoimmunity may now be at risk for developing autoimmune disease.

This is a big, big statement. The idea that so many chemicals, pesticides, heavy metals, and viruses are burdening our mast cells that we can be struck with autoimmune disease even if we do not carry any of the genes that predispose us to autoimmunity is almost revolutionary. Still, the idea is not completely unprecedented. We already know that some environmental triggers to autoimmunity are so potent that one does not need to have predisposing genes to be vulnerable to disease: recent research shows that smoking almost always doubles the odds of developing rheumatoid arthritis in women who have not inherited the well-established genes for the disease.

The standing worst-case scenario assumption has long been that 25 percent of people carry some genetic susceptibility to autoimmune disease. Even if every single one of that vulnerable group developed an autoimmune disease, we'd still be looking at a ceiling of, say, 75 million Americans developing autoimmune disease at some point in the future, around triple the current rate. Scientists have long assumed that the other 225 million Americans would remain largely invulnerable to autoimmune diseases. Given that current rates of autoimmune diseases have tripled in the last thirty to forty years and that levels of dozens of known autoimmune-stimulating chemicals and heavy metals have been rising in human breast milk, blood, and urine every few years, the idea that 75 million Americans might be suffering with lupus or multiple sclerosis or some other autoimmune disease by 2050 is not far-fetched.

If Fairweather and her colleagues' discovery is correct—that autoimmune disease, when stimulated through the mast cell interaction, does not require any genetic predisposition to be set in motion—then the ceiling on how many people in the United States stand at risk for developing autoimmune disease is far higher than the 75 million (or 25 percent of) Americans who carry the genetic predisposition to autoimmunity. There is, in fact, no ceiling at all.

To bring this point home, Fairweather poses the scenario of a woman who does not possess any genetic autoimmune-disease predisposition who, in the afternoon, takes a walk with her two-year-old down the sidewalk of their townhouse complex, rounds a corner, and walks right into a cloud of atrazine herbicide being sprayed on the crabgrass in the community. Meanwhile, unbeknown to her, her two-year-old is coming down with a coxsackie-virus she picked up at daycare, and Mom just shared the end of a Popsicle with her, so the virus is beginning to work on her mast cells as well. Mom sets out cheese nachos for lunch, served from their plastic wrapper fresh from the microwave, estrogen-disruptor laden, and some strawberries heavily sprayed with insecticides. At this point, our young mom's mast cells are being hit nonstop, overwhelmed by the pesticides she's taking in through her skin, the virus through her nose and mouth, the chemicals and additives through her food. A triple whammy. All these cause mast cells to stay turned on for far too long. The cytokines, running amok, begin to signal the immune system to target the body's own tissue and organs and fire away. A similar triple whammy might occur when the immune system gets hit with a virus, a vaccine, and heavy metal exposure in one fell swoop.

For someone who does possess the genes for autoimmune disease, or who already suffers from autoimmunity, the process of cytokines running haywire might just happen all that more quickly, with each mega combo of environmental hits exacerbating his or her disease.

As we begin to understand better how different molecules and genes interact to set autoimmune disease in motion—whether it is John Harley's discovery of the Epstein-Barr virus causing molecular mistakes that lead to lupus, or Fairweather's mast cells being overstimulated and leading to autoimmune disease—we splice together more of the clues we need to decode the mysteries of the human immune system. However slowly, practitioners at the front lines of diagnosing these diseases are formulating clearer guidelines about what to look for in patients, and researchers are better able to develop lab tests for biomarkers that provide telltale clues as to what combination of potential triggers to autoimmune disease might already make up each patient's barrel.

As this understanding emerges, researchers are likewise better able to test for certain biological markers in the immune system that may signal trouble long before disease strikes—as well as work toward novel interventions. Around the world, as the number of patients suffering from these diseases surges—and few efforts are made, meanwhile, to eliminate the very pollutants that trigger these diseases in the first place—scientists are starting to put their muscle into developing cures that are so outside the box they seem like something straight from a sci-fi movie.

CHAPTER FIVE

THE AUTOIMMUNE DISEASE DETECTIVES: ERA OF THE MAVERICKS

On an unseasonably windy October Sunday in 2006, four hundred multiple sclerosis patients are gathered at the Maryland chapter of the Multiple Sclerosis Society's annual conference in Towson, Maryland, to hear scientists discuss hopeful research for MS. Outside, the first fall leaves bluster past the hotel lobby windows like bright, pantomiming hands. But inside the banquet room all eyes are riveted on a short film clip playing on a screen in the front of the room. In the scene a white rat, paralyzed from the waist down, struggles repeatedly to use his front legs to drag the lower half of his body along behind him. Try as he might, he can't budge an inch.

As the clip ends, the silence in the Sheraton ballroom grows eerie but for the sound of the Oz-like winds picking up again. Too many patients in this ballroom, myself included, know all too well what it feels like to muster every ounce of grit and muscle you possess in the hope your legs will hold your weight, only to lose that struggle over and over again. Everybody in this room knows just what the rat is dreaming of, if rats do dream.

The short film ends. A second begins. The same rat that, moments ago, was unable to move is now racing around a shallow-sided plastic box with the vigor of a rodent triathlete. Call him Regeneration Rat, call him Robo Rodent, call him the Rebound King. He is one of a group of thirteen rodents recently cured of paralysis in a groundbreaking stem-cell study at Johns Hopkins Medical Institutions.

The audience bursts into enthusiastic applause. One gets the impression that, if they could, the folks who are dependent on wheelchairs, walkers, or canes would be on their feet by now instead of hooting cowboylike bravos and clapping from their seats, letting their voices and hands convey the standing ovation that their bodies cannot.

The researcher they are lauding is the slightly sheepish but smiling Dr. Douglas Kerr, associate professor of neurology at the Johns Hopkins University School of Medicine, and principal investigator on this groundbreaking stem-cell study that recently rocked the scientific world. Whether by disposition or by training, Kerr is reluctant to accept the wave of admiration coming his way. He lowers his hands to stem the tide of applause, eager to explain to the crowd how, utilizing embryonic mouse stem cells in a novel set of strategic scientific steps, he has been able to regenerate the damaged axonal nerves and myelin sheaths in paralyzed rats.

"Is this the first time that paralysis has been cured in adult mammals?" a man in the audience calls out from his wheelchair, near the back of the ballroom.

"The first time," Kerr answers, duly aware that the breakthrough offers a long-overdue gleam of hope on what often seems a bleak scientific horizon for the growing number of Americans facing multiple sclerosis, Guillain-Barré syndrome, chronic inflammatory demyelinating polyneuropathy, transverse myelitis, and a host of other neurological autoimmune diseases in which the body attacks its own nervous system, leading to weakness, numbness, and, in some cases, paralysis in the limbs.

•••

There is a well-loved joke in scientific research in which a veteran lab researcher calls his grown son in order to share with him some astonishing news. "Son," he says, "we are turning old rats into new rats in the lab!" His son replies, "Great dad—call me when you can turn old people into young rats."

The point is well taken. Curing rats is a far cry from curing humans, and yet because rats, like mice, share remarkably similar neurological and immune systems to ours, it is with rodents that most medical research begins.

The story of how Kerr and his team came to cure paralyzed rats began in 1998 in Douglas Kerr's lab on the fifth floor of the Johns Hopkins Bloomberg School of Public Health. At the time, Kerr's meager research team consisted only of himself and two others. Today, taped across the door to his lab, along with photos of Kerr with his wife and two young daughters costumed as a bee-keeper and bees for Halloween, are pictures of him with his current research staff—which has burgeoned into a team of twenty. The latter photos speak to the kind of teamwork mentality that any pioneering scientific endeavor such as this one requires. In the center picture, taken in Kerr's family room, his lab staff poses together sporting goofy hats—straw hats with flowers, caps with cascading pink rose petals, panamas, and fedoras. One researcher holds a stuffed Elmo to his chest. They are laughing; they exude the aura of a family.

In the lab today, country music plays softly in the background. A half-consumed chocolate bar sits on a stool top. Beakers and bottles covered with aluminum foil fill the shelves of the glass and blue metal cabinets that line the walls, and a glass vase holds purple orchids. It is in this lab that the forty-year-old Kerr has developed what he likens to a step-by-step cookbook recipe on how to use embryonic stem cells to restore lost nerve function in paralyzed mammals. Kerr's impetus to practice what he terms "science for a cure" began early on in his career when he worked as both a researcher and clinician treating many patients—especially kids—with neurological autoimmune diseases such as multiple sclerosis, a chronic central nervous system autoimmune disease that can cause blurred vision, poor coordination, slurred speech, numbness, acute fatigue, and, in its more extreme forms, paralysis. He also tended many patients with transverse myelitis, an MS-related auto-immune disease of the central nervous system that causes severe paralysis and other neurological disabilities.

In his fourth year of residency at Johns Hopkins in 1999, Kerr treated an eleven-month-old baby named Morgan Gertz, who was suffering from transverse myelitis. Kerr grew discouraged when current treatment therapies "couldn't do a thing for Morgan." Re-search into neurological autoimmune diseases wasn't moving fast enough to help one whit. Morgan died. The loss of Morgan Gertz, coupled with similar losses, "broke my heart," says Kerr. When Kerr became a father for the first time at the age of thirty-three, he began to appreciate even more viscerally what it was like for a dis-abled person—child or parent—to be unable to partake fully in the small milestones of growing up or raising children. "When I see those small moments aren't possible for a patient because of their autoimmune disease, it becomes even more poignant," he says.

Today, a picture of Morgan Gertz sits on Kerr's desk, and an-other is on his office wall "to remind myself and every person who works in this lab why we're here," says Kerr. "I feel very strongly that I have to be these patients' advocate."

Until very recently Kerr's pursuit to cure paralysis with em-bryonic stem cells—by attempting to grow brand-new nerve path-ways throughout the adult body—was viewed by most scientists as little more than a pipe-dream hypothesis too far-fetched to warrant the research effort. The accepted science has long held that neural pathways can only grow during our initial development when we are still fetuses in the womb. After we finish developing in the womb, new nerves cannot grow in the body. Likewise, once those nerves are damaged they cannot be regrown—and most certainly not in an adult. Well aware that pursuing a plan to regenerate nerve pathways in adult mammals would mean skepticism from fellow researchers and years of patience, if it were to work at all, Kerr nevertheless pursued his experiments.

Step one involved taking mouse embryonic stem cells—which,

at the earliest stages of development are known as "undifferenti-ated" stem cells—and "differentiating" them into motor neuron cells. In development, undifferentiated embryonic stem cells be-come differentiated as they take on the distinct, necessary roles needed to create specific organs and tissue. Undifferentiated stem cells are kind of like college freshmen who haven't yet decided what subject they want to major in. Some go on to become heart tissue cells, others skin cells—and some become motor neurons. During our development in the womb, motor neuron cells are responsible for creating the complex nervous system that runs like a superhigh-way throughout our bodies, connecting our brain, cerebellum, and spinal cord to every nerve in our skin, limbs, fingers, toes, organs, and muscles. Kerr had to find a way to prompt these undifferenti-ated mouse embryonic stem cells to differentiate into motor neuron cells in such a way that they would go on to create axonal nerves covered with myelin sheaths—a fatty insulating tissue—that to-gether make up the elaborate electrical highway that constitutes the nervous system.

Under Kerr's microscope, undifferentiated stem cells don't look like much; a group of fifty thousand appears no bigger than a speck of table salt. To the naked eye, they are invisible. But these small cells are integral to human life. When the axonal nerves and myelin sheaths become damaged we become—in simplest terms—a bit like marionette puppets without any strings: nothing connects the brain and the toes, the central nervous system and the muscles in our arms or legs. Or, imagine the body as an electrical system. If you turn on the light switch in your bedroom, the electric current races through the wiring behind the walls and around to the socket where the lamp is plugged in, then into the lamp cord, where it races up to light the bulb. If you damage that wiring or cut too deeply into the plastic coating around the wire, your light won't turn on. Damage the myelin sheaths or axons that run from the spinal cord down into the legs and toes and your toes won't move; you won't feel the floor beneath your feet.

These myelin sheaths and axonal nerves are of critical impor-tance in MS and transverse myelitis research. Much MS research is focused on an autoimmune process in which immune fighter T cells, which are only supposed to attack foreign pathogens and invaders, mistakenly attack and damage myelin. The process of demyelination interrupts the electrical impulses that run through these nerve fibers, causing weakness and paralysis. More recently, however, researchers have discovered that B cells are also involved in the autoimmune response to MS. Instead of targeting myelin, B cells—which T cells signal to attack foreign antigens—can directly attack axons. In transverse myelitis, demyelination and injury to bundles of axonal nerves occurs in focal areas of the spinal cord, often leading to permanent and severe paralysis.

Kerr knew that if he were to succeed in stimulating the regrowth of axonal nerves and myelin sheaths—the kind of growth that happens naturally during a mammal's fetal development—he would need to give each embryonic motor neuron cell the strength, power, and precise signals necessary to tell it exactly where to go in the nervous system and what axonal nerves to redevelop once it landed there. You might call it a "smart cell." If such a plan succeeded, one could theoretically repair the damaged nerves in MS, transverse myelitis, Guillain-Barré syndrome, chronic inflammatory demyelinating polyneuropathy, and acute disseminated encephalomyelitis—all neurological autoimmune diseases in which the myelin sheaths and axonal nerves are compromised.

Kerr's first step was to collaborate with other researchers at Columbia University who had succeeded in prompting mouse embryonic stem cells to become specialized motor neurons by adding growth factors—known as "retinoic acid" and "Sonic hedgehog proteins"—to undifferentiated stem cells to induce them to specialize into motor neuron cells, the same cells that, when we develop inside the womb, assume their proper place in the spinal cord and, from there, are responsible for the growth of our axonal nerves and the myelin that sheaths them.

Once Kerr's team succeeded in prompting undifferentiated embryonic mouse stem cells to become differentiated motor neuron cells, they had to figure out a way to make these newly differentiated motor neuron cells do their natural job—to grow brand-new nerves from the spinal cord down into the legs. Kerr's lab team took these motor neurons and injected them into the paralyzed rats' spinal cords, hoping they would begin to grow new nerves. The experiment failed; once Kerr's team transplanted these hard-won motor neuron cells into the rats' spinal cords, the motor neuron cells died, without exception. "We found that if we just transplanted motor neurons into the spinal cord and did nothing else, then the surrounding neighborhood in the spinal cord—the white matter surrounding the spinal fluid, which is full of other, healthy myelinated axons—would see these motor neurons as foreign and reject them," Kerr says. The motor neuron cells expired. Kerr had to find a way to make the neighborhood recognize the transplanted motor neuron cells as friendly so that the motor neurons would be allowed to generate new nerves.

In 2001, Kerr and his team achieved this second step by treating the newly created motor neurons with additional growth factors that told the surrounding white matter that the motor neurons emitted the kinds of growth hormones that they excrete during development—even though they weren't. The trick, as Kerr terms it, worked—and it worked beautifully. The transplanted cells survived in the rat. Step two was complete.

But there was another problem. Although Kerr's team had succeeded in creating new motor neurons and in getting the adult body to accept them, the transplanted motor neuron cells didn't do what he had hoped they would once the successful transplant was completed. The transplanted cells did grow new axonal nerves, but these only ran up and down the spinal cord. They didn't reach out from the spinal column and shoot new axonal nerves into the arms and legs, which is where they needed to go if they were going to help the rats use their paralyzed limbs again.

In order to coax the nerves to grow out into the paralyzed legs, Kerr had to introduce two last chemicals into his nerve-regenerating cocktail: chemicals that told the myelinated axons that these newly birthed nerves were exactly the same as those that wire the body during fetal development. Now, says Kerr, "We got wild growth of myelin. We looked at this in our lab animals to see whether axons could now grow out of the spinal cord and we found that they did." Check off step three.

Kerr hoped that once the newly developing peripheral nerves were free to move out into the limbs, they would know what to do—they might even, he hoped, regrow along the exact same channels that they do in original fetal development, allowing the repair to happen of its own accord, as if from memory. That, however, turned out to be far from the case. The axons did not grow where they needed to—instead they wandered around aimlessly. They seemed to be struggling to find out where to go, choosing one path and then another fruitlessly, only to give up and ultimately stop growing altogether. The original wiring of the nervous system in utero is staggeringly complex, and the cues that allow the nervous system to become wired are turned off completely after development. They no longer exist in the grown mammal. The question loomed: How could Kerr re-create those original cues in an adult mammal?

The developmental cues that are necessary for "wiring" the body for the first time act as signposts in the developing fetus. Placed along the nerves in the limbs of the body, they tell myelinated axons during development whether to go left or right. These signposts are basically proteins on the surface of cells, and they wave like flags in the wind during development so that when the myelinated axon gets there it's like a signal flag telling the axon which direction to head in to connect with the right muscle and, conversely, which direction to avoid. Together, these axons pave the road with the nerves that will form the intricate highway of the nervous system.

Kerr realized he had none of these signposts in place. And so it made sense—if frustratingly so—that the axons would then meander aimlessly and never reach muscle. Which is exactly what they did.

Kerr and his colleagues realized they had to apply some bait in or near the muscle—something that they knew that motor neurons liked and that they would respond to—so that the motor neurons would grow toward that source. Step four began to become clear.

Kerr applied a particular molecule that other researchers have found acts as just this sort of signpost during fetal development to the area where he wanted the newly growing axonal nerve to go. When the axonal nerve detects that particular molecule—known as GDNF—it is attracted to it and grows toward it. GDNF binds to a receptor that's on the surface of the axon—and when it does, it turns on the neuron so that it continues growing in that direction.

Once those signposts were placed like bait in the paralyzed rat's muscle, the axon started to get highly motivated. It began to move right toward the paralyzed muscle.

It was a goosebump-raising moment in the lab. The smart cell was working.

"I was looking right at the axonal nerves moving straight into the paralyzed muscle tissue, but still, I didn't trust myself," says Kerr, recalling the exact moment when he looked through his microscope and found that the stem-cell axons had actually reached the muscle tissue throughout the animal's legs. As the newly generated axonal nerves reached the paralyzed muscle tissue, the muscle began to twitch. Kerr stared at what he was seeing under the microscope in a state of disbelief: "I thought, wow, this is amazing that we've gotten this far, that we've gotten all these steps together—but I still didn't trust what I was seeing with my own eyes. It didn't seem possible."

By 2003, getting motor neurons to reanimate paralyzed muscle in mice had already consumed five years of Kerr's life, with a staff of nearly a dozen often working largely around the clock. Kerr—who, when he needs to unwind from the constant pace of lab research, relaxes by tooling about on weather.gov and explaining the science behind worldwide weather patterns to staffers—felt it critical to confirm those five years of work by doing a massive blind study in 150 rats.

Kerr wanted to be absolutely sure that his cocktail was a success, especially before word of his work stirred the hopes of any patients. Several patients who were involved in advocacy work for transverse myelitis had been keeping abreast of his stem-cell research. One young woman in particular, Cody Unser, the daughter of ex–racecar driver Al Unser, Jr., had been deeply involved in raising funds to help find a cure for TM, and Kerr had come to know her well.

COOKING UP A CURE FOR PARALYSIS

In February of 1999, Cody Unser had been at sixth-grade basketball practice in Albuquerque, New Mexico, when she began to feel excessively tired and have trouble catching her breath. Her legs felt heavy, numb, tingly. She developed a mind-bending headache. After being evaluated at the local hospital, Cody was sent home, but the next morning she couldn't sit up or get out of bed. She was paralyzed from the chest down. She saw half a dozen doctors who were not completely sure of her diagnosis. Eventually she was told she might have transverse myelitis.

Cody first came to Doug Kerr during his last year of residency in 1999, seeking him out because of his reputation in cutting-edge TM research. At that point, Cody says, "I had visited so many doctors who treated me like just another number, one more faceless patient with TM who they couldn't help. But Doug was so compassionate. He reassured us that he was going to do everything he could to try to find a cure." On one of their visits, Cody says, "he took my mom and me into his lab and showed us his stem-cell research. I felt I was in the hands of a miracle worker."

Despite being paralyzed and in a wheelchair, by eighth grade Cody had created the Cody Unser First Step Foundation to help establish a TM research consortium spearheaded by Johns Hopkins Hospital. "My experiences taught me that there were many doctors out there who didn't know all they should about TM and that there were researchers in the TM field who weren't sharing information. There had to be more awareness and collaboration. We wanted to get doctors talking about TM." Today, Cody Unser, now twenty-one years old, has spent the last eight years of her life in a wheelchair. She follows Kerr's work closely. Her hope, she says, is "plain and simple: for paralysis to be history, for everyone to walk again."

"Seeing Cody's strength and courage has been a driving force for me from the day I first met her," says Kerr. "I feel that she and I are a team determined to help her walk again. And we are both sure that we'll succeed."

In 2003, with some trepidation coupled with inspiration from patients like Cody, Kerr, working on his standard five hours of sleep a night, set to work to prove his theory right. His team treated 15 of the 150 paralyzed rats with the entire recipe for axonal nerve growth, including all the necessary growth factors and signposts that had proven effective in the lab. In order to test the cocktail's effectiveness, the remaining 135 rats were split into groups and each treated with only a partial cocktail. For instance, one group of rats was treated with the transplanted motor neuron cells with all the growth factors, but they were not given the signposts that told the motor neurons where to go. Other groups lacked a different single, essential ingredient from the recipe as well.

In order to ensure accurate findings, Kerr had each paralyzed rat coded with a different number so that even he would not know which rats had been treated with which protocols. Then the key to that code—which rat had been given which treatment and, moreover, which rat had been given the full treatment—was set aside where no one could access it. Kerr was blind as to which of the identical rats had been given the entire nerve-regenerating cocktail. The researchers carefully followed and evaluated the rats for the next six months. After three months, they began to see signs that some animals were recovering. They didn't know which group was showing signs of greater mobility, but a few animals were starting to move limbs that had been completely paralyzed before.

"Of course we were hoping that these rats were in the group in which we'd replicated our findings," Kerr says. "My worst fear was that it would turn out to be one or two rats in each of our partially treated groups that were getting better—and we'd never know why."

After a total of six months, the almost unimaginable happened: 13 of the 150 rats were now scurrying around like healthy rodents. It was an astonishing sight. In February 2005 the entire group of researchers gathered in Kerr's lab to break the code. They started reading off each rat's code and looking to the original cipher to see which rats had been treated with which protocol. If all thirteen of the now healthy rats belonged to the group of fifteen that had been treated with Kerr's complete nerve-regeneration cocktail, it would mean that he had developed a revolutionary approach to make motor neurons reach out their "wires" from the spinal cord and move into paralyzed muscle, retracing complex pathways of nerve development that had been long shut off—recreating in an adult mammal the neural development that originally takes place in the womb.

When it became clear, only a few minutes into the process, that five of the recovered rats all belonged to the group that had been treated with Kerr's entire cocktail for curing paralysis, the excitement in the lab became palpable. As they continued to read off the codes, each additional recovered rat also turned out to belong to the same fully treated group. When they read the code on the thirteenth and last cured rat and found that it, too, belonged in the group that had been fully treated with Kerr's cocktail, people began to shout and jump up and down, hugging and clutching one another. A staffer grabbed a bottle of champagne that had been left in a lab fridge after a recent staff celebration. Kerr called his wife to tell her over the din that his dream had come true. Adult paralyzed rats—treated in a large-scale, fully controlled, blind study—were running around their cages again as if they had never been paralyzed at all.

"That's your eureka moment," says Kerr. "It's an amazing moment when you say to yourself, 'We did it in the most rigorous way possible, we blinded ourselves, and we found that we had it right.' "

Next, Kerr and his team will use the same basic framework to attempt to cure fifty pigs, looking to show safety and efficacy. Within five years he hopes to move on to human trials. One thing he will be looking to answer in his pig study is the question of distance: it's one thing to grow new axons the short fourteen centimeters it takes to travel from a rat's spine to his feet. But what about the greater length nerves must run from a pig's spine to its toes? And what about the distance motor neurons have to travel in, say, a six-foot-tall man, whose longest nerve spans a full three feet?

Kerr is hoping to start clinical trials in paralyzed adults within five years—before 2012—if all goes well in his study on pigs. Still, there are formidable hurdles given that embryonic stem cells remain a political no-no in today's federal funding arena. Although researchers have tried to use already-differentiated stem cells—taken from umbilical-cord blood, thus negating the need to use controversial embryonic stem cells—experiments striving to use this line of stem cells to regrow nerves have failed. Efforts are in the works to use stem cells from amniotic fluid, but many researchers say they would be seriously surprised if amniotic stem cells have all the capability of an undifferentiated embryonic stem cell, which has unlimited potential.

Some states, like California, have passed their own propositions to circumvent the federal ban on stem-cell research. And in Maryland, in 2007, legislators allotted $15 million for stem-cell research—including embryonic stem cells. About fifty Hopkins researchers, including Kerr's group, have entered grant proposals hoping for some of the $100,000 to $500,000 grants being offered. But to get from where Kerr is now in his research to clinical trials "will take millions of dollars," says Kerr. "With the current political climate, it's not clear where that money will come from. We know that the federal government will not help. Drug companies are reluctant to step in because of patent issues—and because each of these diseases, taken individually, does not afflict a large enough number of patients. We go month to month hoping that something will happen with funding that will allow us to keep going."

Although the idea of using embryonic stem cells for research is one that each scientist, politician, and voter must wrestle with for him- or herself, when the question arises among the four hundred sufferers of multiple sclerosis at the annual MS meeting where Kerr recently detailed his work on stem cells, their position is unanimous: embryonic stem cells hold the potential promise for them to live normal lives as mothers and fathers. Certainly embryonic stem cells are most promising when growing as an embryo inside a woman's body, but once embryonic stem cells that are by-products of in vitro lab fertilization are discarded, they no longer hold any glimmer of promise at all.

Beyond the hurdle of embryonic stem-cell funding, even if researchers succeed in regrowing axons in paralyzed humans with multiple sclerosis, or in those with Guillain-Barré who have not had good recoveries, or in patients with chronic inflammatory demyelinating polyneuropathy, a cousin to Guillain-Barré in which demyelination persists, they still face the issue of how to keep the hyperactive immune system that is the hallmark of these autoimmune diseases in check and prevent it from going after and damaging the myelin and axonal nerves time and again—after an initial stem-cell treatment. One might have one's nerves restored only to lose those connections each time the original neurological autoimmune disease flares.

It may be that stem-cell therapy will emerge as a kind of co-cure, along with therapies and lifestyle changes that help to keep the immune system from malfunctioning in the first place. Little by little, preventive therapies are being developed. "In five or ten years we're going to have good ways to tamp down the immune system and keep severe paralysis from happening—ways that do not carry the severe side effects of many of the drugs in use today," Kerr says. But, he ponders, "What about those people who are already in a wheelchair? Or who are struck suddenly and without warning by autoimmune disease and end up paralyzed before treatment to stop severe damage can even begin? We need to be able to give these mothers and husbands and children and grandparents back the lives they deserve to have. Then we can use newly developed immune-system therapies to help keep the immune system from attacking their nervous system again."

Kerr looks thoughtful for a moment before telling me about newborn infants he works with who suffer from what is known as spinal muscular atrophy. These babies have a fatal genetic flaw and do not develop a normal nervous system—and there is no way to help them. Inevitably, they die. But what if? What if, Kerr asks, we could help reconnect motor neurons to grow axonal nerves along their neural pathways according to normal developmental cues—which are still in place in newborns—so that they could develop a normal nervous system? Live normal lives? What if he could help these infants' mothers and fathers keep their newborn children healthy and safe and alive?

What if, he asks, we can help mothers and fathers and children who have been hit with neurological autoimmune disease lead the lives they, as families, dream of leading? What if Cody Unser could get out of her wheelchair and live her dream of being able to take that first step? "I feel that my career should be judged by whether I can deliver on this hope," Kerr tells me, his green eyes probing and earnest. "If I can't then I should be judged a failure." He reflects for a moment on his recent friendship with deceased actor Christopher Reeve, who, he says, "used to call me on a regular basis to see where we were with our stem-cell study—not just for his own sake, but for those he knew would survive after him. If I can look in the mirror when I'm seventy-five and say that I saved those babies who weren't born with developed neurological systems, or that I helped parents or children be the parents and children they dream of being, that's it for me, I'll die a happy man."

Still, the day when you can go to your doctor for a stem-cell injection to regenerate damaged nerves and expect to quickly re-grow your axons and myelin sheaths is years off—and there are numerous scientific and political hurdles to surmount along the way. In the meantime, scientists around the globe are researching ways to prevent the immune system from attacking itself in the first place—as well as to achieve more accurate and faster diagnosis for autoimmune diseases of every sort. One of the most dramatic breakthroughs in this research centers on trying to detect distinct blood biomarkers that will alert clinicians years before symptoms begin that a patient's immune system is on the verge of attacking his or her own body and destroying vital bodily systems.

THE BLOOD DETECTIVES

Imagine a future in which your regular checkup includes state-of-the-art blood tests that can predict with striking accuracy whether ten years down the road you'll develop rheumatoid arthritis, lupus, multiple sclerosis, Sjögren's disease, Addison's disease, or type 1 diabetes. If your lab tests do prove positive for specific patterns of antibodies that predict you have, say, an 80 percent or better chance of developing one of these autoimmune diseases, your physician quickly reassures you: worry not. With finely tuned, cutting-edge intervention she can treat you in advance of any severe symptoms of disease appearing and prevent your immune cells from ever turning on you.

It may sound farfetched—not unlike the capabilities of Dr. McCoy's handheld tricorder scanner in the futuristic *Star Trek* TV series, which could detect *Enterprise* crew members' hidden medical ailments in a matter of seconds. Yet in labs around the world, the ability to take blood samples and use blood biomarkers to predict autoimmune disease far in advance of a patient's falling ill is a rapidly evolving science—and a most promising one. In scientific breakthroughs that smack of *Star Trek* special effects, scientists from top medical research institutes have begun to identify the precise autoantibodies that foretell autoimmune disease in patients' bloodstreams as early as ten years in advance of illness, potentially paving the way for preventing these diseases from causing devastating damage in the first place.

One of the scientists voyaging into this new territory is Dr. Hal Scofield, an associate member of the Arthritis and Immunology Research Program at the Oklahoma Medical Research Foundation (OMRF). Scofield serves as a professor in the Department of Medicine as well as an adjunct associate professor in the Department of Pathology at the University of Oklahoma Health Sciences Center, where he works with Dr. John Harley, chief of OMRF's Arthritis and Immunology Research Program. Along with Harley, Scofield is coauthor of one of the most definitive works on prediagnostic biomarkers for lupus—work that has opened up a whole new window for researchers into how early autoantibodies can portend what might be happening deep in the immune system long before a single lupus symptom rears its ugly head.

One of the inherent difficulties in detecting what type of autoantibodies people may carry in their blood before they fall ill is finding a sufficient test group. Where in the world can a researcher hope to find a group of individuals with autoimmune disease who also just happen to have had their blood taken, frozen, and safely stored away for the past twenty years—allowing researchers to examine that blood to determine whether they developed autoantibodies years prior to falling sick or not?

As it turns out, there is just such a place. About twenty years ago, in the mid 1980s, when HIV (which is not an autoimmune disease) was first rapidly on the rise in the United States, the U.S. Army decided to take blood from all military personnel, both when they enlisted and each time they were deployed overseas, and to store those samples away. No one exactly knew what they planned to do with so many blood samples, but given the AIDS crisis brewing around the globe, it just seemed like a good idea at the time. The blood samples were stored at the Department of Defense Serum Repository in Silver Spring, Maryland. By 2003 the repository possessed 30 million blood samples taken from more than 5 million U.S. Armed Forces personnel—all stashed away in large silver walk-in freezers. It was a researcher's dream, the kind of treasure trove that no one but the army could possibly have stockpiled, given the deep pockets of the Department of Defense versus the dwindling sum doled out for the typical autoimmune-disease research grant. The repository also provided a logistical dream come true for researchers: every enlisted person's record can easily be traced back through time—unlike most civilian records, which are usually on file with a plethora of different physicians and hospitals and often can't ever be properly reconstructed in full.

Led by John Harley, in the late 1990s Judi James, a member of the Arthritis and Immunology division at Oklahoma Medical Research Foundation, along with Hal Scofield, began to ask themselves if, using this incredible resource, they might be able to determine whether the blood of army personnel who had ultimately acquired the autoimmune disease lupus would show the presence of any particular combination or pattern of antibodies that were not present in healthy personnel.

James and Scofield—who had both been closely mentored by Harley early in their careers at Oklahoma—had good reason to believe that this might not be a farfetched idea. In the 1980s other researchers working with infants born with a rare disease known as neonatal lupus had noted a fascinating but unsettling health pattern among these newborns' mothers that had led them to ask a similar question.

Babies born with neonatal lupus, a disease in which the immune system attacks the tissue of one or multiple organs in the baby's own body, have a lupuslike rash and very slow heartbeats—often as low as thirty to forty beats a minute. Sometimes they are born with heart block. Yet mothers of infants with neonatal lupus are often surprisingly quite healthy and free of lupus at the time that they give birth. Over time, however, researchers working with infants with neonatal lupus began to notice that four or five years down the road, mothers who had been seemingly healthy at the time of giving birth were routinely developing either lupus or lupus-related Sjögren's disease, an autoimmune disease in which sufferers experience symptoms such as dry eyes, dry mouth, and difficulty swallowing. Curious as to whether this could have been predicted, scientists took blood samples from twenty-one mothers of babies with neonatal lupus—including those mothers who had no symptoms of any disease—looking for specific autoantibodies that were indicative of lupus and Sjögren's. They discovered that these autoantibodies were present in all of the mothers who had given birth to babies with neonatal lupus. Indeed, over the next ten years, eighteen of these mothers went on to develop symptoms of lupus or Sjögren's. Evidently, these mothers were carrying the autoantibodies indicative of lupus and Sjögren's years before falling ill.

In 2000, the three Oklahoma researchers, along with researchers at the Walter Reed Army Medical Center, began working with stockpiled blood samples sitting at the Department of Defense Serum Repository. They set out to compare the blood work of 132 servicemen and women who were initially healthy but who later developed lupus with personnel who did not develop lupus. They were searching for a group of five different antibodies that, individually, go by names such as anti-nRNP, anti-Sm, anti-double-stranded DNA, anti-Ro, and anti-La antibodies.

Collectively known as ANA, or antinuclear antibodies, these antibodies are able to bind with the nuclei of tissue and organ cells and inflict damage. When clinicians test a patient who has lupus-like symptoms, they look for one or more in this array of autoantibodies to help in their diagnosis. While it's no surprise that patients already suffering from lupus would test positive for one or more of these ANA, it is another thing altogether to discover that these autoantibodies can exist in someone who is feeling perfectly fine, long before he or she feels the first twinges of malaise.

And yet that is exactly what Scofield, Harley, and James found to be the case. In 2003, they published a landmark study showing that of those servicemen and women who did develop lupus, 88 percent had at least one autoantibody to lupus ten years prior to diagnosis.

Although unaffected military personnel who never developed lupus also occasionally showed abnormal immune responses, in their cases, the autoantibodies appeared in a fleeting manner; they emerged only to disappear quickly again. Among those who developed lupus, the story was quite different. Their immune systems continued to create an increasing number of different autoantibodies right up until a few months before the onset of lupus symptoms. Looking at the bloodwork of these 132 people, a pattern emerged not unlike that of a progressive drum roll announcing the full-fledged arrival of the illness itself. Typically, one or two autoantibodies appeared ten years prior to disease, more appeared two to five years prior to disease, and several more appeared like a final drum roll just a few months before the patient experienced the first symptoms of lupus.

Scofield, a fifth-generation Texan from the whistle-stop town of Lewisville who retains a slight Texan twang despite two decades in Oklahoma City, cautions that he and other lupus researchers are still a long way from being able to pinpoint a specific pattern of autoantibodies that is 100 percent predictive of a person's developing lupus. Possessing autoantibodies that are indicative of a particular illness such as lupus doesn't necessarily mean that you're going to develop that disease. The most definitive thing that researchers can say at this point, believes Scofield, is this: "Those who are destined to go on to get lupus have these autoantibodies in their blood long before they get the disease, and normal people who don't have lupus don't have these autoantibodies very often, and so we do have the chance to go on and predict who might get disease." But scientists don't have all the kinks worked out quite yet.

It's still science in the making. Scofield points out that "When two people in the waiting room in our clinic sit next to each other and realize that they have lupus, often the only thing they have in common is the name of their disease. Their symptoms are different, and the autoantibodies they test positive for may be different as well." In short, which autoantibodies appear when and in what sequence or number varies a lot from patient to patient.

Nevertheless, says Scofield, "If we can further determine this exact pattern then the exciting part is that you can identify patients before the onset of disease." Armed with that information, doctors will be able to counsel patients who stand at a significantly heightened risk for developing a specific autoimmune disease about what symptoms to watch out for so that they can receive earlier treatment when symptoms do begin to appear. Early intervention could go a long way toward helping patients to sidestep some of the serious risks that come with lupus, including the life-threatening complications of kidney failure and major organ damage.

Scofield, Harley, James, and their colleagues are currently

working to elucidate more specific patterns to predict more definitively who will have lupus. Using the blood samples of a new, larger cohort of three hundred army personnel who developed lupus, they hope to detect the precise pattern of autoantibodies and ferret out the difference between patterns that are surefire predictors of the disease versus configurations of autoantibodies that don't necessarily mean you're at risk of developing lupus at all.

Similar research is going on in other diseases as well, such as rheumatoid arthritis. In a 2004 study, researchers looked at blood donors who later developed rheumatoid arthritis. About half the patients had autoantibodies for the disease an average of four and a half years before diagnosis. Patients who had the marker also ended up with a more severe form of the disease than those who did not. A Swedish study of rheumatoid arthritis published in 2003 found similar results.

Although lab researchers are working hard to elucidate biomarkers that predict disease years in advance of patients' developing autoimmunity, the irony is that many autoimmune-disease patients still struggle to receive an accurate diagnosis even when they have been terribly ill for years. The gap between what is happening in today's top diagnostic research labs and the diagnostic struggles that most patients experience in their doctors' offices is vast.

CAN WE PREDICT WHO WILL DEVELOP TYPE 1 DIABETES?

Nowhere is the ability to predict who will have an autoimmune disease more advanced than in type 1 diabetes research. Here, scientists have been able to identify prediagnostic markers for the disease with staggering accuracy. Type 1 diabetes is an autoimmune disease in which the immune system attacks the healthy beta cells—the cells that produce insulin—in the pancreas. When this happens, the body does not produce adequate insulin, the hormone our body needs to help our cells to absorb glucose. And that means that the body cannot balance its blood sugar. Untreated, type 1 diabetes is quickly fatal. People with type 1 diabetes need to take insulin artificially on a regular basis through injections or pumps. Even so, kidney disease, heart disease, and neuropathy are all common with long-term diabetes.

The disease is particularly troubling to autoimmune-disease researchers because of the rate at which it has been skyrocketing in children in recent years. More than a million Americans suffer from type 1 diabetes, and each year thirty-five thousand children are newly afflicted with the illness. A recent 2006 study—the largest surveillance effort on diabetes in youth conducted in the United States to date—found that 1 in 648 children and young adults under the age of nineteen now has type 1 diabetes—a staggering number. Worldwide studies confirm that even in babies and children aged four and under, rates have been increasing by 6 percent a year.

Knowing that, each year, so many children are being born who will develop type 1 diabetes has been a unique motivator for researchers to identify at-risk children in time to stop the disease in its tracks. Although scientists agree that some combination of genetics, toxins, viral hits, and diet are at play in the development of type 1 diabetes, predicting which children might be most at risk has been, until very recently, a pipe dream.

Older, traditional assays, or tests, determine risk for type 1 diabetes by identifying what are called islet cell antibodies. Islet cell antibodies are produced when the body's immune system fails to recognize insulin-generating islet cells produced by the pancreas as natural to the body and attacks them as if they were dangerous foreign substances, suddenly decreasing the body's ability to produce the insulin that helps cells absorb glucose. High levels of islet cell antibodies show that the body is destroying the islet cells in the pancreas.

Tests developed in the mid-1990s found that a combination of two newly recognized autoantibodies—GAD65 and IA-2—could also predict type 1 diabetes over time. However, researchers found that—as with prediagnostic lupus biomarkers—there were some patients who were positive for some of these biochemical markers but still did not develop type 1 diabetes. In 2005, Dr. Massimo Pietropaolo, a native Italian who came to America in 1990 to study as a research fellow in medicine at Harvard Medical School and who now serves as director of the Laboratory of Immunogenetics at the Brehm Center for Type 1 Diabetes Research and Analysis at the University of Michigan, set out to study the effectiveness of combining both the older islet cell antibody test with the two newer biochemical tests to predict who will develop type 1 diabetes.

Pietropaolo, who began the work while an associate professor of pediatrics, medicine, and immunology at the University of Pittsburgh School of Medicine, looked at both levels of islet cell antibodies and newer biochemical markers of autoantibodies in 1,484 first-degree relatives of people with type 1 diabetes. Those who tested positive for GAD65 and IA-2 autoantibodies had a 14 percent risk of developing type 1 diabetes after 10 years. However, those who displayed those two autoantibodies along with islet cell antibodies had an 80 percent risk of developing the disease after just 6.7 years. The surprise, says Pietropaolo, was that "by using these older assays in combination with the newer tests, we were able to more accurately predict type 1 diabetes in the family members of those with type 1 diabetes." His results delivered the highest level of accuracy ever achieved in not only predicting type 1 diabetes, but any autoimmune disease.

In addition, family members who tested positive for a fourth newly recognized biomarker developed type 1 diabetes more quickly than others. Pietropaolo, whose work is funded by the National Institutes of Health, suspects that having this new biomarker may predict a more rapidly developing form of the disease in first-degree relatives of patients with type 1 diabetes. In 2005, Pietropaolo began more in-depth studies, looking at all these prediagnostic biomarkers to predict who will develop type 1 diabetes and when. Results have been exciting. "We can now predict with accuracy type 1 diabetes in first-degree relatives of type 1 diabetic patients," he says. "This allows us to consider novel intervention strategies in an effort to delay or even prevent overt disease in those individuals who are at greatest risk of developing type 1 diabetes."

In other autoimmune diseases, the race has only recently begun to recognize antibodies that confirm diagnosis after symptoms have already occurred—and researchers remain years away from using such newly understood blood biomarkers to predict who may or may not develop disease. In multiple sclerosis—a disease that has traditionally been difficult to diagnose conclusively—recognizing what protein patterns signal that the body is at work against itself is just evolving, as researchers struggle to find a distinct pattern of proteins and antibodies that is highly indicative of disease. In an array of recent studies over the past two years, researchers have found a distinct fingerprint of individual proteins that can differentiate people with MS from healthy people. This suggests that, over time, scientists may be able to develop a blood test that could help them to identify the earliest changes that represent MS and aid in speeding up diagnosis as well as treatment. Other breakthroughs in MS diagnostics include a recent Yale study in which investigators isolated several newly recognized antibodies that were shown to interact with a form of myelin found in MS and state-of-the-art eye exams that use four different tests to find abnormalities in the retina and damage to optic-nerve fibers, often the spot where MS damage first occurs.

Other researchers, including Douglas Kerr at Hopkins, are looking at elevated levels of specific proteins not in the blood, but in the spinal fluid of MS patients, to help confirm diagnosis. Kerr has found that levels of a particular protein, interleukin-6, or IL-6, are dramatically elevated in the spinal fluid of patients with transverse myelitis. Interleukin-6 is a pro-inflammatory cytokine, a messenger that cells of the immune system use to communicate with one another. One of the cell types injured by high levels of the protein IL-6 includes oligodendrocytes, which help to produce the protective myelin sheath around nerve cells. Kerr's team found that the level of IL-6 proteins directly correlated with the severity of paralysis in patients.

Additional proteins and antibodies related to multiple sclerosis are being isolated in labs across the country—raising the question as to whether or not, one day soon, a map of blood biomarkers may emerge that predicts disease years in advance in multiple sclerosis, just as in lupus and type 1 diabetes.

As newer technologies are developed, researchers are on the cusp of being able to measure increasingly complex combinations of unique proteins and antibodies at one time. Such measurements may provide clinicians with the ability to study large groups of people to see how predictive these patterns of biomarkers are in determining who develops a disease and how long it takes for symptoms to appear. As we improve our ability to see what biomarkers of disease predict actual disease, researchers can begin to look at patient-specific therapies and develop prevention trials.

THE GENETIC LINK

Genetic testing provides yet another key to identifying who is most likely to be afflicted by these diseases. Researchers believe that our genes determine roughly 30 percent of one's risk of developing autoimmunity, with the remaining risk being attributable to environmental factors. All of the twenty thousand genes that scientists (at latest count) believe we are born with are encoded in our DNA from the moment of conception. Our cells read these genes in order to build proteins in our bodies. Proteins carry out the various cellular processes that make our bodily systems function. What genes we have determine what protein sequences we create and what enzymes we produce—which, in turn, determine how our cells will behave in an array of challenging circumstances. Small defects in genes—and in protein codes—can make a whopping difference in how the cells in our bodies act. By understanding which genes precipitate a specific disease we can better understand the process by which disease is kick-started. But it's a complex task: not only do we have an estimated twenty thousand genes, but each of these genes can have multiple, complex, individual variations. One gene might have only the slightest modification in terms of the proteins it expresses, but that small difference will lead to dramatic changes in the way our body functions.

As with all gene research, efforts to decipher how specific genes influence our susceptibility to an array of autoimmune diseases is stepping up around the country. In two related 2006 studies, researchers at the University of Texas Southwestern Medical Center recently found defective genes in mice that contribute to triggering lupus. One of the two studies determined that a defective version of a gene known as *Ly108* rendered mice susceptible to lupus. The defective version of the gene impairs one of the most basic steps in the development of immune-system cells. When it is functioning normally, the body destroys any immune-system cells that, by mistake, have started to produce antibodies against the body. But in mice with a defective *Ly108* gene, those rogue self-attacking cells escape detection, allowing them to attack the body's healthy cells, resulting in the disease. If researchers are able to demonstrate that the same genetic defect found in the mouse model also creates susceptibility in human lupus, it might open ways to block the disease by developing new drugs that block the activation of a defective *Ly108* gene.

In a separate lupus study from UT Southwestern, researchers describe the role of a mutated gene called *Tlr7*, which interacts with *Ly108* in triggering lupus by causing another component of the immune system to malfunction. The gene turns out to affect the body's ability to alert the immune system to an invading germ. The research team, led by Dr. Edward Wakeland, professor of immunology and director of UT Southwestern's Center for Immunology, discovered that mice that died of lupus in their study carried twice the normal amount of the mutated receptor gene *Tlr7*. Interestingly, for lupus to occur, the lupus-causing versions of *Tlr7* and *Ly108* both have to be present. If you put both genes together, you create a fatal form of lupus—the mouse dies.

Although these genes are in mice and not humans, chances are that they will shed light on the genetics of lupus in people. Already, genes that have been linked in mice to type 1 diabetes and rheumatoid arthritis have turned out to influence the same diseases in humans. Ultimately, understanding how small differences in our genetic expressions can lead to disease may help doctors to tailor lupus treatments to individual patients, since the cause of each individual patient's disease may differ, and the genes that work together to help precipitate disease in one person may be different from those that lead to genetic susceptibility in another.

At the Oklahoma Medical Research Foundation, John Harley has played an instrumental role in identifying a pair of genes in humans that may be responsible for genetic susceptibility to lupus. His lab has also created the Lupus Multiplex Repository and Registry, the world's largest collection of blood and tissue samples from families in which more than one member suffers from lupus, in order to help researchers investigate more genetic links to lupus in people—and to see which combination of genes is most likely to result in disease. Likewise, a 2007 genome study searching for MS genes pinpointed two gene variants as heritable risk factors for multiple sclerosis.

Already, the technology we have to look at how genetic codes influence disease is opening up new avenues of scientific questioning. For example, researchers have shown that mutations of several genes are strongly associated with Crohn's disease. Surprisingly, one type of mutation appears actually to be protective—helping to prevent people from acquiring Crohn's or ulcerative colitis, both types of inflammatory bowel disease. Lupus researchers are likewise discovering that there are certain strains of mice that—even if exposed to high levels of what are traditionally thought to be lupus-causing agents—still don't develop disease. The idea that a gene might be protective against disease—meaning that those with a specific gene don't get the disease—is a twist on the traditional thinking of the genetics of disease, opening up inquiry into what we might think of as the genetics of health.

THE GENDER EQUATION

One clear-cut genetic difference that weighs in heavily on who will have autoimmune disease is the most obvious of all—gender. Women account for nearly 80 percent of the 23.5 million Americans with autoimmune disease. Women also tend to have higher antibody levels than males and mount more robust immune responses to antigens. Hormonal shifts in pregnancy, menopause, and aging are associated with fluctuations in the course of autoimmune disease. Think back to Jan Pankey, who started taking birth-control pills and developed full-fledged antiphospholipid antibody syndrome shortly after starting their use. Birth-control pills didn't cause Jan's sudden plunge into autoimmunity, but increased hormonal levels no doubt helped to fill her barrel so that when she met up with those chemically noxious smoke clouds crossing into Montana something in her immune system just snapped. Indeed, research shows that many women who develop lupus do so a few months after giving birth to a child—a time when hormone levels undergo swift and dramatic changes.

Yet the precise ways in which sex hormones influence autoimmune disease remain largely unknown. What researchers do know is that sex hormone balance is a crucial factor in the optimum regulation of immune and inflammatory responses and that hormones such as estrogen that women produce modulate the activity of proteins in our bodies, leading in ways we do not yet fully understand to a more reactive autoimmune response.

At the Mayo Clinic in Rochester, Minnesota, researchers have made some headway in explaining how the genetic difference between the sexes plays a role in why women develop multiple sclerosis almost twice as often as men. Their findings suggest that how much of the protein interferon gamma—a cytokine that signals the immune system to start the immune response—a person produces appears to be a key variable in understanding who gets MS and who doesn't and especially in explaining why women develop MS more often than men. If you have a gene that produces high levels of interferon-gamma, or signaling proteins that tell the immune system to get active fast, it may predispose you to developing MS. Under this scenario men get MS less often because men, in general, are less likely to have a gene variant that is related to higher secretion of these cytokines. Research by scientists at the Cleveland Clinic and elsewhere have also shown that women and men naturally produce different levels of interferon-gamma and that higher levels of interferon-gamma can intensify the MS damage processes and make the disease worse. The fact that men have a lower frequency of the interferon-gamma genetic variant may be part of the reason why men are generally protected from MS.

A PATIENT'S DIAGNOSTIC PORTRAIT

Scientific discovery is often made up of many, many dots that together create a pointillist picture. In the future a patient's diagnostic portrait may consist of putting together a number of these dots, small glimmers of information that, when we step back to view them, create an impressionist portrait of a disease-in-the-making. In the next decade it is possible that clinicians will be able to examine a patient's specific pattern of autoantibodies to see if he or she fits more precise, established predisease patterns; be attuned to the genes that predispose a patient to a particular autoimmune disease (taking into account gender); ascertain a patient's viral load by testing for autoantibodies against viruses such as Epstein-Barr and cocksackie B that are known to be implicated in one's risk of developing diseases such as lupus and diabetes; examine a patient's diet to see if it is likely to be adding to the stress on the immune system because of the food choices a patient routinely makes; and test for the chemical and toxic "body burden" a patient is carrying by screening blood, hair samples, and urine (and, in breast-feeding women, their breast milk). This type of patient portrait is certainly likely to lead doctors to make what Hal Scofield calls "some good predictions" that a patient's immune system is being triggered in the wrong way and that he or she totters on the verge of disease.

Physicians can then warn patients about the adverse health course they are on and intervene with lifestyle changes and medications with the intention of averting an array of life-altering and debilitating diseases.

Think of LaShekia Chatman of Buffalo, New York. What if LaSheika had been able to go into a physician's office and, as part of a routine adolescent checkup, be tested for all known autoantibodies for lupus with an eye toward seeing whether she was developing the specific "drum roll" pattern that precedes the disease; for Epstein-Barr autoantibodies to see if she might be experiencing a case of molecular mimicry; and for heavy metal and other environmental chemical levels through her blood, urine, and hair? With prior knowledge that her barrel already sat right at the brim with a telltale pattern of lupus autoantibodies, Epstein-Barr antibodies, and a plethora of chemicals and metals absorbed into her body from her Buffalo neighborhood, could treatment have been started to prevent lupus as well as scleroderma from doing such devastating damage to her by the age of twenty, stealing away her chance to live a normal life?

THE HIGH COST OF PREVENTIVE TREATMENTS

Such a scenario is still years off, of course. Indeed, Michelle Petri, clinical director of the Johns Hopkins Lupus Center, who is currently spearheading an international task force to revise clinicians' criteria for diagnosing lupus, isn't sure such pretesting will ever be truly viable. She cautions that this kind of antibody and genetic testing would pose a tremendous cost to our health-care system if we began to use it widely on patients who were not yet showing overt signs of illness, a cost our already overburdened health-care system certainly could not bear.

Meanwhile, there remain pressing ethical questions. Although a discussion of medical ethics falls outside the scope of this book—certainly whole books have been written on the topic by experts in the field—it's important to consider the risks of preventive testing and treatments. For example, many of the drugs prescribed as preventive medicine come with dangerous side effects. A physician treating someone who shows all the signs of being on the verge of disease but who is still enjoying relatively good health in his or her day-to-day life would have to think twice before intervening with the sledgehammer treatments available today that damp down whole aspects of the immune system without discriminating between the good and the bad. Furthermore, if we can test for genetic predisposition and detect the earliest biomarkers of disease before patients fall ill, will health- and life-insurance companies cover such patients? Will companies hire them? When we consider that autoimmune disease may show up in individuals who are not genetically predisposed, the complexities surrounding any attempt to predict disease multiply.

Predicting who is going to be sick is a highly promising field of scientific inquiry, but deciding when to test for prediagnostic biomarkers and intervene with such patients promises to be dangerously tricky. The physicians' creed is "First, do no harm." Currently on the market for treatment of rheumatoid arthritis and Crohn's disease are classes of drugs that remove or inactivate certain immune activity, such as tumor necrosis factor, or TNF. Tumor necrosis factor, which belongs to a group of proteins that communicate with cells, is essential in maintaining cell life and death decisions and control of T-cell populations. The thought has been that if you could prevent TNF from signaling the release of joint-damaging substances in diseases like rheumatoid arthritis, you could go a long way in treating the disease. These anti-TNF therapies go by names that consumers recognize as Remicade and Enbrel. Anti-TNF therapy, which has been used most broadly to treat rheumatoid arthritis with hopes that it would prove to be the bright new promise for suffering patients, has turned out to pack a nasty surprise. These drugs do help to stave off joint destruction, but in the process TNF blockers also cause rheumatoid arthritis and psoriasis patients to have several-fold-higher rates of lymphoma (a type of cancer). According to FDA officials, Remicade and Enbrel use have a "probable or possible" link to the development of lymphoma, and studies show that several patients' lymphomas regressed once treatment with these medications was discontinued. In other rheumatoid arthritis patients, TNF therapy actually kickstarts new forms of autoimmunity that mimic multiple sclerosis, autoimmune hemolytic anemia, type 1 diabetes, lupus, and psoriasis. Also used in the treatment of Crohn's, anti-TNF therapy has been linked to the development of other autoimmune diseases, such as lupus. Once we muck about with one aspect of the immune system, we may derail other important immune-cell functions. All too often the cure is worse than the disease.

A similar story arises with Tysabri, a drug used to treat multiple sclerosis that the U.S. Food and Drug Administration fast-tracked for approval in November 2004. Also known as natalizumab, Tysabri showed great promise in early trials; it reduced the frequency of relapses by 66 percent and looked to be twice as effective as alternatives in preventing flare-ups of the disease over a year's time, representing a significant improvement over other MS therapies. It was certainly a far more attractive alternative than low-dose chemotherapy, which has often been used to treat MS in the past. The success of Tysabri, which was also being tested for efficacy in treating Crohn's disease and rheumatoid arthritis, is based on its ability to bind to a protein on immune-system cells, preventing them from traveling to the brain, where they can then pass into the nervous system and cause the brain and spine lesions that lead to MS symptoms. The drug, which is administered intravenously once a month in a doctor's office—making it a better alternative to drugs that require daily injections—appeared to be safe and well tolerated, although there was no information about long-term safety.

But within months of Tysabri's approval it became clear that the drug posed rarely seen but potentially fatal side effects. Some patients taking the drug developed a rare infection—progressive multifocal leukoencephalopathy, or PML—and two patients died. Anita Louise Smith was one of these patients. Smith had enrolled in an experimental drug trial for treating multiple sclerosis with Tysabri in 2002 in Colorado. Although Smith had been diagnosed with

MS, she had not yet developed debilitating symptoms. Tysabri was a promise that she could reduce the chances of being ravaged by the disease by keeping her MS from progressing. But in 2005, Smith died at the age of forty-six from PML, an infection that usually affects people whose immune systems are compromised. In Smith's case, her infection was linked to her use of Tysabri in combination with another drug, Avonex, which also helps to prevent immune cells from entering the brain. It appeared that Tysabri's mechanism of action—blocking the entry of immune cells into the nervous system by blocking their entry into the brain—might also make patients more vulnerable to infection. The FDA withdrew Tysabri only three months after its approval. By that time Tysabri had come to seem less impressive for other reasons as well: its ability to halt episodes of MS relapse, while notable, was generally not much better than what was seen, over time, with other available drugs. The risk of relapse dropped from an average of two relapses every three years using other approved MS drugs such as Copaxone, Rebif, Betaseron, and Avonex—all of which reduce flare-ups or minimize the appearance of lesions in the brain—to one every three years with Tysabri. The question was simple but grave: Would a physician want to expose someone to the risk of death for the sake of eliminating one relapse every three years? For some patients the answer might be yes, but for many others, like Anita Louise Smith's family, the answer would certainly have been no.

Today, researchers are working to tease out whether the fatal brain infections associated with Tysabri might have something to do with the fact that the patients who experienced them were receiving Tysabri along with Avonex. There were no cases of PML among the five hundred patients who took Tysabri alone for multiple sclerosis or the two thousand who have taken it in clinical studies for Crohn's disease or rheumatoid arthritis. On June 5, 2006, the U.S. Food and Drug Administration approved the reintroduction of Tysabri as treatment for relapsing forms of multiple sclerosis. Investigators suspect, for the time being, that it could be that the two drugs together had an additive effect preventing immune-system fighter cells from entering the brain—working in tandem to open the door to brain infection. Still, no one is sure. Which is the point: when working with the inscrutable immune system, investigators are often working partially blind: they don't understand nearly enough about how one pathway of immune cell interactions impacts another to predict what will happen when they alter one of these pathways. Science tends to be murky that way, but as any immunologist will tell you, perhaps in no field is it messier than in autoimmune-disease drug research. When we attempt to develop therapies to keep the immune system from attacking itself, it is impossible to guess whether all other functioning parts of the immune system will remain uncompromised in the process—and only long-term clinical trials can provide the answer.

All of which leaves autoimmune-disease sufferers with dicey options. The multiple sclerosis drugs Avonex, Rebif, and Betaseron can lead to rare liver problems, Copaxone can lead to severe allergic reaction. For those with rheumatoid arthritis, Remicade and Enbrel can lead to a greatly elevated risk of lymphoma, serious infections, and tuberculosis; Celebrex and Vioxx are overwhelmingly linked to cardiac problems. Those suffering from Crohn's disease can choose between methotrexate, which can be toxic to the liver, and prednisone, which can also lead to potentially fatal infections because it suppresses the entire immune system. Not a pretty picture.

Newer therapies are emerging as more promising, perhaps the most impressive of which is Rituxan, also known as rituximab, now being used to treat those with multiple sclerosis and other autoimmune diseases. Rituxan works by preventing signals from being transmitted that set B cells in motion to react against the body's own tissue. So far, early studies in MS populations are promising, indicating that Rituxan does lead to rapid depletion of self-reactive B cells. The drug, which has been used for nine years as a cancer drug to treat non-Hodgkins lymphoma, can cause serious side effects in lymphoma patients, including liver problems, but these side effects do not seem prevalent in those with multiple sclerosis—at least not in the nearly two years in which Rituxan has been studied. Some studies show that Rituxan not only helps to stop MS disease progression, but helps patients to recover some of the neurological function that they lost due to MS in earlier months and years. Rheumatologists are also using rituximab (under the name MabThera) to treat patients with rheumatoid arthritis. In a study of 156 patients who had not responded to TNF inhibitors such as Enbrel (which works by tamping down T-cell activity), patients taking MabThera reported an improvement in their physical well-being and ability to perform daily tasks, as well as a slowing down of joint damage. For some patients, their disease went into remission.

In lupus trials, the Rituxan story is less rosy: in 2006 the FDA issued a warning following two deaths from viral infections of lupus patients who were using Rituxan "off label"—meaning that they had been prescribed the drug even though it has not yet been approved for lupus. Doctors and analysts are unsure about cause and effect and may never know the truth; lupus patients have compromised immune systems, and it's impossible to say whether Rituxan alone was responsible for these infections. Two clinical trials using Rituxan to treat lupus patients are now under way. So far, Rituxan has an overall record that is better than many other newer drugs, but how promising the drug turns out to be will only be truly known after it has been in use in patients with autoimmune disease for the next five to ten years.

Meanwhile, as drug companies see a worldwide trend in which rates of lupus are doubling and tripling, there is a horse race just breaking out of the starting gate to see who can be the first one to gain approval to make and market the first new lupus drug in many decades. At this writing, there are currently three other drugs in late-stage lupus trials in addition to Rituxan. These include Orencia, a rheumatoid arthritis drug new to the market that researchers hope will help lupus patients; LymphoStat-B, which has had some success in reducing lupus disease activity; and CellCept, a drug in use for organ-transplant recipients, now being tested in lupus patients with severe kidney disease—but which also carries an increased risk of lymphoma because of the way it suppresses the entire immune system.

"I FELT LIKE A TICKING TIME BOMB"

For many patients, that horse race is regrettably late out of the gate. Joy England, a thirty-two-year-old mom from Georgetown, Texas, began her struggle to find out what was happening to her in 1999, when she was twenty-four years old. Sore joints and a flulike fatigue that never abated led her to seek out the help of her family practitioner. England's doctor took her ailments seriously from the get-go—four people on England's mother's side had rheumatoid arthritis, and her mother had diabetes. Her doctor ran an antinuclear antibodies test, or ANA. England's ANA factors were moderately high, but her doctor reassured her that healthy people sometimes have comparable ANA counts and nothing comes of it at all. They could only wait and see whether this might turn into something more worrisome for Joy.

A committed athlete who, up until her illness, had been running on nearby park trails six days a week and working nine hours a day at a job she loved, traveling as a representative for a teachers' association, England felt she was getting weaker by the day. "I woke up with joint pain and fatigue and I went to bed with it being worse than when I woke up," she says. She went on the Internet and found out that a high ANA count could be indicative of lupus, rheumatoid arthritis, and scleroderma, as well as a number of other autoimmune diseases—but that testing for specific antibodies unique to each of those diseases is still imperfect, and many patients aren't diagnosed until long after their symptoms become more severe. England had recently become engaged to a firefighter who worked twenty-four-hour shifts. When he was working and she was alone for long stretches of time, she says, "I would lie on the couch in my apartment and ask myself how could this be happening to me—a twenty-four-year-old runner with a great job, so in love for the first time in my life and planning my wedding?"

Six months later, England's doctor sent her to a rheumatologist. The rheumatologist ran another ANA panel but could not find a pattern that bespoke any particular autoimmune disease, be it lupus, scleroderma, or rheumatoid arthritis. He was hesitant to start any medications, well aware of the significant health risks and side effects associated with most drugs used to treat autoimmunity. That, in conjunction with the fact that they did not yet know what disease it was they were going to need to treat, made it imprudent to commence with sledgehammer medications. Still, he told Joy that her high ANA titer was worrisome and would likely turn out to be indicative of an autoimmune disease down the road. Meanwhile he prescribed Advil four times a day and told her that they would keep a keen eye on the situation.

For the next year Joy lived, she says, in diagnostic purgatory—waiting, on one hand, to discover what might be wrong with her as her symptoms steadily worsened, and on the other hand planning for the "wedding moment I'd wanted and waited for." At one point, she jokes, she was carrying a color-coded binder full of the details for her wedding and a second binder with all the information she was gathering on autoimmune diseases.

Around the time Joy and her fiancé decided to move into his house together, along with her schnauzer, Buster, and David's Dalmatian, Lucky. Many nights, she would listen to the fire scanner David had had installed in the house, enabling Joy to hear what was happening, live, when David was in the midst of fighting a fire. While David was fighting actual fires, Joy was fighting what she likened to her own fire, only this one was happening from within. She would often lie on the sofa with Buster and Lucky next to her for company, sleepless from the constant pain in her hot, swollen, inflamed joints, unable to even shift her weight—her distress exacerbated by the sheer anxiety of not knowing what was happening to her body. "I would watch a television show and see people my age running through a field and it would suddenly hit me that I might never be able to run again."

Joy was taking more and more sick days, unable to manage the joint aches and weakness, though she had to force herself to go into work as often as she could because she needed the health insurance. She was retested for autoantibodies but results remained inconclusive. She had been struggling to manage symptoms with-

out any diagnosis for a year and a half and she was steadily deteriorating. The Advil wasn't helping. Because her symptoms were
intensifying, her rheumatologist started her on a nonsteroidal anti-
inflammatory medicine, Relafen, used often in treating arthritis. It
didn't do much for Joy. Whatever autoimmune disease it was, it
was continuing to progress. "I felt like a ticking time bomb, and we
had no way of doing anything to defuse it," England says. "My
doctor and I knew that eventually I would fall into one of these
autoimmune-disease categories, but meanwhile there was nothing
we could do to keep my body from attacking itself. We could only
watch and wait for the other shoe to drop."

After Joy and David's wedding, Joy—who was advised not to
use birth-control pills because of the link between estrogen and
autoimmune disease in women—found herself unexpectedly pregnant. She was frightened, but during the pregnancy she found, surprisingly, that her symptoms improved—as can sometimes happen
in autoimmune disease. But after her daughter Emily was born,
Joy's health started going downhill fast.

Over the next several months, Joy's joint pain and swelling
became so intense that it was hard for her to get out of bed and lift
her newborn daughter from her crib. Her white blood cell count
fell very low. Then she developed a rash across her back that looked
like a raging case of teen acne. She put some acne cream on it but
it didn't go away. She went to her dermatologist, who decided to
biopsy the eruptions. The biopsy revealed that Joy did, indeed,
have systemic lupus. At that point Joy England was finally given
the lupus label. Her rheumatologist put her back on Relafen and
began treating her with Plaquenil, a medication used for the treatment of malaria that is also useful in treating lupus and rheumatoid
arthritis, although how Plaquenil helps with inflammation in autoimmune disease is still not well understood.

But it wasn't enough. By then, Joy England had gone largely
untreated for lupus for four years. She continued to have severe
flares every other month and was frequently put on prednisone for
a month at a time. She would feel better for a short time, only to
flare again. Her rheumatologist worried about the ramifications of

having her on a roller coaster of prednisone and decided to try Imuran, a chemotherapy medication that suppresses the immune system in general, which he and Joy had been hoping to avoid since it carries with it a heightened risk of lymphoma and leukemia. She stayed on Imuran for fifteen months. At that point she seemed stable enough that her doctor began to wean her off it, but suddenly she had another severe flare—her joints swelled and she developed pleurisy, an inflammation of the lining of the lungs. She began having severe migraines. And so she began another course of prednisone.

Joy and her rheumatologist often discuss new drugs coming down the pike that might be helpful in lupus—a disease for which no new drug has been approved for forty years—but clinical trials are only now in the works, and the potential health risks and side effects of the new drugs are far from known. "My doctor told me that if I were an older patient he might try me on a new drug that's being tested in clinical trials in lupus patients, like Rituxan," Joy says. "But I'm a young mom, and the jury on these drugs isn't yet in and it isn't going to be in for years. None of us want to take the chance that I might be that one patient who develops a rare, fatal viral infection."

Joy says she's perplexed as to why researchers haven't done more sooner to help lupus patients. "I always worry about the long-term damage that being in this constant state of inflammation is doing—damage that can't be reversed and could have been prevented. To have a drug that would target just the autoimmune process that is causing lupus without knocking out my entire immune system would make all the difference for me." It is very difficult, she says, "having a young child and being on an immunosuppressant drug. My daughter is in day care, and if she gets sick for a few days then I usually get it and I get sick for weeks—which brings on a flare and then I need more immune-suppressing drugs. It's a vicious cycle." Joy and David always talked about a big family when they first fell in love, but they know it would be extremely risky given how Joy's disease flared after the birth of their daughter. As her husband David says, "I'd rather have Joy here than two children and no wife—and we have one child who needs her mom."

"It makes me angry," Joy says. "Motherhood is something I truly love, and I want my daughter to have a brother or sister. If I knew there were drugs available that could safely help me to be stable then I would feel I could go off them, get pregnant, have a baby, and then go right back on. But that's not the case, and it's probably not going to be the case for a long time." To do what she can to aid the lupus cause, England raises money for the Alliance for Lupus Research and finds corporate sponsors to support the Austin lupus walk. Meanwhile, she has never gone for a run since the summer eight years ago when her illness began. She is limited as a mom—she can't run after her daughter, she can't be in the sun with her at the swimming pool or on the soccer field because sunshine can provoke a flare. And when she does flare, she is often in bed, unable to be the mom she once imagined she would be.

One can only wonder: What if Joy England's condition had developed at some future time when doctors would not only be able to better detect complex diagnostic biomarker patterns that foretell disease earlier on, but when drugs finally arrive on the market that will help to block only the cells and autoantibodies involved in autoimmunity without targeting the entire immune system? How many Joy Englands might then be able to go on and live their lives as the mothers, wives, athletes, and career women they always dreamed of being—without being broken down by years of pain and suffering?

THE ROAD TO REGENERATION

These diseases will not be felled by a single magic bullet. It will take exploring numerous avenues and eclectic approaches. For those with rheumatoid diseases such as lupus and rheumatoid arthritis, one set of drugs might prove most useful, while for those with neurological autoimmune diseases, other approaches may prevail. One such vanguard venture in the works for those with neurological autoimmune diseases is now under way at Johns Hopkins Hospital, under the direction of Dr. Ahmet Hoke, associate professor and director of the Division of Neuromuscular Diseases of the Department of Neurology and Neuroscience. In his lab on the fifth floor of the pathology building of Johns Hopkins Hospital, Hoke—who is also my own neurologist—recently discovered that a unique growth factor produced naturally by our nerve cells has a surprising ability to regenerate nerves in the body after they've been damaged by diseases such as multiple sclerosis, transverse myelitis, Guillain-Barré syndrome, and chronic inflammatory demyelinating polyneuropathy.

Once nerves have been impaired, regeneration is difficult. This is especially true in humans, versus lab mice, given the long distance between our spinal cords and the extremities where nerve damage so often occurs. To regenerate nerves in our arms and legs, axons have to shoot out from the spinal cord and travel as much as three feet in a human to get to a foot or a toe that no longer moves. While investigating one growth factor, called pleiotrophin, that has been around for a while—though no one has known its exact effect—Hoke uncovered something surprising. Pleiotrophin has a particularly robust ability to increase the growth of motor neurons and appears to aid in regenerating axons over long distances, which then allows damaged muscle to move again. In experiments in lab mice, even very low doses of pleiotrophin, or PTN, significantly enhanced the regeneration of myelinated axons, leading Hoke to hope that PTN may lead to novel treatment options for neurological autoimmune disease.

This is significant because most available therapies for those who have peripheral neuropathy, or damaged nerves in the peripheral limbs of their bodies, are designed to control painful symptoms, not to treat the underlying nerve degeneration. Others are protective therapies—such as Rituxan, which researchers hope will prevent autoimmune-disease relapses—but protective therapies do not help nerves to regenerate. "Pleiotrophin looks to be a unique growth factor that can cover long distances quickly," says Hoke. "Uncovering its potential may lead to the development of growth factor–like drugs that will improve the intrinsic ability of neurons to regenerate and speed the growth of damaged axons in the body—without the side effects that come with drugs that tamp down T-cell and B-cell interactions."

Clearly, making use of prediagnostic biomarker technology to determine who will eventually be struck with an autoimmune disease will only be useful if that technology is not only foolproof, but if we possess fail-safe and side-effect-free interventions to offer to those who are informed by their doctors that they sit at the precarious edge of disease. No one should ever take a relatively healthy patient—such as Anita Louise Smith—and give to her a drug that might cause a fatal complication.

Still, should funding dollars increase for these diseases, helping scientists to achieve treatments that target specific molecular processes precisely and safely, the ability to scourge out disease before it wreaks destruction would allow 23.5 million Americans to live their lives without the devastating lifestyle changes that come with the onset of autoimmunity. Over time, such technology would also eventually mean savings in health-care dollars; no small matter given that autoimmune diseases now represent a yearly health-care burden of more than $120 billion, compared to the yearly health-care burden of $70 billion for direct medical costs for cancer.

THE DIABETES CURE: TURNING OVER PARADIGMS

At Massachusetts General Hospital, Dr. Denise Faustman, associate professor of medicine at Harvard Medical School and director of the Massachusetts General Hospital Immunobiology Laboratory, may well be on the verge of developing just such a cure for type 1 diabetes. Humor has helped Faustman along what has proven to be a rocky road over the past several years as she developed a revolutionary approach to targeting and destroying errant immune cells in laboratory mice.

In 2001 and 2003, Faustman published two highly controversial studies in top journals. One paper in the journal *Science* demonstrated that a forty-day treatment targeted to kill off only the very specific defective cells that cause the autoimmune destruction of healthy beta cells in the pancreas could effectively stop type 1 diabetes in its tracks. In Faustman's experiments, 75 to 85 percent of mice were permanently cured of type 1 diabetes—an unheard-of outcome for any autoimmune disease research of its kind. The finding was remarkable: mice suffering from end-stage type 1 diabetes were not only permanently cured, their pancreases spontaneously regenerated and their blood-sugar levels returned to normal. The research would pit scientist against scientist and cause many researchers to reexamine their long-held assumptions about how autoimmune-disease treatments might be revolutionized in the future.

Faustman first decided to pursue research after years of working as a clinician treating patients with type 1 diabetes. In her seventh year of residency, she realized that she spent most of her time delivering a laundry list of bad news to patients about the progress of their disease: bodily systems that were breaking down, amputations that needed to be performed, and other grim tidings that it was her personal daily duty, as resident, to deliver. She wanted to be able to tell those suffering something good and was disturbed by the uneasy feeling that she wasn't "making a dent" in anyone's disease. By 1987 Faustman had done an abrupt about-face and was heading up a program to try to cure diabetes in lab mice at Harvard Medical School.

Over the next fifteen years, Faustman struggled, with a dedicated crew of eleven PhDs, to identify the exact group of pathological T cells that were misbehaving in type 1 diabetes and destroying islet cells in the pancreas. These errant T cells, she found, produced completely different proteins within their cells than did normal cells. In fact, these rogue T cells ought not to have been circulating in the body in the first place.

Normally, our bone marrow and thymus produce millions of T cells, which are the foot soldiers that work diligently to serve the immune system. All of these T cells have different random receptors on them that are equipped to recognize millions of pathogens that might enter the body—and destroy them. But many T cells are "born" faulty when they are first produced in the bone marrow; they mistakenly react to the body itself, rather than to outside pathogens: they are "autoreactive." In normal circumstances 99 percent or more of these friendly-fire-prone T cells are killed off quite efficiently; the body recognizes them as autoreactive—long before they escape out of the bone marrow—because they have a protein sequence on their surfaces different from the good kind of T cells that help to defend us from invading foes. This faulty protein sequence on errant T cells is a signal to the immune system that these T cells should be destroyed before they have a chance to turn on us.

The specific group of dangerous T cells that Faustman discovered were mistakenly escaping the bone marrow weren't being read as autoreactive when they should have been. Instead, they eluded discovery and snuck into the blood along with other healthy T cells.

The fact that Faustman was able to uncover and identify this specific group of flawed autoreactive T cells escaping out of the bone marrow was hugely promising. She began to wonder: What if she could kill only the misbehaving T cells in the pancreas and in the bone marrow—thus eliminating them from the body—in the same way that antibiotics would kill bacteria? Antibiotics are able to kill off bacteria in the body because the antibiotic interferes with different proteins that are unique to the bacteria, causing them to die—without interfering with any other cells. Faustman was determined to find a way to interfere with only the misguided T cells, singling them out and killing them off by recognizing the protein sequence unique to them and leaving the other T cells intact, creating something akin to an antibiotic for autoimmune disease.

Faustman's approach offered a distinct advantage over much of the current treatment in autoimmunity, which is usually more broadly immunosuppressive—meaning it tinkers with all T cells or all B cells in order to try to keep the autoimmune reaction from occurring. The problem with such broad-spectrum therapies, Faustman knew, is that they suppress the good cells as well as the bad, which often meddles with other important functions of immune cells in the body, causing other diseases.

Faustman wanted to avoid that by being more selective. Luckily, the same defect that allows autoreactive T cells to escape from the bone marrow also results in a flaw on the surface of these T cells that allows them to be singled out and destroyed. Autoreactive T cells are more susceptible to the action of a signaling protein, known as TNF-alpha, which initiates the process of cell death only in defective T cells. Faustman's lab was able to use TNF-alpha to kill off only those cells. This was an entirely novel concept: many drugs on the market used to treat autoimmunity are aimed at inactivating TNF-alpha. But Faustman's data suggested the opposite. Perhaps select forms of autoimmunity, including type 1 diabetes, needed more TNF-alpha to eradicate these erratic T cells.

The thing that astonished Faustman and her team the most, however, was that when you killed off just the incorrectly functioning T cells, it not only stopped the disease, it allowed the body to regenerate the insulin-producing islet cells, reversing the disease entirely.

The very idea that by killing off the fugitive T cells that cause type 1 diabetes damage you could encourage a healthy pancreas to regenerate was considered so far-fetched that Faustman's team was met with scathing skepticism from most of the scientific community. Scientists throughout the world openly questioned her claims. Despite her breakthrough, Faustman could not convince drug companies or major diabetes foundations to offer research funding. In 2003, two fellow colleagues at Joslin Diabetes Center—not on Faustman's research team—sent a letter to the *New York Times,* which had run an article describing Faustman's work, deeming the claim that she was the first scientist to cure diabetes in mice "patently false." The researchers also apologized to patients with diabetes "on behalf of Dr. Faustman" for "having their expectations cruelly raised." Although the *New York Times* did not publish the letter, it was posted on the Joslin Diabetes Center website and distributed by e-mail by the Juvenile Diabetes Research Foundation. Ironically, three competing lab teams from the University of Chicago, Washington University in St. Louis, and Joslin Diabetes Center were provided with Juvenile Diabetes Research Foundation grants to try to duplicate Faustman's data, while Faustman, who had also applied for funding to continue her work, received none. Faustman's research hung on by its fingernails.

In 2004, the three other labs set out to test the validity of Faustman's finding that severely diabetic mice can recover on their own if researchers squelch the immune-system attack that is causing the disease through this very specific destruction of only defective T cells. All three labs followed Dr. Faustman's procedures and, after three years of work, each study came up with similar results to Faustman's: you could cure diabetes in mice using the protocol of killing only the autoimmune-disease-causing T cells in the pancreas. In every experiment a significant proportion—slightly less than half of the mice in these three studies—were cured, suggesting that even severely diabetic mice who have experienced significant damage to the pancreas over time still have the capacity to regenerate new beta cells if the autoreactive T cells can be eliminated.

CAN THE MOUSE CURE BE APPLIED TO HUMANS?

Faustman—like most mavericks who manage to create a new paradigm—has learned to be tough and sanguine in the face of years of scientific opprobrium. She smiles, recounting that when her original 2001 paper was first published, "We were not allowed to use the word 'regenerate' because it was not accepted that regeneration could happen. People thought that you are born with one pancreas and it can't regenerate—therefore we had to be wrong. But in science, if you dig hard enough, you can find something new."

Faustman jokes about having had to develop what she calls "scientific maturity" about the "sibling-like rivalry" scientists display in order to compete for funding. She feels that this adversarial approach to getting research dollars only serves to circumvent progress. "I thought when we developed this breakthrough that people would be excited," she laughs. "But I learned the hard way that if you break open a new avenue in science you won't be invited to every cocktail party. National and international research is not set up for sharing and promoting each other's ideas and helping each other along. It's set up so that researchers fight for limited funding, which does not allow for the kind of collaborative thinking that accelerates the delivery of new ideas to the public. But we in our lab wanted to share our work with every lab that was interested in doing follow-up studies to ours, to help them along in duplicating our protocol—with the hope that we might go further faster in curing this disease."

Indeed, there is now considerable evidence that the same T-cell defect found in diabetic mice is physiologically identical to that found in diabetic humans. Moreover, worldwide research has found evidence of similar cell errors in a number of human autoimmune diseases similar to those seen in type 1 diabetes—meaning this target-the-fugitive-T-cell approach has the potential to impact the treatment of other autoimmune diseases, including multiple sclerosis, Crohn's disease, scleroderma, Hashimoto's, Sjögren's syndrome, and lupus.

Faustman, along with Harvard colleague David Nathan, will soon launch a clinical trial in humans, funded by a private $11.5 million grant—provided by Lee Iacocca's Iacocca Foundation. Iacocca, Faustman says—with words bathed in the kind of laughter that comes only on the heels of hard knocks—"likens this to what happened in the transportation industry when the car threatened to replace the horse and buggy. When the paradigm is changed in a way that affects others in the field negatively, it upsets a lot of people. Industry calls it 'disruptive technology.'" She laughs more deeply. "Our work in diabetes has turned out to be disruptive technology."

Faustman and Nathan's clinical trial will involve three components. First, they are working to develop a laboratory test that will allow them to determine the level of defective cells in a patient's blood rapidly and accurately. This test will enable physicians to identify patients who are most likely to benefit from treatment and can also be used to provide evidence of the success of the treatment. If the number of defective cells is lower after treatment, then researchers will know that they are succeeding in eradicating defective cells from the pancreas. In a second phase of the study, researchers will inject diabetic volunteers with a compound called BCG, which, like the compound given to mice to kill off errant T cells, stimulates the human immune system in a way that eliminates only the faulty T cells that attack beta cells. The study, which will include forty patient volunteers, will be double-blind—patients will either receive a placebo (no drug) or BCG. The researchers will evaluate whether BCG reduces the number of defective cells that attack and kill the insulin-producing cells in type 1 diabetics. Using blood tests to determine how many defective cells are still active, Faustman and Nathan will be able to see whether the mouse cure is working in humans. The clinical trial is already approved by the FDA. Faustman hopes that by 2012 her lab will have enough data to enable them to launch multicenter clinical trials around the country. Her goal in such a wide-scale clinical trial will be to find the exact dosing that can best kill off the renegade T cells that cause type 1 diabetes in the average patient. By 2017, she says, she hopes to have a "good therapeutic window" on what would be a standard dose to cure type 1 diabetes in your local doctor's office. She smiles. "Better yet, by then I will hopefully have come up with even better ideas."

CHAPTER SIX

SHIELDING YOUR IMMUNE SYSTEM: RETHINKING FOOD, STRESS, AND EVERYDAY CHEMICALS

When Gerard Mullin was forty-three years old, he was already a who's who in medicine. He was head of the Gastroenterology and Hepatology Division at North Shore University Hospital in Manhasset, New York, and had contributed scores of papers to top medical journals on two particularly difficult-to-treat autoimmune diseases of the digestive tract, Crohn's disease and ulcerative colitis. Mullin was an expert on both of these inflammatory bowel diseases—which afflict 1 million Americans, one hundred thousand of whom are children—and patients lined up to see him for the kid-glove care he gave to their cases. The obligatory ten minutes most physicians spend per patient often became an hour of discussing drug strategies and counseling patients on how to manage life-derailing symptoms, including abdominal pain from severe inflammation of the digestive tract, diarrhea, and rectal bleeding. It was nothing for Mullin to call a patient over the weekend to see how he or she might be faring on a new medication.

Then, in September 2003, without warning, the unexpected

happened: Mullin went from being an autoimmune-disease specialist to being a forty-three-year-old patient with a roaring autoimmune disease of his own almost overnight.

During the summer leading up to that September, Mullin had
been unusually stressed out. In addition to working grueling hours
because of hospital staffing shortages, he was caring for two dying
parents. He began to experience minuscule muscle twitches in his
arms and legs. A colleague suggested that Mullin have a spinal tap
to rule out multiple sclerosis—although the likelihood of MS, given
his atypical symptoms, was remote. Still, hospital doctors often
over-test colleagues; it is not unusual for one doctor to send another for a wide battery of potentially unnecessary hospital tests
"just to rule everything out."

During the spinal tap, or lumbar puncture, a terrible medical
mishap occurred: the lumbar puncture was made into what physicians refer to as the danger zone—the cauda equina—a group of
nerve roots that send and receive messages to and from the lower
abdominal organs and down into the legs. When these nerves are
damaged, sensation to the legs can be seriously impaired. Not yet
aware of what had happened, Mullin left the procedure experiencing excruciating pain. The puncture into his spine began bleeding.
Something was terribly wrong. His brother drove him to the emergency room at New York Presbyterian Hospital/Weill Cornell
Medical Center where he was hospitalized until the bleeding
stopped. Physicians treating him told him that they could only hope
that the pain would lessen with time as the area began to heal.
There was nothing more they could do.

But a new problem developed while he was in the hospital.
The puncture began seeping spinal fluid, and Mullin developed debilitating headaches. In October 2003 he underwent a procedure to
have the leak patched. But in a second corrective procedure in February 2004, blood was mistakenly injected back into the spinal
fluid while he was being treated under local anesthesia, sparking a
rapid autoimmune reaction that would nearly cost Mullin his life.
Since blood does not normally enter the cerebrospinal fluid, the
body viewed these new, circulating blood proteins as potentially

dangerous invaders that they needed to destroy. Mullin's immune system sent out autoantibodies to wipe out these blood proteins—but in the process these same autoantibodies also targeted the innermost layers of the sac that surrounded Mullin's spinal cord and the already inflamed nerve root of the cauda equina. Known as arachnoiditis, this devastating autoimmune disorder can lead to paralysis in the legs and turn life threatening as it attacks nerves throughout the lower organs of the body, even shutting down the bladder and bowels. (If the name arachnoiditis makes you imagine "land of the spiders," that's no coincidence: the nerve network that the immune system begins to demyelinate looks something like a spider web's intricate fibers spanning out from the lower spinal cord.)

Mullin's case was no exception. The burning pain down the back of both legs was constant. He was too dizzy to stand. He had poor control over his bladder and bowels. On April 18, 2004, two months after having had the leak patched, his heart began to beat irregularly and he began to bleed heavily through his gastrointestinal tract. Doctors started him on a third course of extremely high-dose steroids in hopes that it would help to stop the bleeding and the damage to his nerves. But he continued to worsen. He was put on a ventilator in intensive care. Mullin's blood pressure fell so low the hospital staff couldn't get a reading. Doctors managed to resuscitate Mullin with injections of cardiac medications and massive plasma and blood infusions. That evening he was told that his heart was so weak he might not live through the night.

But he did. The following day, doctors were finally able to stop the gastrointestinal bleeding and regulate Mullin's heartbeat and blood pressure. He was released one week later on heavy doses of oral steroids. The pain remained untenable. His arachnoiditis—which keeps most sufferers in a wheelchair—was so severe he couldn't walk across a room without feeling as if his back and legs were aflame, yet there was nothing more that modern medicine could do for Gerry Mullin. He was bedridden, on full disability, and the future was bleak. "I had become just another hard-to-treat patient that doctors didn't know what to do with," he says, looking back. "They'd run out of answers. I was unmarried, disabled, living alone, unemployed, and for the first time staring at the colder, uncaring side of modern medicine that patients so often complain about."

Those seven months of hell taught Gerry Mullin a lot. Like many physicians who find out in an all-too-chilling manner what it's like to be lying helpless in a hospital bed rather than standing in a white coat over bedridden patients, Mullin became a changed man. There had to be something more—beyond conventional medical approaches and drugs—that he could do to help himself. Meanwhile, his father had passed away, and his mother, who lived an hour and a half away, was very near to dying. Mullin was unable to get to her bedside, but he talked to his mother often. Growing up, she had owned a health-food store in the small town of Pompton Lakes, New Jersey, which had offered an array of health foods and supplements decades before health-food stores became part of mainstream America. She had been well known in their community for her vast knowledge about how a healthy diet and dietary supplements can affect overall wellness. Over the years she had often chastised her son for focusing only on pharmaceutical drugs when treating patients. "You're going too medical on me, Gerry," she would warn him, encouraging him to offer patients more holistic treatment options. She believed in the wisdom of Sir William Osler, the Canadian physician revered as the father of modern medicine, who said that "the good physician treats the disease: the great physician treats the patient who has the disease." Diet and nutrition were, she felt, essential.

DISCOVERING THAT FOOD IS MEDICINE

Over the next several months—his laptop perched on his bed—Mullin prodigiously researched how a carefully manipulated diet along with dietary supplements has been shown in some studies to lessen the autoimmune reaction by helping to dampen down the production of cytokines—the signaling molecules that tell the immune system to react to an invader and that, if they become uncontrolled, can prompt the production of autoantibodies which attack in a friendly-fire assault, resulting in autoimmune disease. As a physician, Mullin was able to sign up for online conferences and courses in an emerging field of research being called "integrative medicine." He became, he says, "very educated" on what a food-as-medicine approach can do to affect autoimmune activity in the body. He consulted several other like-minded physicians who specialized in alternative and complementary care. Together, the medical experts devised a carefully thought out dietary and supplementation plan to augment the conventional therapy with steroids that Mullin was using. Mullin began to consume a completely whole-foods diet coupled with nutritional supplements, with the hope that it would help to temper the autoimmune response that was raging through the nerves in the lower half of his body.

Over the next eight months Mullin's constant pain and weakness began to ebb. His near-constant dizziness and heart-rate swings diminished. By December 2004, Mullin was able to get into a car and drive for the first time in fifteen months. His first priority was to see his mother, who had been hospitalized. He shared with her his belief that a holistic approach to his illness had allowed him to take back his life. He had decided, he told his mom, to pursue a PhD in nutrition to augment his medical degree. "She never said, 'I told you so,'" Mullin recalls. "She just said she thought it was about time." A few weeks later, she died.

Today, Mullin appears to be the portrait of health. It is hard to believe, watching him make in-patient rounds at Johns Hopkins Hospital, where he serves as director of Integrative GI Nutrition Services, that he spent more than a year disabled from a neurological autoimmune disease. He now regularly employs a holistic method to help keep his own autoimmune disease in check and feels it's critical to offer the autoimmune-disease patients he sees each week complementary approaches to treatment in addition to traditional drug therapies. His papers on how vitamin D helps to prevent autoimmune disease are as likely to appear in *Nutrition in*

Clinical Practice as his papers on T-cell activity in Crohn's disease have been in *Inflammatory Bowel Diseases*. He now serves as a fellow at Dr. Andrew Weil's program in integrative medicine at the University of Arizona.

"The idea that we should rely solely on drug therapies to help autoimmune-disease patients is antiquated," Mullin posits as we enter his Hopkins office, where photos of his nieces and nephews sit on the windowsill and complementary health tomes line bookshelves. He sits down at his desk, his large hands clicking on the keyboard and moving the computer mouse with lightning speed, taking me on a virtual tour of research papers linking special diets and supplements to better outcomes for autoimmune-disease patients. "Drugs alone should no longer suffice as quality care," he sighs, rubbing his hand over his three-day stubble of beard. "We know so much about the potential for special diets and supplementation to help modulate autoimmune disease and we have to help patients reap those benefits." Still, the majority of doctors do not understand the role that diet plays in helping to ameliorate autoimmune disease. "Even in the field of inflammatory bowel disease the firm belief is that diet plays no role," Mullin says, his fingers steepled in front of his face in a gesture that belies his frustration. "Yet we have clear data showing that changing an autoimmune-disease patient's diet and adding in simple supplements can dramatically change the course of his or her illness."

Not surprisingly, in the medical world, Mullin is still something of a lone ranger—though the landscape of traditional American medicine is slowly changing. Today, complementary and alternative medical centers are being developed at several top medical institutes—Hopkins, Harvard, Duke, Yale, and Stanford among them—largely driven by consumer demand. Many patients who suffer from autoimmunity are already trying dietary, supplement, and herbal approaches. Today, 21 percent of patients with autoimmune inflammatory bowel disease use complementary and alternative approaches to treat their disease. Consumers in general in the United

States spend nearly $21 billion annually on nutritional supplements alone—$4 billion more than what they spend each year on going to the movies and video rentals combined.

Even so, the vast majority—61 percent—of American patients don't feel comfortable discussing the alternative therapies they use with their physicians. Nor does the typical physician probe about diet or supplements when seeing a patient during a routine visit. Few physicians are well versed in cutting-edge nutritional research or are comfortable stepping outside of the traditional drug-the-disease box of treating patients. In what is known as allopathic medicine, physicians are trained to seek out "the differential diagnosis"—a disease name that alerts the doctor to what disease the patient has from a larger group of disorders with similar symptoms. Often, the doctor doing the diagnosing is a specialist—trained to look specifically at the neurological, gastrointestinal, or rheumatological aspects of disease—but certainly not all bodily systems together. Once the disease has a label, specific disorders and overt symptoms can be treated with pharmaceuticals that may or may not have their own symptom-producing side effects. The goal is to match symptoms to a specific disease and then prescribe the most appropriate drug.

Having a specialist is a good thing—it's usually an experienced specialist who can diagnose more quickly and accurately and ensure a patient has the best that modern conventional medicine has to offer. But on the downside, specialists are less likely to think of the body as an interconnected, holistic system. Physicians who focus solely on a drug-the-disease approach often miss the interrelationships of the patients' genetic background and predispositions, their history of infection, the burden of environmental chemicals and heavy metals that they may carry within, and their eating habits. In fact, a 2007 study of fifty-six second-year gastrointestinal fellows from top academic institutions in the United States bears this out all too well: 70 percent of the fellows reported having had no rotation in inpatient nutrition at all, and 87 percent had never been assessed for competency in nutrition. And yet these were subspecialty doctors in training from the nation's top hospitals who would be specifically treating those with diseases of the gut. Counseling autoimmune patients about helping to quiet the inflammatory response through nutrition, in addition to drug therapies, necessitates a paradigm shift in medicine—toward seeing a patient's complex biology as a dynamic, fluid, interlocking system where small and seemingly insignificant changes to the system, including shifts in diet, can dramatically influence the well-being of the whole patient.

What exactly does a special diet that can help to subdue the autoimmune response look like? As anyone who likes to browse in bookstores knows, consuming a healthy diet is a topic that fills whole bookshop aisles and magazine stands. But oddly enough—despite the fact that nearly 24 million Americans suffer from autoimmune diseases and that number is steadily on the rise—there is not yet a recognized diet focused on combating autoimmunity through nutrition.

Before discussing what an anti-autoimmune diet should consist of, it might be helpful to consider why our current diet is so harmful to our immune system in the first place.

THE RISE IN FACTORY-MADE FOODS

One of the most significant ways that foreign antigens, which may trigger the immune system to overreact, can enter the body is through what we eat. In the past hundred years we've completely changed what we digest as food. We've gone from a whole-foods diet—one in which we digested whole grains, fruits, vegetables, poultry, and livestock produced locally or on our own land—to a processed-food diet. This processed-food diet often consists of highly preserved bread products, doughnuts, prepackaged coffee cakes, and cereals laden with sugar for breakfast. (Think of it: one bowl of Cocoa Puffs has the same amount of sugar as a 50-gram bag of Hershey's Kisses, and a bowl of Corn Pops is the sugar equivalent of eating a Kit Kat bar.) Chips, multi-dye-colored cheese Goldfish, and pretzels in foil-lined bags, along with processed meats, fill the typical lunch box. Dinner often comes from a box or prepackaged bag from the freezer, and snacks and sodas—of which there are a plethora to choose from in our snack culture—serve as pick-me-ups in between.

What fresh foods we do consume—unless organic—are sprayed liberally with pesticides and fungicides. Nonorganic poultry and meats are packed with hormones and antibiotics, not to mention often full of PCBs, mercury, and other chemicals that accumulate up the food chain in the cows, pigs, lambs, and chickens we consume. Processed meats are preserved with nitrates. Patient studies show that higher intake of nitrates and nitrites is associated with a higher risk of developing type 1 diabetes. Grocery-store chicken comes to us having been raised on feed laced not only with hormones and antibiotics but chemical dyes to give the meat a more attractive hue. Indeed, today farmers can select from fifteen different shades of yellow dyes, in a range from light yellow to bright orange, to add to chicken feed in order to make egg yolks the perfect color. Known as tartrazine, or FD&C yellow no. 5, yellow dye is present in thousands of other foods and drugs and has been linked in research studies to higher rates of asthma and allergic reactions. There is also evidence it may trigger lupus symptoms in some patients.

Today, only 10 percent of all American adults consume enough healthy foods for their diet to qualify as "good," according to researchers at the USDA Center for Nutrition Policy and Promotion. When you look at recent studies on what Americans do get in their diet, it is pretty grim: U.S. soft drink consumption has grown 135 percent since 1977; 75 percent of preschoolers in America are not getting the daily recommended amount of fiber in their diet; fewer than 11 percent of Americans consume the USDA recommended five servings of fruits and vegetables a day; junk foods such as chips, snacks, desserts, and soft drinks now constitute 30 percent of the American daily food intake. Fruits and vegetables no longer pack the nutritional wallop they once did; their nutrient value has declined as much as 38 percent since 1950. One reason is that farmers tend to select produce breeds that are faster growing, bigger, and more pest resistant—meaning crops have inadequate time to make or absorb nutrients during their shortened growing season. Likewise, the soil in which crops are grown is contaminated with far more mercury, PCBs, and other noxious industrial fallout than it was half a century ago. Acid rain has taken its toll as well: American soil has lost as much as 75 percent of its calcium during the past century, which also compromises a crop's nutrient intake and growth.

Processed foods are just as troubling. When we hear phrases such as "food manufacturing" or "food processing," few of us have a visual picture of what that really means or how many chemicals, preservatives, and additives work their way into the foods we eat as they're processed and packaged on manufacturing assembly lines. "Processed food" basically means any food that you can buy in a can, jar, packet, or bottle that has been produced in some kind of factory as part of a bulk manufacturing process. Most processed foods would quickly spoil if kept on a shelf for very long. In order to make sure that won't happen, raw food ingredients are processed at very high heats. This causes grains, fruits, and vegetables to lose most of their vitamins, minerals, and fiber, as well as other nutrients. Preservatives are then added in order to prevent germs from proliferating in the food while it sits in the jar or package on the supermarket shelf. That way, your food won't spoil or be covered with mold when you tear open the plastic packaging a week or a month or even a year down the road. Preservatives make sure that insects and germs find the food too toxic for them, so bacteria won't grow on the marshmallows in your kids' Lucky Charms and ants won't find that package of chocolate cupcakes in your cupboard the least bit attractive.

Centuries ago, salt, sugar, and vinegar were among the first food preservatives. Today, industrial food manufacturers have at their disposal an endless variety of chemical ways to preserve food, including benzoates, BHA, BHT, FD&C dyes, MSG, nitrates, nitrites, parabens, and sulfites. The final step in food processing is the addition of vitamins and minerals, to make up for what was lost during the initial heat-stripping phase. In an ironic sense, food processing might be defined thus: taking a food from nature, removing everything natural from it, then adding preservatives, dyes, bleaches, flavors, emulsifiers, and stabilizers to make it taste, look, feel, and smell like what it was originally supposed to be, but no longer is. The resemblance is there, but little else remains.

Those of us who grew up in the wake of the 1950s food-processing revolution probably know exactly what a non-whole-food diet is like. My own mother, mom of four, was, like most fashionable housewives of the 1960s and 1970s swept up in the great processed-food sensation that swept the nation, offering housewives every conceivable convenience food from Tasty Baking Company's Tastykakes to Oscar Meyer wieners. And who can forget "Cold or hot, Spam hits the spot!" It was the age of Cap'n Crunch for breakfast, bologna and Velveeta on Wonder Bread with barbecue chips and Twinkies for lunch, and Hamburger Helper for dinner. (As kids, we once found a half-eaten Twinkie under one of my brother's beds that had been there for nearly a year, and it still looked exactly as it had the day he opened the package, with the outline of his bite mark still perfectly intact. It was so full of preservatives even the ants that feasted on nearby forgotten banana peels wouldn't touch it.) During our childhood, if it didn't come in a package, it wasn't newfangled, it didn't have that zing of being remarkably, modernly American.

Immigrants to America also fall under the spell of our processed foods. Studies show that almost 40 percent of newly arrived immigrants quickly change their diet to add in more prepackaged highly processed foods and snacks, eating fewer vegetables and fruit and less fish, rice, and beans. Not surprisingly, autoimmune inflammatory bowel diseases are more common in Western countries such as the United States, the United Kingdom, and Scandinavia—where rates of Crohn's disease have been rising—and less common in southern Europe, Asia, and Africa. But what is especially striking is that South Asian immigrants who move to Western countries soon show an increased incidence of autoimmune inflammatory bowel diseases like Crohn's disease and ulcerative colitis.

Clearly, the diet most Americans favor is a far cry from the whole-foods diet that Gerry Mullin and other complementary and alternative-minded physicians believe might help to rebalance an overreactive immune system. Indeed, for individuals who are genetically susceptible to autoimmunity, eating a diet full of chemicals, dyes, pesticides, and the like may be tantamount to swallowing tiny doses of antigens that the body does not recognize as safe and may, over time, help nudge the immune system toward an autoimmune response. This shift from a whole-foods diet to a processed-food diet over the past sixty years is a critical factor in pushing autoimmune disease rates ever upward.

THE AUTOIMMUNE DIET

As more studies are published on how specific foods and supplements can modulate the autoimmune response, a comprehensive anti-autoimmune-disease diet plan is slowly emerging. Increasingly, top specialists are suggesting whole-food diet guidelines to their patients. No single recommendation fits all patients, and none of the following should be construed as medical advice. Every single dietary step should be checked with one's personal physician, and anyone considering following a special diet and/or taking supplements should first share the plan with his or her health-care provider. Another caveat: not all supplement manufacturers are the same, and some supplements manufactured both in the United States and abroad have been found to contain traces of heavy metals and other harmful ingredients.

An essential first step for anyone suffering from autoimmune disease is to ensure that his or her gastrointestinal tract is thriving. Although the disease one might be suffering from might affect a completely different system of the body—and it might seem absurd to consider worrying about what's going into one's stomach when one can't walk without a cane due to multiple sclerosis—the health of the GI tract is inextricably linked to what's transpiring elsewhere in the body.

A healthy intestine allows only digested nutrients to pass into the bloodstream. In patients with immune and inflammatory-based illnesses, the body's intestinal lining often becomes impaired, thus permitting larger molecules, such as bacteria and undigested foods, to slip through. In the bloodstream, these foreign items can trigger an immune reaction, making the body think that it's under attack and prompting the body's immune system to lash out to battle those foreign pathogens.

Even for people who are not ill, eating a Western diet high in carbohydrates, fats, and sugary foods causes the balance of microflora in the gut to change dramatically, creating an overgrowth of bad bacteria and yeast, says Mullin. This directly damages the intestinal wall. To understand how this happens, consider the carefully interconnected parts of the intestine. The human bowel is lined with millions of projections called villi that facilitate the efficient absorption of nutrients. These villi are covered in cells that are constantly being shed and renewed—around a thousand billion cells are shed from them every day. Our intestines also have tiny gaps in the lining. In healthy individuals, as the villi are renewed, the body secretes a substance to plug the gaps, thus sealing the gut and preventing antigens from leaking into the bloodstream. These sealed gaps serve the critical purpose of keeping foreign antigens from being able to escape. But when the intestinal flora lacks sufficient good bacteria from a healthy whole-foods diet, or when we consume foods that can produce an allergic sensitivity in some people—as do many chemicals, artificial preservatives, and dyes—inflammation develops in the lining of the intestine. That inflammation breaks these seals, the gaps widen, and antigens leak out. Those antigens can rev up the immune system. Believing itself to be under attack, the immune system releases cytokines, which rally the production of antibodies that go after those added antigens circulating through the body. If food components or bacteria that escape through that intestinal barrier share a similar protein sequence to a virus or other patho-

genic microorganism that the immune system de
can generate an immune response, leading to a
action.

"Untreated gut permeability can perpetuate the a
reaction," says Mullin. "One of the most important things
autoimmune patients can do is to cleanse the GI tract through diet
to make sure that they're not letting antigens into their body
through the gut and worsening their immune-driven disease." The
first step is to work with your physician to test for pathogens in the
gut—bacteria, yeast, and parasites—all of which can be tested for
through high-quality stool tests, coupled with a lactulose breath
test for bacterial overgrowth. (One word here on parasites: Although some recent studies show that having a certain type of par-
asite may actually keep the immune system busy and help to keep
people from getting sick with autoimmune disease, this is only true
in the case of certain harmless parasites, such as pig whipworms,
which do not harm people. Most common parasitic infections
found in Americans such as giardia and *Entamoeba histolytica* and
Blastocystis hominis infection can and do cause severe health problems.) Interestingly, laboratory studies show that when rats with a
predisposition to Crohn's disease have their GI tracts sterilized, so
that they have no gut permeability and no bad bacteria or parasites, they are no longer susceptible to Crohn's and they do not
develop the disease.

The second step is to make sure that you are not consuming
any potential allergens or foods to which you may be sensitive. For
those who are facing severe autoimmune disease, this is best done
by going on a complete elimination diet, with the help of your physician. Mullin recommends beginning such an elimination diet by
consuming only hypoallergenic protein powders such as whey protein or rice protein—which will give you all of the essential nutrients—for a period of three days and then slowly adding in limited
foods such as rice, chicken, turkey, and vegetables (see below) for a
period of up to eight weeks. Patients keep a journal and take note
of any type of reaction (bloating, abdominal discomfort, rashes,
headaches, and any worsening of their autoimmune-disease symp-

ͻms). Gradually, with continued careful monitoring, a wider variety of foods can be added to the diet as well.

In research on those with Crohn's disease, elimination diets helped symptoms to abate in a third of patients who tried them. Irritable bowel syndrome, or IBS—a gastrointestinal syndrome characterized by abdominal pain and cycles of intense diarrhea and constipation—has been found to be inflammatory in nature, says Mullin. In a recent scientific paradigm shift, IBS is now becoming classified as an inflammatory bowel disorder—though whether it is autoimmune in nature and there are autoantibodies involved that attack the body tissue itself has not yet been fully investigated or answered. It is, however, says Mullin, a very good question to ask. Could it be that an overgrowth of bacteria in the small intestine— which is often found to be an issue in patients with irritable bowel syndrome—triggers the inflammatory response in the same way that bacteria triggers the autoimmune response in Crohn's disease and ulcerative colitis? We may yet find, posits Mullin, that in irritable bowel syndrome, the body sees the bacterial overgrowth occuring in the small intestines as foreign, and as the immune system strikes out against that infection, the immune system generates not just inflammation but sets off an autoimmune response against the gut.

Meanwhile, patients with irritable bowel syndrome—which affects one in five women in America—respond profoundly to changes in their day-to-day diet. In one study, 75 percent of patients with irritable bowel syndrome found that their symptoms improved with dietary changes alone. Clearly, for someone suffering from an inflammatory bowel disorder, shifting toward a diet that eliminates foods that increase inflammation can help to repair the gut and reestablish the balance of healthy intestinal microflora. Individuals who want more information about elimination diets should have no difficulty finding it. Literally scores of books have been written on elimination diets, and many are available on the Internet. But be sure to discuss any such plan with your doctor.

It may also prove helpful to undergo testing for food allergies and food sensitivities. Food allergies (versus sensitivities or intolerances) are divided into two major categories: IgE mediated and T-cell mediated allergies. IgE allergic reactions are immediate; after being exposed to the food, your body quickly overproduces what is called immunoglobulin E antibodies, or IgE. You begin to experience fairly immediate symptoms—tingling of the extremities, wheezing, coughing, tightening of the throat, nausea, abdominal cramps, and diarrhea—within hours of having ingested the food. More severe anaphylaxis (a sudden, severe, potentially fatal systemic allergic reaction that can involve the skin, respiratory tract, gastrointestinal tract, and cardiovascular system) can occur after eating nuts, shellfish, fish, peanuts, and tree nuts. A second type of food allergy—known as a T-cell mediated allergy—occurs when T cells within the intestinal mucosa see a food as foreign and the immune system reacts to the presence of that food. T-cell mediated food allergies—which are more common in children—usually occur four to twenty-eight hours after ingestion of a food.

As if all this weren't complex enough, allergists are now examining the possibility of a third type of hyperreactive response to food, referred to as an IgG food sensitivity. With IgG food sensitivities, the body slowly begins to produce immunoglobulin G antibodies, and the resulting symptoms—which can take up to three days to appear—can be more subtle and more difficult to detect than an IgE reaction. Many patients remain unaware of their food sensitivities—after all, if you are frequently consuming a food you're having a delayed sensitivity to, then you'll never notice a direct correlation. Although the concept of IgG food sensitivities is still controversial, many doctors believe that IgG mediated food reactions increase inflammation in the body and can worsen disease symptoms. Many autoimmune experts believe food sensitivities may be even more prevalent in autoimmune-disease patients, who tend to have higher rates of allergies in general. In fact, in one new study at Children's Hospital and Regional Medical Center and the University of Washington, researchers found that allergic reactions may contribute to the triggering of autoimmune diseases, though they are not yet sure of the mechanism by which this occurs. Studies confirm that for some patients with rheumatoid arthritis, food sensitivities worsen their symptoms, and avoidance of these foods helps their symptoms to abate. For this reason, Mullin recommends asking your doctor to run blood tests that will help to pick up not only foods to which you have an allergic reaction, but also foods to which you might be sensitive or intolerant.

What follows is a short list of foods that Mullin and many nutritionists believe may help to quiet down autoimmune activity. In terms of a general diet, consider eating a low-inflammatory diet of range-fed beef, lamb, chicken, and turkey; fish with a low mercury content (wild salmon, mackerel, sardines, flounder, red snapper, and tilapia); hormone-free eggs; all vegetables (avoiding eggplant and tomatoes); avocados; all fresh fruits; unsweetened yogurt (if you are not dairy allergic or sensitive); freshly made whole-grain breads from alternative nongluten grains; brown rice; beans; nuts, seeds, and sprouts; and raw honey or stevia (in moderation); organic butter; olive, flaxseed, cod liver, and sesame oils; and seasonings such as rosemary, thyme, and oregano.

Conversely, avoid wheat, rye, and barley (these contain gluten, which can be a common source of food sensitivities and cause severe reactions in those with the autoimmune disorder, celiac disease), refined carbohydrates, including potato chips, donuts, pastries, commercial cereals, and commercial breads (especially white breads); potatoes and eggplant (which have inflammatory properties); fast food, hydrogenated oils; safflower, sunflower, cottonseed, and corn oils; instant foods; microwaved foods (heating food in the microwave can deplete it of essential nutrients); canned fruit; lunch meats with nitrates; commercial salad dressings; artificial flavors, colorings, and MSG; aspartame, high-fructose corn syrup, and sucralose; yeast; genetically modified grains; and commercially fried foods.

In one recent study of seven hundred children between the ages of seven and eighteen living on the island of Crete, those who consumed a diet rich in fish; fruits such as red grapes, oranges, and apples; fresh vegetables twice a day; olive oil; and nuts three times a week were significantly less likely to suffer from allergic responses, including allergic asthma, allergic rhinitis, and skin allergies.

CHOOSING ORGANIC FOODS

As you shop for healthy foods, buy organic. One recent study brings home how genetically vulnerable some of us may be to the damaging effects of exposure to pesticides. Investigators recently looked at 130 Latinas and their newborns living in California's Salinas Valley, an agricultural community where organophosphate pesticides are widely used. Overall, 82 percent of the women had had some exposure to pesticides while they were pregnant—mostly because they were living with agricultural workers.

Researchers looked at blood samples taken from these women and measured them for levels of an enzyme known as paraoxonase 1, or PON1, which is able to break down the toxic metabolites of organophosphate pesticides. That's an important function for your body to have: those who have a certain type of the PON1 enzyme are much more protected against the damaging health effects of pesticides. Having this protective feature of the PON1 enzyme depends on whether you have the Q or R form of the PON1 gene. People with what is known as the QQ genotype have two copies of the Q variant of the PON1 enzyme (one from each parent), which is significantly less efficient at helping the body to detoxify following exposure to organophosphate pesticides. People with the RR genotype have two copies of the R variant of the PON1 gene, producing a PON1 enzyme that is more resistant to pesticide exposure because the enzyme helps to break down and eliminate pesticides from the body.

The PON1 enzyme also varies by ethnicity. Approximately 50 percent of whites have the QQ genotype, compared with 25 to 35 percent of the Latino population and 10 to 20 percent of African Americans—making Caucasians most susceptible to the ill effects of pesticides.

In studies of mice, those that lacked the PON1 enzyme died

after being exposed to low levels of organophosphate pesticides, while the same low dose of pesticides elicited no symptoms in mice that possessed normal levels of the enzyme. That's how important an enzyme it is—and whether or not you have it in healthy abundance matters a lot in how exposure to pesticides will affect you.

Infants are at particular risk of not being able to break down pesticides, since the level of PON1 enzyme in newborns is one-third of what it is in adults, and it takes six months to two years for a baby to develop mature levels of PON1. In looking at infants born to Latinas who were exposed to these pesticides, researchers found that infants who inherited the QQ genotype were 50 times more susceptible to pesticide exposure than newborns with the RR genotype, because babies with the QQ genotype do not possess the ability to break down the toxic metabolites. This is particularly frightening given that animal studies show that exposure to organophosphates tampers heavily with normal neurodevelopment, and studies in infants show that pesticide exposure is related to abnormal reflexes as early as in the first few days of life. Combined exposure to mixtures of pesticides is also related to significantly higher rates of asthma in children under the age of two. Most to the point, as we have seen in earlier chapters, organophosphate pesticides—which are also endocrine disruptors—are linked in animal studies to risks of developing the autoimmune disease lupus, and farmers who mix their own pesticides stand a greater likelihood of developing lupus. Although researchers are only now beginning to look at how such genetic differences to susceptibility to pesticides lead to the development of autoimmunity in humans, the glimmers of knowledge we already have are very sobering indeed: some infants do not possess the genetic ability to break down and detoxify their bodies after exposure to pesticides; infants have lower levels of these enzymes in general; pesticides are implicated in the development of neurological disorders and autoimmune disease; and autoimmune-disease rates, as well as other immune-mediated disorders such as asthma and allergies, are rising rapidly among children. The idea that some individuals might be more immune to the effects of environmental contaminants—while others, given their genetic codes, are the proverbial canaries in the mine—is rarely taken into account when government agencies examine environmental exposures to chemical agents and establish safety rules about their use. Until we see change in this arena, buy pesticide-free fruits and vegetables for yourself and for your children.

Indeed, one recent study funded in part by the Centers for Disease Control and Prevention found that eating organic foods substantially lowers children's dietary exposure to organophosphate pesticides. Investigators measured the exposure to several organophosphate pesticides in twenty-three children between the ages of three and eleven over a fifteen-day period. They had children eat a conventional, nonorganic diet for three days, followed by a five-day diet of all organic foods, and then a seven-day diet of conventional nonorganic foods. During the five days in which children ate an organic diet there was a "dramatic and immediate" drop in their levels of pesticides, going as low as zero during the organic food phase. Pesticide levels increased five- or sixfold—and in some cases substantially more—when children began to eat a nonorganic diet again.

Remember to also wash all fruits and vegetables well—even organic ones—before you eat them. According to new data from the Centers for Disease Control and Prevention, produce accounts for 12 percent of all food-borne illnesses—a number that has been on the rise of late. Illnesses from leafy greens such as spinach and lettuce have been particularly worrisome: between 1996 and 2006, there were twenty-four such outbreaks, according to FDA records. Unlike the meat, egg, milk, and processed-food industries, the fresh produce industry is not regulated or monitored for safety by government agencies.

Food-borne illnesses have been linked to developing Guillain-Barré syndrome, the worsening of Crohn's disease, and sparking autoimmune disease flares. To avoid food contamination, use common sense: wash produce including leafy greens well (one autoimmune disease specialist suggests washing all leafy greens three times); be sure to refrigerate all cut, peeled, or cooked fresh fruits and vegetables within two hours; wash cutting boards and peelers well; use separate cutting boards for produce versus meats; throw away fruits or vegetables that have touched raw meat, poultry, seafood, or their juices; and cut away bruised or damaged portions of fruits and vegetables before eating them.

THE QUEST FOR SAFE FOODS AND SUPPLEMENTS

It's important to read labels and carefully choose foods that are chemical and additive free, and if you choose to use dietary supplements, ask your doctor to corroborate that they are from a reputable source. Several past cluster outbreaks of autoimmune disease still haunt scientists because of the rapid and insidious way in which thousands of individuals were struck ill with autoimmune reactions seemingly overnight, not from contact with unseen chemicals but from impurities in the processed food products, drugs, and supplements they consumed.

In May 1981, for instance, food product salesmen in Spain sold a rapeseed oil to stores that, unbeknownst to them, contained trace ingredients derived from an oil diverted from industrial use. The oil derivatives were erroneously used while the oil was being refined into a consumer product. This rapeseed oil made it to the tables of tens of thousands of consumers, and "toxic oil syndrome" burst onto the scene. Twenty thousand individuals fell ill with a lupuslike autoimmune disease, and 1,200 people died.

Keeping track of the vast array of food additives in use by the food manufacturing industry today and making sure that they don't contain traces of harmful chemicals is a heady job. Food processing (for foods other than meat, poultry, and egg products) is regulated by the Food and Drug Administration, or FDA. FDA inspectors are responsible for visiting between sixty and eighty thousand facilities in any given year. The FDA devotes several hundred inspectors and laboratory personnel to this activity nationwide, and state and local governments also inspect food processing plants with varying frequencies and under varying standards, attempting to ensure that product ingredients are safe and free of chemical impurities.

But inspectors can't be everywhere all the time. Food, drug, and supplement manufacturers sometimes make seemingly minute changes in the use or combination of chemicals that can result in dire consequences for consumers—some of which, in the past, have led to frightening overnight autoimmune cluster epidemics.

Such was the case, for example, in 1989 with an outbreak of eosinophilia-myalgia syndrome (EMS), an autoimmune cluster epidemic that caused severe fatigue, muscle pain, and weakness to the point that patients were rendered unable to function. EMS affected thousands of individuals around the world after a manufacturer made a minuscule change in the manufacturing of an amino acid food supplement, L-tryptophan. Unbeknownst to the manufacturer, the changes led to an increase in trace chemical impurities in the product and resulted in thousands of individuals who took the supplement falling ill with EMS. Similarly, in 1998, hundreds of Haitian children died from autoimmune pediatric renal failure, with others suffering permanent comas after ingesting a commonly used children's acetaminophen cough syrup that had been defectively manufactured with trace amounts of diethylene glycol, a toxic substance.

Some researchers believe that such contamination of our food supply, or other consumer products, happens when large commercial networks operate without sufficiently tight oversight or when businesses are not knowledgeable about the consequences of making even minor alterations in manufacturing processes. One high-level researcher, who prefers to talk off the record, cautions that, without proper oversight and improved regulation, we may well see more such food- and additive-related clusters in the future, both in epidemic and sporadic form. The FDA itself has rather lax regulations for food products. And many of our food products are now imported from countries where regulations are even more lenient. This researcher plays out a frightening scenario that he hopes never to see. "Let's say a manufacturer decides to change how they manufacture a food-coloring additive in a children's cereal." Bear in mind, he explains, that even a very minor change in manufacturing techniques and trace ingredients can cause molecular changes in something like a food additive to occur—creating a "neo-antigen," or a new target for the immune system to potentially recognize as foreign. "That change might seem insignificant to the manufacturer," he explains, "yet it might have a very severe impact, resulting in an autoimmune response in a subset of children who are genetically predisposed to autoimmunity." Now let's say that the fact that these children are getting sick from a causative agent in the cereal—the food coloring—goes unappreciated for some time. After all, it's a cereal that these kids have been eating for years. "We could have thousands of kids who are exposed to the cereal falling ill or even dying before we remotely begin to figure out that this is another autoimmune cluster epidemic in motion."

Several scientists are now working under the auspices of the World Health Organization to create an autoimmunity task force that, if given adequate dollars, would serve as a worldwide monitoring group to educate against manufacturing practices that are most likely to put populations at risk. Such a watchdog group would also act as a rapid response team, investigating outbreaks in time to prevent widespread problems.

If you decide to take supplements and vitamins, choose them with special care, and go over all of them with a qualified nutritionist or with your doctor if he/she is knowledgeable about cutting-edge studies on food-as-medicine. A good specialist recognizes that so-called natural remedies are drugs. After all, aspirin was originally derived from willow bark, and the anticancer chemotherapeutic agent Taxol was derived from the bark of the Pacific yew tree. Natural products can be very potent indeed, and some natural products are turning out to have a surprisingly profound effect in helping to quell an overenthusiastic autoimmune response. Supplements and vitamins that are currently being studied in autoimmune disease research include:

ANTIOXIDANTS. In the normal process of metabolism, cells produce unstable oxygen molecules. These unstable molecules—known as free radicals—damage cells. Exposure to pollutants can increase free radicals, as can smoking and the use of cooking oils that become overheated. Antioxidants help to repair the damage done by free radicals.

Oxidative damage has been linked to the development of antibodies in lupus, and one recent study that followed the diet of twenty-five thousand individuals for nine years found that those who developed rheumatoid arthritis consumed 40 percent fewer antioxidants. Another study found low levels of antioxidants in patients with rheumatoid arthritis or lupus. Lab tests show that antioxidants help to decrease inflammation, which plays a role in many autoimmune diseases. Antioxidants are most easily available in the fruits and vegetables we eat. Blue-green algae (available at most health-food stores) contains omega fatty acids and the antioxidant phycocyanin and works similarly to a nonsteroidal anti-inflammatory drug like ibuprofen. Cranberries, blueberries, cherries, and blackberries are jam-packed with antioxidants called anthocyanins and polyphenols, which also have anti-inflammatory qualities. Leafy greens such as kale and spinach contain lutein, another superantioxidant. Cocoa carries flavonoids, particularly potent antioxidants that can zap free radicals and protect against inflammation. (The best way to consume cocoa is to add plain cocoa powder—preferably non-Dutched cocoa; Dutched cocoa is treated with an alkali during processing—into chili or other Southwestern recipes, thus avoiding the sugar in chocolate bars. If you eat chocolate, make sure it's dark or extra dark chocolate with 60 to 80 percent cocoa solids and that it has low sugar content.) Small red beans, kidney beans, and black beans are also packed with antioxidants.

Antioxidants can also be found in supplement and vitamin form. One particular antioxidant currently under study, alpha lipoic acid, has been shown to help in the treatment of multiple sclerosis by balancing T-cell activity and has also been found to help lessen symptoms in those with diabetic neuropathy. Alpha lipoic acid has such a profound effect, says Mullin, because it penetrates into the central nervous system, offering protection from the kind of free-radical damage that is often seen in multiple sclerosis and other neurological autoimmune diseases.

Again, work carefully with your doctor and/or nutritionist. Just because a supplement or vitamin is rich in antioxidants doesn't mean gobbling handfuls of it will be at all useful or prudent. Research on antioxidants and autoimmune disease is still new—as is research into antioxidants in general. For example, one highly controversial study suggested that people who consume high amounts of vitamin A may face an increased risk of certain illnesses. Vitamin E has also been the source of recent controversy. Figuring out what is salient and solid research is not easy—which is why it's so important to work with a health-care professional who stays completely up to date on the latest data on food and supplements as medicine.

ESSENTIAL FATTY ACIDS. There are two families of essential fatty acids, or EFAs: omega-3 and omega-6. High consumption of omega-6 can increase inflammation; in contrast, omega-3 fatty acids have strong anti-inflammatory properties. Omega-3 is most readily available through the consumption of fish and shellfish. Wild salmon, North Atlantic mackerel, sardines, flounder, sole, scallops, shrimp, pollack, red snapper, and tilapia are best because they all have a low mercury content. Avoid farmed salmon, which has a high PCB content, and high-mercury fish such as king mackerel, marlin, orange roughy, shark, swordfish, tilefish, and tuna. Essential fatty acids are also available in omega-3 rich eggs and flaxseed, as well as in supplement form. A growing number of studies show omega-3 to be beneficial in the prevention and management of Crohn's disease, ulcerative colitis, and rheumatoid arthritis. In one fascinating study, investigators at the Cleveland Clinic found that a nutritional supplement enriched with both fish oil and antioxidants reduced reliance on traditional therapies for people with ulcerative colitis, and that patients taking this oral supplement were less likely to need steroid therapy. Other research shows that higher dietary intake of omega-3 fatty acids is associated with a lowered risk of autoimmunity in children who are at genetic risk of type 1 diabetes.

VITAMIN D. A striking body of data shows that having higher levels of vitamin D in the blood may lower the risk of developing multiple sclerosis significantly. Researchers from the Harvard School of Public Health examined more than 7 million U.S. military personnel who had serum samples stored in the Department of Defense Serum Repository and correlated each individual's vitamin D levels. Those who had high levels of vitamin D were least likely to develop the disease later on in life. Likewise, a study of nearly thirty thousand women in their fifties and sixties found that the likelihood of having rheumatoid arthritis went down as dietary vitamin D intake increased.

Other studies show that vitamin D can be protective against not only multiple sclerosis but inflammatory bowel disease. According to Mullin, 75 percent of Crohn's patients are deficient in vitamin D. There is growing evidence that vitamin D plays a central role in rebalancing T-cell activity, which is why it is proving to be such an important adjunct to the treatment of autoimmune diseases such as MS and Crohn's disease. One provocative investigation looked at forty-two thousand people to determine why those born in the month of May have a 13 percent increased risk of developing multiple sclerosis (while being born in November carries a 19 percent *decreased* risk). The study concluded that the mother's exposure to the sun—which directly affects a pregnant woman's vitamin D levels and therefore that of her fetus—may influence the immune system even in the womb. Vitamin D occurs naturally in fish, but is most efficiently produced in the body by exposure to sunlight. Daily use of sunscreen and sunblock, however, can interfere with our absorption of vitamin D, says Mullin, making supplementation all the more critical. Juices fortified with vitamin D can also boost exposure, as can taking supplements.

CURCUMIN. According to a recent study from the National Institutes of Health, turmeric, an ancient spice long used in traditional Asian medicine, may hold promise for the prevention of rheumatoid arthritis and osteoporosis. Scientists tested the extract of curcumin—

found in this common spice—to see if it could help to stave off rheumatoid arthritis in lab animals. Turmeric, a key ingredient in curry, has been used for centuries by practitioners of Ayurvedic medicine to treat inflammatory disorders, and turmeric extract containing curcumin (not to be confused with cumin, a spice commonly associated with Moroccan cooking) is available in most health-food stores as a dietary supplement for the treatment and prevention of rheumatoid arthritis. NIH researchers found that curcumin completely inhibited the onset of rheumatoid arthritis in animals by working to keep inflammatory proteins from being released and preventing destruction in the joints. The daily dose of curcumin administered was roughly equivalent to 120 curry dinners—so future uses of curcumin in humans will revolve around supplementation rather than dietary intake. Meanwhile, clinical trials are currently planned to test turmeric supplements in suppressing rheumatoid arthritis in humans. Other investigations show that two grams of curcumin a day helps to control ulcerative colitis.

SEA ANEMONE EXTRACT. In what sounds like something straight out of *Twenty Thousand Leagues Under the Sea,* researchers from the University of California, Irvine recently found that natural compounds derived from a Cuban sea anemone extract—referred to as SL5—block the autoimmune disease response in type 1 diabetes and rheumatoid arthritis. In one set of tests using blood samples from type 1 diabetes patients and joint fluid from people with rheumatoid arthritis, the researchers found that the extract suppressed cytokine overproduction at a level similar to that seen with pharmacological drugs—without affecting other critical cells that fight infection.

RUE SHRUB PLANT. The same University of California, Irvine researchers working with sea anemone extract have likewise found that a compound from the rue shrub plant—known as PAP-1—delayed the onset and reduced the incidence of disease in diabetic rats and helped to improve the joint function of rats with rheumatoid arthritis. Research into both the rue plant, a small evergreen shrub also

known as the herb of grace, and sea anemone extract beg
ago when researchers at the University of California, Irvin
across a report that described the beneficial effect of a scorpion
on a patient with multiple sclerosis. They began to ask thems
about other natural substances that might, in a more control
manner, be able to influence T-cell and cytokine activity.

It remains to be seen if PAP-1 will work in people as well as i
does in lab animals. Meanwhile, such discoveries speak to the importance of protecting our plant and animal biodiversity. Ironically,
many of the same factors that are precipitating today's autoimmunity epidemic—environmental degradation and chemical pollution
both on land and at sea—are threatening to extinguish plant and
animal species that may one day turn out to hold the very cures we
seek for autoimmune disease.

GLUCOSAMINE. More familiar to many of us, glucosamine, the over-
the-counter natural product that has been touted to help with joint
and cartilage problems associated with arthritis, may also provide
some relief to individuals with multiple sclerosis. Using a mouse
model of MS, neurologists recently found that doses of glucosamine
similar to those commonly taken as supplements dramatically delayed the onset of MS symptoms and improved the ability of lab
animals to walk and move. Researchers believe that glucosamine
may prove useful in human trials for those suffering from MS.

PROBIOTICS. One area in which a great deal of research has been
done in autoimmune-disease patients is that of probiotic supplementation. Preparations of living microbial cells that are commonly
referred to as "friendly bacteria" are prescribed to repair the gut in
patients with inflammatory autoimmune diseases such as Crohn's
disease and ulcerative colitis. Ten years ago the concept that a food
ingredient such as probiotics—commonly found in yogurt—could
aid in fighting autoimmune disease was scoffed at by most medical
professionals. Yet today you can find more than three hundred
studies on PubMed linking probiotics to the treatment of inflammatory bowel disease. It has become well accepted, says Mullin,

in years
came
sting
lves
ed

inflammatory bowel disease and in-
decade an increasing number of
ing the mix of bacteria, probiotics
se autoimmune diseases of the gut sig-

is full of bacteria—most of it beneficial. But
e set of these healthy bacteria can interfere with
and fighting off illness and inflammation. In inflam-
wel disease studies, researchers reintroduce these positive
and allow them to repopulate the gut. Like other natural
ements—such as vitamin D and antioxidants, which modulate
ro-inflammatory cytokines—probiotics often produce their own
anti-inflammatory chemicals. Indeed, recent research finds that
therapy with the probiotic *Lactobacillus reuteri* directly modulates
pro-inflammatory cytokine production in mice, and a recent paper
published in the *American Journal of Gastroenterology* showed that
the majority of patients taking a probiotic mixture of eight bacteria,
known as VSL#3, for six weeks improved their ulcerative colitis.
The proper balance of intestinal flora also plays a strong role in
preventing gut permeability, which can spark the body toward an
allergic or autoimmune response. Researchers believe this is why
supplementation with probiotics has also shown promising results
in treating the symptoms of rheumatoid arthritis.

For Gerry Mullin, a combination of probiotics, antioxidants,
omega-3s, a whole-foods diet, and herbal approaches—coupled
with "prayer and determination"—proved critical in taming and
changing the course of his disease.

As consumers begin to demand more options for difficult-to-treat
autoimmune diseases, biotech companies are increasingly turning
toward what industry and consumers refer to as "nutraceuticals"—
supplements that they hope will compete with prescription drugs.
Likewise, research institutes that have long specialized in conventional, Westernized medical care are starting to investigate whether
plant extracts and herbal preparations may yield promising results

for patients. The Mayo Clinic, for instance, recently announced that they are decoding—using "sophisticated data mining techniques"—ancient, historical herbal texts to help develop potential new drugs for the future. Using nontraditional, ancient medical information taken from seventeenth-century texts, they have pinpointed certain herbal extracts to be "invaluable sources of healing agents."

At other institutions around the country, researchers are now studying an array of supplements and natural remedies that may ameliorate autoimmune activity and inflammation, including green tea extract (recently found to be a potent anti-inflammatory that provides therapeutic benefits to people with rheumatoid arthritis), grape seed extract, evening primrose oil, avocado/soybean extract, willow bark, ginger, devil's claw (a South African plant long touted for its anti-inflammatory properties), cat's claw (a Peruvian remedy found in the cat's claw vine), and boswellia (a remedy extracted from a tree that grows in India).

Again, anyone wanting to try any supplement, nutrient, or vitamin should be cautious. Almost every day conflicting studies emerge on the properties of various foods and supplements. One day, vitamin E is good; the next, we find out that the benefits of vitamin E supplements have been oversold. Large doses of some supplements such as vitamin A, vitamin B_6 and vitamin E may even be harmful. If you are concerned about a particular nutrient or supplement, in addition to discussing it with your health-care provider, peruse the National Institutes of Health Office of Dietary Supplements website for data on a wide range of dietary supplements and their risks and safety (www.ods.od.nih.gov). You can also download the USDA's free nutrient database software (go to www.ars.usda.gov/ba/bhnrc/ndl and hit Download Software) to get in-depth information about the nutrients and vitamins present in the food you eat. The site gives you a detailed breakdown of nearly seven thousand common foods. Plug in an item, from a cup of arugula to a turkey sandwich, and the program gives you an analysis of more than thirty nutrients. It also covers many kinds of processed and fast foods in greater detail than you'll find on most packages or menus.

A similar resource is available for helping you to make choices about what type of seafood to eat and how much. Go to http://www.gotmercury.org and enter your weight and the quantity and type of seafood you will eat during the coming week, then hit Calculate. The calculator will tell you whether your exposure to mercury through consuming a particular fish in a specific amount at your given weight constitutes a low, moderate, or high toxicity risk, based on current EPA standards.

UNDERSTANDING THE STRESS CONNECTION

We've all heard by now that stress is toxic to our immune system. "First-Year College Students Who Feel Lonely Have a Weaker Immune Response to the Flu-Shot," "Asthmatic Responses to Allergens Worsen During Stressful Times," "Marital Strain Increases Women's Risk of Death, Heart Disease," and "Arguments Slow the Body's Ability to Heal from Wounds" are all recent newspaper headlines that warn that stressful events can derail the basic function of our immune cells. Even stressful events that happened in our childhood can take a costly long-term toll on our health: people who experience significant traumas as children have an increased risk of developing immune-system problems as adults, including lowered white blood cell counts and elevated biomarkers of inflammation. Likewise, stressful events as adults—getting divorced, being physically assaulted, losing a job—take a toll on physical health even many years after the fact. One recent study found that those who had suffered more serious, negative life events had a 25-percent higher chance of dying within the next eight years.

In autoimmune disease, the link between stress and disease is profound. Stressful events are associated with an increased risk of having MS relapses, and periods of high stress are linked to the onset and worsening of rheumatoid arthritis. One startling study bears this out all too starkly: parents who have suffered the loss of a child are 50 percent more likely to develop multiple sclerosis than parents who've never lost a child—and the risk of developing MS spikes highest among those parents who lost a child unexpectedly.

What happens in our immune systems to cause this cellular cascade where psychological stress can lead to a malfunctioning immune system? When we are stressed, our adrenal glands produce several hormones, including adrenaline and cortisol. The stress response starts in the hypothalamus, a part of the brain that also regulates body temperature, respiration, hunger, sleep cycle, sexual function, and blood pressure. In addition to all that, the hypothalamus works as a kind of on-duty internal alarm system, constantly surveying the world around us, trying to ferret out any signs of impending danger. When something stressful—something that feels potentially unsafe—occurs, the hypothalamus sends an instant warning alert to the adrenal glands, which in turn flood our bloodstream with adrenaline. Adrenaline increases our heart rate and sends more blood into our muscles and added oxygen to our brains to keep us quick on our feet and help focus our attention on the crisis at hand.

The hypothalamus also sends a signal to the pituitary gland in the brain, which triggers the adrenal gland to flush the body with the stress hormone cortisol. In a short-term stressful situation—when you suddenly have to veer away from an oncoming car on the highway, or leap to scoop up a toddler who is about to tumble down the stairs, or flee from a house that's on fire—coritsol is critical to survival, preparing us for "fight or flight," helping us to take action with the energy, determination, and speed that such a situation requires. This hormonal rush can happen all in the few seconds it might take to slam on the brakes of your SUV to keep from hitting a stray dog meandering across the highway. When the stressful event ends, your adrenals send the message back to your hypothalamus to tell it to stop producing extra cortisol and adrenaline so that your heart rate, breathing, and perspiration levels can subside to normal. That's how the stress response is meant to work: it gets turned on when needed—and then it gets turned off quickly.

However, under chronically demanding conditions—the kind

of unrelenting psychological stressors that are the standard menu of modern life such as looming bills, fraught relationships, worries over children, caregiving for elderly parents, work crunches, and nonstop schedules, or all of the above rolled into one—heightened levels of cortisol are repeatedly pumped through the body. These stressors are rarely as life threatening as a car collision, but we can feel so anxious and overwhelmed in the face of them that the body really can't tell whether it's dealing with an actual emergency or not. Unfortunately, it just doesn't take very much to switch on the stress response. A deadline crunch or having a spat with your mother can both trigger it into overdrive.

Cortisol plays a central role in the immune system's responses and activity. The immune system's response is so potent that it requires intricate regulation to ensure that it is not too powerful and yet is strong enough to do the job of keeping the body safe. Under stress, cortisol mobilizes all major types of immune cells to battle stations in the body—primarily along the lymph nodes. That's great when we are trying to fight off infections and other diseases. But when stress turns chronic and an increased number of immune cells are ushered to sentry posts in the body too frequently, it can put too much wear and tear on the immune system. Overwhelmed by stress hormones and chemicals, immune cells never get a chance to recover from the constant barrage of cortisol, making us incapable of responding to new stress with even a slight burst of cortisol. We're all tapped out. The faucet is leaking a steady stream of cortisol, yes, but we can't get a full-force stream when we desperately need one. Our immune cells become so beleaguered that they become less able to react quickly to clear away pathogens—which is why research shows that you're more likely to catch colds and infections if you're in a troubled marriage.

Prolonged levels of heightened cortisol can not only lead to an underfunctioning immune reaction, but can also indirectly stimulate an autoimmune response. Stress hormones and chemicals travel to the immune system through the bloodstream and nerves and can dramatically alter how immune cells work. Cortisol helps to regulate our immune-system response not only by turning on the immune response, but also by turning it off. When cortisol keeps being pumped out because of daily anxieties and stressors, we stop producing sufficient cortisol to signal the immune response to turn off. This increases the likelihood that the immune system will go into erratic overdrive, that mistakes will be made and autoantibodies will attack the body itself.

In numerous studies, people who experience grinding, ongoing stress show higher levels of inflammatory cytokines in their blood compared to nonstressed individuals. One research study found that those experiencing chronic stress had higher levels of interleukin-6, or IL-6, which are pro-inflammatory cytokines that act as signaling messengers between cells of the immune system and which can whip up the immune cells to turn against the body itself. You might remember that this is the same inflammatory cytokine that Douglas Kerr, associate professor of neurology at Johns Hopkins School of Medicine, found in elevated levels in the spinal fluid of MS patients. Indeed, Kerr found that in patients with MS and transverse myelitis, the level of IL-6 proteins in their blood closely correlated with the severity of their paralysis. The same cytokine activity now being measured to help diagnose MS is also present in higher levels in those going through chronic stress.

Of course, one might ask which came first, the chicken or the egg? Is stress a contributing factor that leads to disease—or does disease lead to stress? The answer is both. For patients with autoimmune disease, stress produces a vicious cycle. Chronic illness is in and of itself an ongoing stressful event. In one recent report on what helps to secure human happiness, psychologists found that although those who suffer the loss of a spouse experience a great deal of stress, they eventually return to what psychologists refer to as their own personal "set point" of well-being. Over years, they become just as satisfied with life as they were prior to their spouses' dying. But those who experience chronic physical illness or major setbacks in physical well-being tend not to rebound as easily; long-term illness may result in significant, lasting decreases in one's personal sense of life satisfaction.

How could it not? Patients with autoimmune disease often

deal with the stress of not being able to trust what their bodies might do next, the stress of strained relationships, lost income, and frayed social connections. The normal stressors of life that once seemed so significant—a difficult neighbor or the sick dog or the sales presentation looming next week—become insignificant when faced with problems such as how to meet escalating medical debts or how to get up and down the stairs.

Which brings us back to a catch-22 situation. If mental and emotional stress can cause elevated levels of cytokine activity, which can lead to more episodes and flare-ups of autoimmune disease, how can we break this self-defeating cycle? If emotional stress can promote disease, can finding a way to be calmer and less stressed by whatever challenges come our way help to improve our health?

THE BIOLOGY OF EMOTION

One of the most fascinating findings about how our thoughts and emotions influence our health springs from a study of 180 nuns ranging in age from 75 to 103. Researchers had access to their early journal writings and were able to determine who among them had a mostly positive attitude when faced with stressful situations and who had a more negative response to life's slings and arrows. Some nuns were in their nineties and were highly functional with full-time jobs, while others were in their seventies and disabled.

What stood out for researchers was this: the nuns who wrote about their lives with the most positive attitudes at a young age were 2.5 times more likely to be in better health in late life than those nuns who saw life through a darker lens. Since the nuns in what is known as the Nun Study were all eating the same food, were nonsmokers, drank little if any alcohol, lived in similar housing, held similar jobs, were receiving the same medical care, and had the same socioeconomic status, the differences were all the more striking. The healthiest nuns were those whose writing showed a clear sense of humor and ability to adapt to life's stressors—including the normal health challenges that can accompany aging.

Researchers suspect that these nuns didn't live longer, healthier lives because they were never stressed. They lived longer and healthier lives because when they experienced the typical physiological response to stress they were able to recover quickly. By staying primarily at a low baseline of emotional stress, they protected their immune systems from becoming erratic.

For centuries, American medicine has deemed the question of whether our emotions can affect our health as irrelevant. Our two-hundred-year span of medical miracles has led us to revere the technological and scientific approach while giving little thought to the impact that emotions might have on our health. In large part that's because until very recently we have lacked scientific proof that our feelings can influence our physical well-being. In the last two decades, however, researchers have developed technology to see—in real time—how our emotions influence our bodies' cells by changing the chemical and electrical activity in our brains. Slowly, the divide that has long separated mind and body is beginning to erode as the two spheres of study increasingly collide, and researchers are focusing on how our emotions, stress levels, and thought patterns might influence our basic immune cells.

Recently, researchers at Harvard Medical School used standard MRI imaging to show visible differences in the brains of those who regularly practice meditation. Over time, areas of the brain that have to do with sensory processing became thicker in the meditators, and these physical changes profoundly changed the day-to-day modulation of the meditators' heart rates and breathing. Researchers have found that redirecting our thoughts through meditation literally rewires the brain and drastically decreases the level of stress hormones and chemical secretions that can be so damaging to our bodies when we encounter stressful situations or ideas throughout the day.

As with diet, entire sections of bookstores are chock-full of advice on coping with stress through a combination of prayer, meditation, yoga, keeping a positive attitude, proper sleep habits, and exercise. Recent press release headings that sit on my desk as I type these pages announce "An optimistic view can help protect a person's health when faced with family member's death and ill-ness"; "Personality trait may influence immune system response"; "Laughter is good for your heart, according to a new University of Maryland Medical Center study"; "Hotheads may be hurting their hearts"; and "Oscar winners live longer than Oscar nominees." (This latter study is quite intriguing: researchers looked at 762 actors who fell into three groups: those who had won Academy Awards; a group who were nominated but did not win an award; and a third group who were in award-winning films but were not nominated. Oscar winners lived four years longer than the other two groups, with study authors concluding that winning an Oscar may lead to increased feelings of optimism and mastery that influence health throughout the rest of one's life. Of course one might well ask: Did winning an Oscar lead to more optimism and better health, or did feelings of optimism and mastery lead to being a better actor, making these actors more likely to take home an Oscar?)

Whether one uses prayer, meditation, medication, therapy, greater attention to sleep, or exercise to lower stress levels and "unplug" from the strains of modern life, one thing is clear: doing so can have a significant effect on our immune systems. According to Douglas Kerr, stress, depression, and interrupted sleep patterns all have a negative effect on the body: these events "decrease the rate at which stem cells divide and create new stem cells in the bone marrow; they cause stem cells to go quiet." On the other hand, exercise results in a marked increase in the production of stem cells and new motor neurons—those same motor neurons that are so essential for remyelinating myelin sheaths and axonal nerves in neurological autoimmune disease. Likewise, exercise can stimulate injured neurons to regenerate their axons; animals that exercise regenerate significantly more sciatic nerve axons than sedentary animals. Other reports show that children with type 1 diabetes who exercise regularly have improved blood glucose levels compared with those who do not. Another study finds that exercise can improve muscle strength in those suffering from multiple sclerosis.

Of course, when we are suffering from illness, finding the time and energy to recalibrate our stress level is not so easily accomplished. When you can't do something as simple as drive your kids to school or walk the dog around the block, it's hard to be bursting with hope. Your overall sense of well-being and optimism takes a bit of a pummeling. Repetitive flares can leave one fearful—rather than hopeful—about what the next week, month, or years may hold. I know this all too well. Still, some studies suggest that a stress-free mood can persist, despite illness. In one study, researchers asked both chronically ill patients and a group of healthy individuals to record their moods into a handheld digital assistant, such as a Palm, every few hours for one week. The findings were both surprising and hopeful for those who assume that being diagnosed with a chronic illness means being sentenced to a lifetime of stress and anxiety. In many cases the moods of those who faced ongoing health challenges were not very different from those in excellent health. In fact, many patients who were chronically ill underestimated how well they were handling their situations. When asked to imagine the moods they would experience if they had never been ill, these patients estimated that they would be enjoying much better moods than those actually experienced by the healthy participants.

HOW THE "PRECAUTIONARY PRINCIPLE" CAN HELP

Ideally, we would all wake up tomorrow morning to an autogen-free world in which the environment is devoid of chemicals and heavy metals, food is always fresh, organic, and free of contaminants, and we do not have to worry about the plethora of triggers to autoimmune disease that surround us.

But tomorrow's reality looks to be quite the opposite. Each day an average of five new chemicals are put out on the market in the United States without any testing as to whether or not they pose a challenge to the immune system. Although our scientific literacy about links between chemicals, heavy metals, and autoimmunity is growing quickly, it has to date had little impact on federal environmental laws. Today, environmental legislation and regulations that guide the decisions we make about public health and the environment focus on managing current risk (how high a level of trichloroethylene or mercury can humans handle in their bloodstreams before falling ill?) rather than preventing future harm (how do we change manufacturing practices that emit toxic agents into the environment in the first place?).

On the other hand, the precautionary principle, an approach to public health that underscores preventing harm to human health before it happens—and the basis behind much decision-making in European environmental policy—holds that when the health of humans is at stake, it should not be deemed necessary to wait for scientific certainty to take protective action. Had we applied the precautionary principle to global warming, whole pieces of the polar ice caps would not now be crashing into the Arctic Sea.

Although the European Union is moving toward requiring companies to register thousands of chemicals with a new regulatory agency that places the burden on industry to prove that chemicals are safe, rather than on scientists to prove that they are unsafe, that is quite the opposite of the way we do business in the United States. In America, toxicologists at research institutions must demonstrate irrefutable cause and effect in the lab between toxins and human disease—the current scientific standard for burden of proof—which is virtually impossible without subjecting humans directly to toxic agents. As we have seen, almost every study examining the effects of chemicals and heavy metals on human health ends with "further study is needed." We know that the average American carries more than a hundred chemicals in his or her body, yet we can only guess what the long-term health effects are from living with this toxic cocktail of chemicals. We remain caught in the paralysis of analysis.

I often wonder if in seventy years we will have classrooms of students grilling teachers as to why their grandparents and great-grandparents—you and me—weren't more concerned about toxic contamination and the immune system. Didn't we see what we were doing to ourselves, to our foods and water, to future generations, to our children? Didn't we grasp the connection between the environmental contamination and degradation of the world around us and skyrocketing rates of diseases in which the immune system runs amok?

Getting involved in grassroots activities and political action groups and backing politicians who are committed to taking back the environment are critical if we hope to leave the legacy of a cleaner environment to our children's children. But the whole planet is not going to be saved from decades of chemical degradation overnight. In the meantime, we need to find ways to lessen the burden of chemicals and potential triggers with which we may come into contact.

PROTECTING YOUR IMMUNE SYSTEM

Once you know what it is like to live every day with an autoimmune disease and experience what it can take from you, the challenge of preventing relapses and flares and finding a way to be as healthy as possible, given your condition, becomes paramount. When you know that even a small relapse or infection can result in large lifestyle changes or the onset of another new autoimmune disease, finding all possible means of aiding your immune system to achieve optimum working order is essential.

Trying to avoid autoimmune-disease triggers can be overwhelming. After all, it seems as if almost anything you touch or eat carries risks. That cup of coffee from the coffee shop? Watch out for the perfluorooctanoic acid lining the inside of your cup. That orange roughy on your dinner plate? Loaded with mercury and PCBs. The newly dry-cleaned suit you just picked up for your cousin's wedding that's hanging in the backseat of your car? With each breath you're taking in a deep whiff of trichloroethylene. It can all seem overwhelming and frustrating. Where do we begin to clean the small sphere within which we live, work, play, and breathe?

What follows is a list of suggestions for minimizing your—and your family's—exposure to products that may trigger or exacerbate autoimmune disease. Several of these suggestions encourage buying chemical-free products. Doing so not only helps to protect your health but flexes your buying power. If enough Americans refuse to buy chemically laden products, the message to corporations and industry becomes clear: consumers are increasingly educated about how chemicals can affect their immune systems and corporations will have to do business according to the precautionary principle, marketing products that are proven to be safe and chemical free, in order to increase the bottom line.

CLEAN GREEN. Manufacturers of household cleaners are not required to list toxic ingredients on their product labels even if those products contain toxins. The truth is, you have no idea what is in the polish you use to make your dining room table shine or the spray you use to make your windows gleam. Yet, according to a study by the Environmental Protection Agency, the fumes and gases released into our homes by everyday cleaners help to make indoor air five times more polluted than the air we breathe outdoors. This is true not only in pristine areas like northern Maine, but in cities like New York and Los Angeles. In Los Angeles, approximately 108 tons of volatile organic compounds are released daily from household cleaners, personal grooming products, and paints. These domestic emissions are about to overtake car emissions as the primary source of the city's outdoor air pollution.

Some schools and hospitals are replacing chemical-based cleaning agents with natural alternatives. Since September 2006, a state law has required schools in New York to use cleaning products that do not carry any endocrine disruptors, carcinogens, or scents that can trigger reactions such as asthma. Other states may soon encourage similar changes, especially if they hear from enough constituents who support such legislation. Meanwhile, most grocery stores now offer a wide array of safe and toxin-free cleaners (Biokleen, Earth Friendly, and Seventh Generation offer toxin-free product lines). As an alternative, try making your own household cleaners. It's both easy and inexpensive. For furniture polish, mix one part white distilled vinegar, three parts olive oil, and a dash of natural lemon oil. For cleaning glass surfaces, try plain club soda or a mixture of half vinegar and half water in a pump spray bottle. More great household-cleaner recipes abound on the Web (see www.ecomall.com/greenshopping/coamerica.htm).

THINK BEFORE YOU PINK. Our skin is the largest organ of the body—and remarkably porous and adept at absorbing toxins. Cosmetic products are full of a disturbing number of chemicals. According to another study by the Environmental Working Group, in a test of fifteen thousand cosmetic products, almost 80 percent contained harmful impurities that include known or probable carcinogens, pesticides, endocrine disruptors, plasticizers, and degreasers. Despite these impurities, many of these products were nevertheless labeled as "organic" or "natural" because the government does not regulate personal-care-product labeling, and a product need only contain one or two botanical extracts to acquire the "natural" or "organic" label. The FDA has reviewed the safety of only 11 percent of the 10,500 ingredients being used in personal-care products today. Which means the onus is on you to do your own screening. Avoid cosmetics that include parabens (methyl-, ethyl-, propyl-, and butylparabens); phthalates; sodium laureth/sodium laurel sulfate; butyl/ethyl acetate; petrolatum; cocamide DEA/lauramide DEA; diazolidinyl urea; propylene glycol; toluene; synthetic colors and fragrances; and triethanolamine. Likewise, avoid using synthetic perfumes and cologne. Studies show that many perfumes and colognes often contain phthalates and parabens (both of which are known endocrine disruptors). Instead, look for organic products that have joined the Campaign for Safe Cosmetics, such as the Body Shop, Burt's Bees, Kiss My Face, Aubrey Organics, Avalon Natural Products, and TerrEssentials. Or visit thinkbeforeyoupink.org for a list of companies that produce products that are paraben and phthalate free.

AVOID DARK HAIR DYES. As we learned when we went through Becky's day, women who use dark hair dye have three times the risk of developing lupus.

SKIP THE NAIL POLISH. The European Union has been moving aggressively to remove phthalates from nail polish. Phthalates are often used in nail polish so that it doesn't chip as readily. In the United States, where regulators wait for proof before taking action, a few major cosmetic makers are electing to eliminate phthalates from nail polish since they have had to reformulate their products for the overseas market. Some companies are also producing polish that is free of two chemicals that are equally troubling to environmental public health groups: formaldehyde, a preservative, and toluene, a solvent that helps polish to flow more evenly. Nevertheless, the majority of nail products still contain phthalates, formaldehyde, and toluene.

One concern with nail polish is that it is often used by even very young girls, and "play" polishes for children abound. To date, Procter & Gamble, Estée Lauder, and several others have eliminated phthalates from their nail polish. (Ingredient labels on nail polish sold in retail stores must now state whether it contains phthalate as an ingredient, although salon nail polish does not have to.)

WASH YOUR HANDS! A recent study found that people infected with rhinovirus, the cause of half of all colds, contaminate many of the objects they touch, leaving an infectious path for those who follow them. The study, conducted in hotel rooms, showed that an adult with a cold who stayed one night in a hotel room left behind residual virus on everything from television remote controls and telephones to light switches and faucets. The study sheds light on how long viruses can survive on common surfaces such as doorknobs and handrails. Viruses left on surfaces are, say researchers "available for transfer for at least one day."

In order to infect an individual, germs must reach the eyes or the nose—usually by way of our own fingers. More than a third of Americans say they seldom or never wash their hands after coughing or sneezing. The average American washes his or her hands fewer than seven times a day, and 70 percent of Americans wash their hands for less than twenty seconds, the amount of time recommended by the Centers for Disease Control for a hand-washing session. (One trick: wash your hands for as long as it takes to mentally hum your ABCs—that's twenty seconds.) To avoid picking up germs left behind by others who have come before you, wash your hands often, avoid touching your mouth, nose, and eyes, and always wash your hands before eating. When you have to sign forms at the doctor's office or sign a credit card receipt at the store, have your own pen ready and use it. You might also consider bringing a handkerchief when you go out to run errands or head to a doctor's appointment. Hold it over the doorknobs or handles rather than using your bare fingers.

MAKE ENVIRONMENTALLY SOUND, COMMON-SENSE CHOICES. Use your common sense when making any purchase. For instance, next time you buy a car, consider buying a used hybrid; you'll emit less pollution into the environment as well as avoid owning the car during the period of time when the "new car smell" is at its peak as the vehicle releases manufacturing chemicals such as flame retardants and plasticizers. Drive a few extra miles (in your hybrid) to use organic dry cleaners; buy wooden toys rather than plastic ones for your children; avoid installing new carpets (which are loaded with flame retardants). Each time you think about purchasing a new item or using a product, ask yourself, based on what you have learned in these pages, whether using this product in your home will cause more chemicals to slowly leach into your body and into the bodies of those you love. If the answer is yes, search out a greener solution. They are increasingly easy to find.

Each small choice adds up. By making small, carefully calculated—and relatively simple—decisions that help us to lessen or eliminate as many chemicals as possible, we decrease the influx of agents that have the potential to tax our immune systems to the point that our bodies make costly mistakes and disease ensues. When we think of the body's capacity to deal successfully with chemical, viral, heavy metal, and emotional stressors as analogous to a barrel that should never be filled to the point of overflowing, we can begin to see each choice we make as one that matters greatly. Nevertheless, as we make decisions that are important in keeping us healthy, we have to avoid, as best we can, living in a state of mental fear of every potential trigger that might surround us. How optimistically you perceive the world around you also impacts your stress level and your health. As Albert Einstein once said, the most important decision you ever have to make is whether you live in a friendly universe or a hostile one.

In the future, perhaps we will all have made enough educated choices, exercising cumulative veto power as consumers and demanding accountability from government officials and agencies, that that roomful of high school students we imagine talking with their teachers seventy years from now—your great-grandchildren, and mine—won't be pressing teachers as to why we didn't foresee the polluted, disease-laden legacy we were leaving behind. Rather, they will be asking how a generation of scientists, researchers, patients, and concerned parents were prescient enough to come together to stop an autoimmune epidemic in its tracks. There can't be a friendlier universe—or a better legacy—to leave them than that.

AUTOIMMUNE AND RELATED DISEASES

For more information about the diseases on this list of more than one hundred autoimmune and related disorders, please contact the American Autoimmune Related Diseases Association (AARDA) at:

(800) 598-4668
(586) 776-3900
fax: (586) 776-3903
aarda@aol.com
www.aarda.org

The following diseases are known to be autoimmune in nature:

Acute disseminated encephalomyelitis (ADEM)
Acute hemorrhagic leukoencephalitis (Hurst's disease)
Agammaglobulinemia, primary
Alopecia areata
Ankylosing spondylitis
Anti-GBM/anti-TBM disease
Antiphospholipid antibody syndrome (APS)
Autoimmune Addison's disease

Autoimmune aplastic anemia
Autoimmune dysautonomia
Autoimmune hemolytic anemia
Autoimmune hepatitis
Autoimmune hyperlipidemia
Autoimmune inner ear disease (AIED)
Autoimmune interstitial cystitis
Autoimmune lymphoproliferative syndrome (ALPS)
Autoimmune myocarditis
Autoimmune polyglandular syndromes, Types I, II & III
Autoimmune progesterone dermatitis
Autoimmune thrombocytopenic purpura (ATP)
Autoimmune thyroiditis

Balo disease
Behçet's disease
Bullous pemphigoid

Celiac disease-sprue
Chronic inflammatory demyelinating polyneuropathy (CIDP)
Churg-Strauss syndrome
Cicatricial pemphigoid
Cogan's syndrome
Cold agglutinin disease
CREST syndrome
Crohn's disease

Dermatomyositis
Devic's disease (neuromyelitis optica)
Diabetes, type 1
Discoid lupus
Dressler's syndrome

Eosinophilic fasciitis
Essential mixed cryoglobulinemia
Evans syndrome

Glomerulonephritis
Goodpasture's syndrome
Graves' disease
Guillain-Barré syndrome

Hashimoto's thyroiditis
Henoch-Schönlein purpura

IgA nephropathy

Juvenile arthritis

Lambert-Eaton myasthenic syndrome
Lichen planus
Linear IgA disease (LAD)
Lupus nephritis

Microscopic polyangiitis
Mixed connective tissue disease (MCTD)
Multiple sclerosis
Myasthenia gravis

Non-length-dependent small fiber sensory neuropathy

Ocular cicatricial pemphigoid

Palindromic rheumatism
Paraneoplastic cerebellar degeneration
Paroxysmal nocturnal hemoglobinuria (PNH)
Parsonnage-Turner syndrome
Pemphigus vulgaris
Pernicious anemia
POEMS syndrome
Polyarteritis nodosa
Polymyalgia rheumatica
Polymyositis

Primary biliary cirrhosis
Psoriasis
Psoriatic arthritis
Pulmonary fibrosis, idiopathic
Pure red cell aplasia

Raynaud's disease
Reiter's syndrome
Relapsing polychondritis
Rheumatic fever
Rheumatoid arthritis

Sarcoidosis
Schmidt syndrome (autoimmune polyendocrine syndrome)
Scleritis
Scleroderma
Sjögren's syndrome
Systemic lupus erythematosus (SLE)

Testicular autoimmunity
Transverse myelitis

Ulcerative colitis
Undifferentiated connective tissue disease (UCTD)
Uveitis

Vasculitis
Vitiligo
Wegener's granulomatosis

The following disorders have a suspected autoimmune component:

Arteriosclerosis
Autism

Castleman disease
Chagas disease
Chronic fatigue syndrome

Erythema nodosum

Fibrosing alveolitis

Herpes gestationis
Hypogammaglobulinemia

Kawasaki syndrome

Leukocytoclastic vasculitis
Lichen sclerosus
Ligneous conjunctivitis
Lyme disease

Ménière's disease
Mooren's ulcer
Mucha-Habermann disease

Narcolepsy

Pars planitis (peripheral uveitis)
Postmyocardial infarction syndrome
Postpericardiotomy syndrome
Progesterone dermatitis
Pyoderma gangrenosum

Reflex sympathetic dystrophy
Restless leg syndrome

Stiff person syndrome (in some cases)
Subacute bacterial endocarditis (SBE)

Sympathetic ophthálmia

Takayasu's arteritis
Temporal arteritis/giant cell arteritis
Tolosa-Hunt syndrome

The following allergic disorders involve a hypersensitive reaction of the immune system against the body itself:

Allergic asthma
Allergic eczema
Allergic rhinitis
Food allergies

FIBROMYALGIA, CHRONIC FATIGUE SYNDROME, AND THE AUTOIMMUNE CONNECTION

Are fibromyalgia and chronic fatigue syndrome autoimmune in nature? According to Ahmet Hoke, MD, Ph.D, associate professor of neurology and neuroscience at Johns Hopkins Medical Institutions, both fibromyalgia (characterized by chronic widespread muscle pain, fatigue, and multiple tender points) and chronic fatigue syndrome (or CFS, characterized by severe chronic fatigue for six months or longer, sore throat, swollen lymph nodes, muscle pain, and other symptoms) may well be autoimmune diseases. However, in most autoimmune diseases, blood tests and lab markers help clue clinicians in to the fact that an autoimmune disease process is taking place in a patient's body. "We have no lab test that tells us conclusively that a patient has fibromyalgia or CFS," says Hoke. "I wouldn't be surprised if at some point in the future we identify a serologic marker for both of these disorders, but I'm not sure when we'll see it. It's not that the scientific community hasn't been trying; we just have not seen any conclusive blood markers despite doing multiple studies."

Certainly, many patients with autoimmune disease also suffer from fibromyalgia. Julius Birnbaum, MD, who serves as both a neurologist and rheumatology clinician at Johns Hopkins Medical Institutions (and is the only physician in the country trained in both of these disciplines) estimates that 20 percent of lupus patients with musculoskeletal pain also suffer from fibromyalgia. In his clinic at Hopkins, Birnbaum is helping many of these fibromyalgia patients through exciting new therapies. "We find that many patients with fibromyalgia suffer from undiagnosed sleep apnea or unrefreshed sleep—and a significant number of them suffer from undiagnosed Vitamin D deficiency," he emphasizes. By correcting poor sleep patterns and checking for Vitamin D deficiency—which he stresses, should be determined through lab tests that look at vitamin D, 25-hydroxy (total) rather than vitamin D, 1, 25-dihydroxy levels)— Birnbaum is helping many patients to improve. Moreover, he says, "New research into the underlying mechanism behind fibromyalgia shows that fibromyalgia patients may have abnormal connections between pain receptors in the skin and the dorsal horns of the spinal cord—which is the area of the spinal cord where pain becomes amplified. This region of the spinal cord may function differently in these patients than it does in those without fibromyalgia.

Like all areas of burgeoning autoimmune disease research, critical studies into fibromyalgia are creating an emerging picture of what lies behind the disease, as well what can help to combat the disease process so that patients can live healthier lives.

As for CFS, Birnbaum points out that patients who suffer from it have a different pattern of fatigue from those who are already suffering from fatigue as the result of another inflammatory autoimmune disease. In patients with a preexisting inflammatory autoimmune disorder, fatigue may also be from underlying inflammation due to their disease. Therefore, he doesn't diagnose CFS as a sole syndrome in patients who are already suffering from an inflammatory autoimmune disease.

NOTES

CHAPTER ONE: THE RED FLAG DISEASE

22 *Statistically, Jan's chances of having APS at the age of forty-nine:*
Current statistics from the National Center for Health Statistics
state that 14 out of 100,000 women develop ovarian cancer and
that 9 out of 100,000 women develop leukemia. Although antiphospholipid antibody syndrome was discovered relatively recently,
emerging statistics (http:www.hughes-syndrome.org/overview.htm)
reveal that as many as 1 in 500 individuals may actually suffer from
APS. Experts believe that as many as 90 percent of those affected are
women. While the actual frequency of APS in the general population
remains unknown due to a lack of epidemiological data, doctors
estimate that one-fifth of all "young" strokes (defined as occurring
in someone under the age of 45) are due to APS. In obstetrics it is
estimated by some doctors that up to 25 percent of all women with
two or more spontaneous miscarriages have APS. For more information see the above website or www.apsfa.org/faq/faq1.htm 9 (accessed July 18 2007).

22 *In fact, recent studies reveal that antiphospholipid antibodies:* Although antiphospholipid antibodies are found in 2 to 5 percent of

the population, not all those who have these antibodies go on to develop the disease, though many do. Because APS is a recently understood autoimmune disease, researchers are not yet certain they know of all the autoantibodies involved. For more on the complexities of predicting who will have the disease based on autoantibody testing in autoimmune diseases in general, please see chapter 5, "The Autoimmune Disease Detectives."

23 *Four hundred thousand patients:* http://www.nationalmssociety.org/ site/PageServer?pagename=HOM_RES_research_factsheet (accessed May 11, 2007).

23 *One and a half million more:* http://www.lupus.org/education/stats .html (accessed April 11, 2007).

23 *Seven out of every one thousand Americans:* http://oto.wustl.edu/ men/mn1.htm (accessed April 11, 2007).

24 *Four million Americans:* http://www.sjogrens.org (accessed April 11, 2007).

24 *And yet, despite the prevalence:* Roper ASW. Knowledge of autoimmune disease. Report prepared for the American Autoimmune Related Diseases Association, February 2003. Available from the American Autoimmune Related Diseases Association, 22100 Gratiot Avenue, East Detroit, MI 48021-2227, (586) 776-3900, aarda@ aarda.org.

24 *Taken collectively, these diseases:* American Autoimmune Related Diseases Association. Who we are. Press release; 3. Available from the American Autoimmune Related Diseases Association, 22100 Gratiot Avenue, East Detroit, MI 48021-2227, (586) 776-3900, aarda@aarda.org.

24 *the third leading cause of Social Security:* Ibid.; 2.

24 *Autoimmune diseases are the eighth leading cause:* Walsh SJ, Rau LM. Autoimmune diseases: A leading cause of death among young and middle-aged women in the United States. Am J of Pub Health 2000 Sep;90(9):1463–6.

25 *shortening the average patient's lifespan:* On March 16, 2005, I attended a congressional briefing in Washington, D.C., at which Dr. Bhagirath Singh, scientific director of the Canadian Institutes of

Health Research, Institute of Infection and Immunity, presented this statistic.

25   *Not surprisingly, the economic burden:* American Autoimmune Related Diseases Association. Who we are. Press release; 1.

25   *yearly health-care burden of $70 billion:* http://www.cdc.gov/nccd php/publications/factsheets/Prevention/cancer.htm (accessed May 24, 2007).

25   *while 2.2 million women are living with breast cancer:* Marcus AD. Medical student takes on a rare disease—his own: Andy Martin donates tissue, then struggles to grow tumor cells in a lab dish. Wall Street Journal, 2004 Apr 1. Available from http://online.wsj.com/article_email/SB108077194020270691-IBjg4NmlaB3oZuoZXm GaqaAm4.html (accessed May 12, 2007).

25   *and 7.2 million women have coronary disease:* http://www .americanheart.org/downloadable/heart/1166712318459HS_Stats InsideText.pdf (accessed May 12, 2007).

25   *an estimated 9.8 million women are afflicted:* These seven diseases are estimated to affect the following number of Americans: lupus, 1.5 million; scleroderma, 300,000; rheumatoid arthritis, 2.1 million; multiple sclerosis, 400,000; inflammatory bowel disease, 1 million; type 1 diabetes, 300,000 to 500,000; Sjögren's, up to 4 million.

25   *Or, slice these statistics another way:* http://www.cancer.gov/cancer topics/factsheet/Detection/probability-breast-cancer (accessed May 12, 2007).

25   *as many as one in nine women of childbearing years:* Estimates hold that nearly 24 million Americans suffer from autoimmune disease and that three-quarters of these sufferers are women, which means that roughly 18 million women have autoimmune disease in America. There are approximately 164 million American females, which means that roughly one in nine American women suffers from autoimmune disease.

25   *which strike three times as many women:* http://www.aarda.org/ women.php (accessed May 12, 2007).

25   *According to the National Institutes of Health:* http://www.cdc.gov/ cancer/npcr/npcrpdfs/about2004.pdf (accessed May 12, 2007).

25　*the 16 million with coronary disease:* http://www.americanheart
.org/downloadable/heart/1166712318459HS_StatsInsideText.pdf
(accessed May 12, 2007).

25　*Yet few of today's practicing physicians are aware:* National Institutes
of Health, Autoimmune Diseases Coordinating Committee. Progress
in autoimmune diseases research. Report to Congress, 2005 Mar;
foreword by Elias A. Zerhouni, MD. Available from http://www
.niaid.nih.gov/dait/pdf/ADCC_Final.pdf (accessed May 12, 2007).

25　*Mayo Clinic researchers report that the incidence of lupus:* Uramoto
KM et al. Trends in the incidence and mortality of systemic lupus
erythematosus, 1950–1992. Arthritis Rheum. 1999 Jan;42(1):46–
50. Researchers report that over the past four decades, the incidence
of lupus has nearly tripled in the United States, and possible explanations include an increased exposure to environmental triggers, in
addition to an improvement in survival rates among patients and
somewhat improved screening techniques.

26　*Over the past fifty years multiple sclerosis rates:* Midgard R et al.
Incidence of multiple sclerosis in More and Romsdal, Norway from
1950 to 1991. An age-period-cohort analysis. Brain. 1996 Feb;
119(Pt 1):203–11. This study cites that the incidence of multiple
sclerosis in Finland increased "threefold" between 1979 and 1992,
"corroborating the increasing trend reported from Scotland, the
United Kingdom, the Netherlands, Denmark and the western coast
of Norway."

26　*Sweden, where rates of MS:* Sundstrom P et al. Incidence (1988–97)
and prevalence (1997) of multiple sclerosis in Vasterbotten County
in northern Sweden. J Neurol Neurosurg Psychiatry. 2003
Jan;74(1):29–32. Umea University Hospital neurologists report that
MS rates between 1988 and 1997 in Vasterbotten County, Sweden,
were twice as high as incident rates between 1974 to 1988, with "a
yearly 2.6% increase in prevalence between 1990 and 1997 . . . mainly
attributable to a higher incidence [rather] than mortality."

26　*Multiple sclerosis rates in Norway:* Edland A et al. Epidemiology of
multiple sclerosis in the county of Vestfold, eastern Norway: Incidence and prevalence calculations. Acta Neurol Scand 1996 Feb–

Mar;93(2–3):104–9. Hospital researchers report that in the county of Vestfold, eastern Norway, multiple sclerosis rates rose 30 percent between 1963 and 1983. Studies on MS among western Norwegians show a twofold increase in MS during the same period. The study's four authors conclude that the "increase in prevalence of MS in western Norway is due to a real biological change of the disease" and cannot be due solely to better diagnostics. Dahl OP et al. Multiple sclerosis in Nord-Trondelag County, Norway: A prevalence and incidence study. Acta Neurol Scand 2004 Jun;109(6):378–84. In the county of Nord-Trondelag, not only is MS increasing, but researchers write "the prevalence is among the highest ever in Norway."

26 *echoing trends in Germany, Italy, and Greece:* Poser S et al. Increasing incidence of multiple sclerosis in South Lower Saxony, Germany. Neuroepidemiology 1989;8(4):207–13. Researchers from Göttingen University report that in Lower Saxony the prevalence of multiple sclerosis doubled between 1969 and 1986 and write that "new handling of early cases [or better diagnostics] by practicing physicians can hardly explain this significant increase. In consideration of similar reports from all over the world biological exogenous factors are suspected but remain to be identified." Rosati G et al. Incidence of multiple sclerosis in the town of Sassari, Sardinia, 1965 to 1985: Evidence for increasing occurrence of the disease. Neurology 1988 Mar;38(3):384–8. Researchers report that MS rates in Sardinia more than doubled between 1965 and 1973. Piperidou HN et al. Epidemiological data of multiple sclerosis in the province of Evros, Greece. Eur Neurol 2003;49(1):8–12. In the province of Evros, Greece, researchers from the Department of Neurology at Aristotle University report that the prevalence rate of MS increased from about 1 in 100,000 people in 1974 to 39 per 100,000 people in 1999. The authors note that while some of this may be the result of causes other than increasing susceptibility to environmental triggers of disease, this overall rate increase points to "the possibility of a variation in risk [causing] factors of the disease."

26 *Rates of autoimmune thyroiditis have risen steadily:* National Insti-

tutes of Health, Autoimmune Diseases Coordinating Committee. Progress in autoimmune diseases research. Report to Congress, 2005 Mar; 43.

26 *Rates of type 1 diabetes:* EURODIAB ACE Study Group. Variation and trends in incidence of childhood diabetes in Europe. Lancet 2000 Mar 11;355(9207):873–6. Childhood-onset type 1 diabetes is also increasing annually at a rate of 3 percent in children between the ages of five and nine. Researchers emphasize that "the rapid rate of increase in children aged under 5 years is of particular concern," citing that this "rapid increase in incidence is not readily explained by shifts in the frequency of susceptibility genes, and change in environmental factors is a more plausible explanation." Also see Onkamo P et al. Worldwide increase in incidence of type 1 diabetes—the analysis of the data on published incidence trends. Diabetologia 1999 Dec, 42(12):1395–403.

26 *Rates of numerous other autoimmune diseases:* Steen V et al. Incidence of systemic sclerosis in Allegheny County, Pennsylvania. A twenty-year study of hospital-diagnosed cases, 1963–1982. Arthritis Rheum 1997 Mar;40(3):441–5. In this study researchers report that cases of scleroderma (SSc), a progressive autoimmune disease in which blood vessels narrow to the degree that they prevent blood flow to the body's tissues, have doubled over a recent twenty-year period. Authors write that although this trend had to do with improved detection and medical record techniques, higher incidence rates in women suggest that there "may have been a true increase in the incidence of SSc."

Crohn's disease, an inflammatory autoimmune disease of the bowels, virtually unheard of until the 1930s, now afflicts 15 out of 100,000 people in highly industrialized nations such as the United States, England, and the countries of Scandinavia. Researchers cite that "the incidence of Crohn's disease has increased strikingly in many areas" around the world and are especially concerned by the fact that immigrants who move to industrialized nations from less developed countries (where the prevalence of Crohn's disease is quite low) suddenly begin to have Crohn's disease at the elevated rates found in their adopted urban landscape. For more on this see Farrokhyar FA et al.

Critical review of epidemiological studies in inflammatory bowel disease. Scand J Gastroenterol 2001 Jan;36(1):10.

Norwegian researchers report a rising incidence of autoimmune Addison's disease, or autoimmune adrenal insufficiency, a disease in which the body destroys the cells in its own adrenal glands. Autoimmune adrenal failure, they say, has "certainly increased over the last 50 years." See Lovas K and Husebye ES. High prevalence and increasing incidence of Addison's disease in western Norway. Clin Endocrinol (Oxf) 2002 Jun;56(6):787–91.

Other diseases show the same alarming pattern. In a 1990 Pennsylvania study, cases of polymyositis, an autoimmune disease of the muscles, resulting in severe muscle weakness, more than tripled between 1973 and 1982. Oddis CV et al. Incidence of polymyositis-dermatomyositis: A 20-year study of hospital diagnosed cases in Allegheny County, PA 1963–1982. J Rheumatol 1990 Oct;17(10): 1329–34.

26 *Norwegian epidemiologists:* Edland A et al. Epidemiology of multiple sclerosis in the county of Vestfold, eastern Norway: Incidence and prevalence calculations. Acta Neurol Scand 1996 Feb–Mar;93 (2–3):108.

27 *Type 1 diabetes researchers:* EURODIAB ACE Study Group. Variation and trends in incidence of childhood diabetes in Europe. Lancet 2000 Mar 11;355(9207):875.

27 *At the Mayo Clinic researchers:* Uramoto KM et al. Trends in the incidence and mortality of systemic lupus erythematosus, 1950–1992. Arthritis Rheum 1999 Jan;42(1):48.

30 *The average patient with autoimmune disease:* American Autoimmune Related Diseases Association. Who we are. Press release; 4.

30 *Recent surveys conducted:* American Autoimmune Related Diseases Associaton. Autoimmunity: A major women's health issue; 2. This patient information literature notes that according to a 2001 AARDA survey, "over 45 percent of patients with autoimmune diseases have been labeled chronic complainers in the earliest stages of their illness." Available from the American Autoimmune Related Diseases Association, 22100 Gratiot Avenue, East Detroit, MI 48021-2227, (586) 776-3900, aarda@aarda.org.

30   *women with autoimmune disease:* American Autoimmune Related
     Diseases Association. Who we are. Press release; 4.

33   *This presumption—set forth in the early 1900s by Nobel laureate:*
     Others recall Ehrlich's use of the term "horror autotoxicus" differ-
     ently. Zoltan Fehervari and Shimon Sakaguchi relate in a recent
     issue of *Scientific American* that Paul Ehrlich theorized autoimmu-
     nity might be biologically plausible yet was somehow "kept in check
     and therefore did not occur." The medical community misconstrued
     this "two-sided idea," taking from it that autoimmunity was inher-
     ently impossible, thus leading to generations of medical students
     and physicians learning that the body could not and would not at-
     tack itself. Fehervari, Z and Sakaguchi, S. Peacekeepers of the Im-
     mune System. Scientific American, 2006 Oct;57.

37   *One of the more interesting diseases:* Germolec DR and Smith DA.
     Introduction to immunology and autoimmunity. Environ Health
     Perspect 1999 Oct;107(Suppl 5):661–5.

37   *In 2005, Mayo Clinic researchers:* Nicola PJ et al. The risk of con-
     gestive heart failure in rheumatoid arthritis: A population-based
     study over 46 years. Arthritis Rheum 2005 Feb;52(2):412–20.

37   *Other studies show similar elevated risk of heart disease:* Swanberg
     M et al. MHC2TA is associated with differential MHC molecule
     expression and susceptibility to rheumatoid arthritis, multiple scle-
     rosis and myocardial infarction. Nat Genet 2005 May;37(5):486–
     94. Epub 2005 Apr 10.

          Maradit-Kremers H et al. Increased unrecognized coronary
     heart disease and sudden deaths in rheumatoid arthritis: A popula-
     tion-based cohort study. Arthritis Rheum 2005 Feb;52(2):402–11.

37   *Although the exact means by which autoimmune disease:* Germolec
     DR and Smith DA. Introduction to immunology and autoimmunity.
     Environ Health Perspect 1999 Oct;107(Suppl 5):661–5.

38   *Recent studies show that in artherosclerosis:* Lunardi C et al.
     Endothelial cell activation and apoptosis induced by a subset of
     anti-bodies against human cytomegalovirus: Relevance to the patho-
     genesis of atherosclerosis. PLoS ONE 2(5):e473. Doi:10.1371/
     journal.pone.0000473, www.plosone.org/doi/pone.0000473 (ac-
     cessed May 30, 2007). Lunardi C et al. Induction of endothelial cell

damage by hCMV molecular mimicry. Trends Immunol 2005 Jan;26(1):19–24.

CHAPTER TWO: THE INVISIBLE INVADERS

45   *Yet the average participant:* Houlihan J, Wiles J, Thayer K, and Gray S. Body burden: The pollution in people. Environmental Working Group, 2005. Available from http://www.ewg.org.

45   *These chemicals included pesticides:* http://www.ewg.org/reports/bodyburden2 (accessed May 17, 2007).

45   *Shortly after, investigators in the Netherlands:* Papadakis M. Placenta chemical cocktail. Sunday Tasmanian, 2005 Oct 2. Available online from http://chickenlittle.org/news/story.php?id=4474 (accessed July 18, 2007).

47   *One recent study found PBDEs:* Carlton J. Study reveals toxic chemicals in household dust. Wall Street Journal, 2005 Mar 23;D7.

47   *A separate study of seventeen homes:* National Institute of Standards and Technology. Flame retardant exposure linked to house dust. Report, 2004 Dec 29. Available from http://www.nist.gov/public_affairs/releases/PBDE_dust.htm (accessed May 16, 2007).

47   *Babies and toddlers:* Ibid.

47   *They discovered, to their alarm:* Williams F. Toxic breast milk? New York Times Magazine, 2005 Jan 9;23. Herrick T. Toxins in breast milk: Studies explore impact of chemicals on our bodies. Wall Street Journal, 2004 Jan 20. Available from http://www.mindfully.org/Health/2004/Biomonitoring-Breast-Milk 20jan04.htm (accessed July 18, 2007).

47   *In 2003, a study of twenty first-time American mothers:* Ibid. Also see Siddiqi MA. et al. Polybrominated diphenyl ethers (PBDEs): New pollutants—old diseases. Clin Med Res 2003 Oct;1(4):281–90.

47   *Overall, levels of PBDEs:* Agency for Toxic Substances and Disease Registry (ATSDR). Public health statement for polybrominated diphenyl ethers (PBDEs). Available from http://www.atsdr.cdc.gov/toxprofiles.phs68_plode.html (accessed May 16, 2007). When

viewed in September 2004 on the ATSDR website, the Public Health Statement on PBDEs stated: "Recent studies have shown that levels of lower brominated PBDEs in the general population of the United States continue to rise. The U.S. levels are 10–100 times higher than levels in individuals living in Europe." When last viewed in May 2004, the page on PBDEs has since been shortened significantly and this statement is no longer included in the abbreviated version.

47 *Other recent studies show that levels of PBDEs:* He J. et al. Microbial reductive debromination of polybrominated diphenyl ethers (PBDEs). Environ Sci Technol 2006 Jul 15;40(14):4429–34.

48 *Recently, however, investigators have found:* Ibid.

48 *The CDC's website now informs:* The ATSDR Public Health Statement for Polybrominated Diphenyl Ethers states that "preliminary findings from short-term animal studies suggest that some PBDEs might impair the immune system." Available from http://www.atsdr. cdc.gov/toxprofiles/phs68-pbde.html (accessed May 16, 2007).

48 *At breakfast, Becky's favorite no-hassle:* Manufacturers of Teflon say that in order for nonstick pans to emit toxic substances into the air they must be heated to high temperatures (which makes the coating break down and vaporize). DuPont, the maker of Teflon, says that temperatures must exceed 500°F for deterioration to occur and 660°F for significant decomposition. According to the manufacturer, temperatures don't reach 500°F in the course of normal cooking except in the broiler. However, according to the Environmental Working Group, nonstick pans do reach such high temperatures when preheated on high—a common practice in many households. In tests conducted on ordinary gas and electric stoves, Teflon and other nonstick pans topped 700°F in three to five minutes. Certainly, in the case of burning pancakes, the pan is reaching such high temperatures. For more on this and other related articles, see http://www.ewg.org/node/8303 and http://www.ewg.org/reports/toxicteflon (accessed July 18, 2007).

48 *It does not break down:* Based on conversation with Timothy Kropp, Environmental Working Group, September 2005.

49 *In 2005, the Environmental Protection Agency:* Eilperin J. Teflon chemical's potential risk cited. Washington Post, 2005 Jan 13;A4.

49   *In one recent and provocative paper from Stockholm:* Yang Q et al.
      Potent suppression of the adaptive immune response in mice upon
      dietary exposure to the potent peroxisome proliferator, perfluorooc-
      tanoic acid. Int Immunopharmacol 2002 Feb;2(2–3):389–97.

49   *In one recent study—which found that 100 percent:* From the press
      release: "100 percent of pregnant women have at least one kind of
      pesticide in their placenta." EurekAlert! 2007 May 14. Available
      from http://www.eurekalert.org/pub_releases/2007-05/udg-1op051407
      .php (accessed May 28, 2007).

49   *Indeed, if you were to do a search:* For a list of studies, go to PubMed
      and type in "endosulfan and immune system." Or see Kannan K et
      al. Evidence for the induction of apoptosis by endosulfan in a human
      T-cell leukemic line. Mol Cell Biochem 2000 Feb; 205(1–2):53–66.

50   *Every single one of the female mice:* Sobel ES et al. Acceleration of
      autoimmunity by organochlorine pesticides in (NZB x NZW)F1
      mice. Environ Health Perspect 2005 Mar;113(3):323–8. Sobel ES et
      al. Comparison of chlordecone effects on autoimmunity in
      (NZBxNZW)F(1) and BALB/c mice. Toxicology 2006 Feb 1;218(2–
      3):81–9. Epub 2005 Nov 22.

51   *the commonly used pesticide methoxychlor:* Sobel ES et al. Accel-
      eration of autoimmunity by organochlorine pesticides in (NZBx
      NZW)F1 mice. Env Health Persp 2005 Mar;113(3):328. In this
      study, the authors write: "It is worthwhile noting that the lower
      dose of methoxychlor tested (3 mg/pellet, or approximately 1.2 mg/
      kg/day) is 4-fold lower than the NOEL used by the U.S. Environ-
      mental Protection Agency (EPA) in developing an oral reference
      dose for methoxychlor. This suggests that an effect on autoimmu-
      nity might be a sensitive toxic end point (an effect that occurs at
      doses lower than other adverse effects) for methoxychlor, and there-
      fore of particular interest for risk assessment."

51   *Yet occupational studies that link groups of people:* Rosenberg AM
      et al. Prevalence of antinuclear antibodies in a rural population. J
      Toxicol Environ Health A 1999 June;57(4):225–36. In this study
      researchers found that farmers with a history of working with pesti-
      cides were more likely to have a low, but still significant, titer of
      antinuclear antibodies associated with lupus diagnosis.

51 *In one 2007 study, reseachers studied data from over 300,000 death certificates:* Gold LS et al. Systemic autoimmune disease mortality and occupational exposures. Arthritis Rheum 2007 Oct;56(10):3189–3201. This study also reported an association between exposures to asbestos, solvents, and benzene and a higher risk of dying from systemic autoimmune diseases.

51 *In yet another study, rural farmers who reported mixing pesticides:* Cooper GS et al. Occupational risk factors for the development of systemic lupus erythematosus. J Rheumatol 2004 Oct;31(10): 1928–33. In this study, researchers found a strong association (based on small numbers) between mixing pesticides and lupus.

51 *Despite such danger signals:* Colborn T. Our stolen future. New York:Plume, 1996;216.

52 *There is mounting evidence that this air pollution:* Gilmour PS et al. The procoagulant potential of environmental particles (PM10). Occup Environ Med 2005 Mar;62(3):164–71. Powell JJ et al. Evidence for the role of environmental agents in the initiation or progression of autoimmune conditions. Environ Health Perspect Supplements 1999 Oct;107 (Suppl 5):667–72.

52 *mice exposed to fine particles of pollution:* Sun Q et al. Long-term air pollution exposure and acceleration of atherosclerosis and vascular inflammation in an animal model. JAMA 2005 Dec 21; 294(23):3003–10. This study showed a direct cause and effect link between exposure to fine-particle air pollution and the development of atherosclerosis, commonly known as hardening of the arteries. Mice that were fed a high-fat diet and exposed to air with fine particles had 1.5 times more plaque production than mice fed the same diet and exposed to clean filtered air.

52 *All nine people tested by Mount Sinai:* http://www.ewg.org/reports/bodyburden2 (accessed May 17, 2007).

52 *It has long been known to cross the placenta:* Dahlgren J et al. Residential and biological exposure assessment of chemicals from a wood treatment plant. Chemosphere 2007 Apr;67(9):S279–85. Epub 2007 Jan 17; also see Kao WY. Site-specific health risk assessment of dioxins and furans in an industrial region with numerous emission

sources. J Hazard Mater 2006 Nov 30. Epub 2006 Nov 30. For many more studies, search PubMed for "dioxin and cancer."

53 *when female rodents are exposed to dioxin:* Holladay SD. Prenatal immunotoxicant exposure and postnatal autoimmune disease. Environ Health Perspect, 1999 Oct;107(Suppl 5):687–91.

53 *Other research is examining the role everyday exposure to dioxin:* Silverstone AE et al. 2,3,7,8-Tetrachlorodibenzo-p-dioxin may accelerate disease in a murine model of a lupus-like nephritis. Organohalogen Comp 1996;29:156–160.

54 *Indeed, environmental exposures to dioxin and PCBs:* Based on an e-mail correspondence with Allen Silverstone, April 24, 2007.

57 *At the University of Tokyo:* Yurino H et al. Endocrine disruptors (environmental estrogens) enhance autoantibody production by B1 cells. Toxicol Sci 2004 Sep;81(1):139–47.

57 *Other lab research confirms that environmental estrogens:* Iwata M et al. The endocrine disruptors nonylphenol and octylphenol exert direct effects on T cells to suppress Th1 development and enhance Th2 development. Immunology Letters 2004 Jun 15;94(1–2):135–9.

58 *a number of studies show that BPA alters:* Waldman P. Common industrial chemicals in tiny doses raise health issue. Wall Street Journal, 2005 Jul 25;1.

58 *In 2006, researchers found that BPA:* Welshons WV et al. Large effects from small exposures. III. Endocrine mechanisms mediating effects of bisphenol A at levels of human exposure. Endocrinology 2006 Jun;147(6 Suppl):S56–69. Epub 2006 May 11.

58 *Significant effects can be seen at extremely low levels:* Daly D. Hundreds of man-made chemicals—in our air, our water, and our food—could be damaging the most basic building blocks of human development. OnEarth 2006 Winter:24.

58 *None of 11 studies conducted:* Ibid.

58 *In the wake of the mounting data:* National Institutes of Health, Autoimmune Diseases Coordinating Committee. Progress in autoimmune diseases research. Report to Congress, 2005 Mar;31.

59 *As an aside, while urban myth holds:* Public Health News Center, Johns Hopkins Bloomberg School of Public Health. Researcher dis-

pels myth of dioxins and plastic water bottles. Press release, 2004 June 24. Available from http://www.jhsph.edu/publichealthnews/ articles/halden_dioxins.html (accessed May 18, 2007).

59 *Phthalates are also key ingredients:* http://www.thinkbeforeyoupink .org/Pages/CosmeticCompanies.html (accessed May 18, 2007). Also see Waldman P. From an ingredient in cosmetics, toys, a safety concern. Wall Street Journal 2005 Oct 4;A1. In this article, Waldman discusses the fact that the United States does not restrict phthalates and has lobbied the European Union hard in the last few years to avoid burdening manufacturers with new regulations on chemicals.

59 *Like dioxin, bisphenol A, PFOAs, PBDEs, and pesticides, phthalates:* http://www.ewg.org/sites/humantoxome (accessed May 18, 2007).

60 *Most sufferers of any one autoimmune syndrome:* Cooper GS et al. N-acetyl transferase genotypes in relation to risk of developing systemic lupus erythematosus. J Rheumatol 2004 Jan;31(1):76–80; also Freni-Titulaer LW et al. Connective tissue disease in southeastern Georgia: A case-control study of etiologic factors. Am J Epidemiol 1989 Aug;130(2):404–9.

60 *Although Becky is not a frequent user of solvents:* Cooper GS et al. Occupational exposures and autoimmune diseases. Int Immunopharmacol 2002 Feb;2(23):303–13. Aryal BK et al. Meta analysis of systemic sclerosis and exposure to solvents. Am J Ind Med 2001 Sep;40(3):271–4. Garabrant DH et al. Scleroderma and solvent exposure among women. Am J Epidemiol 2003 Mar 15;157(6):493–500. Bovenzi M et al. A case-control study of occupational exposures and systemic sclerosis. Int Arch Occup Environ Health 2004 Jan;77(1):10–6. Epub 2003 Oct 3.

61 *Fibrous bits of nine different synthetics:* Thompson RC et al. Lost at sea: Where is all the plastic? Science 2004 May 7;304(5672):838.

61 *When Becky eats a dinner of mako shark:* Environmental aspects of pharmaceuticals and personal care products. Symposium, American Chemical Society National Meeting; 2004 Aug 22–26; Philadelphia. Available from http://www.scienceblog.com/community/older/2004/ 3/20042309.shtml (accessed May 18, 2007); see Highlights.

62 *blends of certain synthetic compounds:* Crofton KM et al. Thyroid-hormone-disrupting chemicals: Evidence for dose-dependent addi-

tivity or synergism. Environ Health Perspect 2005 Nov;113 (11):1549–54. Bergeron JM et al. PCBs as environmental estrogens: Turtle sex determination as a biomarker of environmental contamination. Environ Health Perspect 1994 Sep;102(9):780–1.

64   *If you were to visit the National Library of Medicine's* TOXMAP: http:// toxmap.nlm.nih.gov/toxmap/main/quickSearch.do;jsessionid=8AD8 DC4EA0E6B4572432B80A581870C7 (accessed May 18, 2007).

64   *In many locations, especially those with porous ground:* Magner M. Pentagon blocks EPA; Deadly solvent still threatens millions. Los Angeles Times, 2006 Mar 29. Available from http://www.stories thatmatter.org/index.php?option=com_content&task=view&id=15 &Itemid=39 (accessed May 18, 2007).

64   *In other cities, including both Tucson and Phoenix:* Kilburn KH and Warshaw RH. Prevalence of symptoms of systematic lupus erythematosus (SLE) and of fluorescent antinuclear antibodies associated with chronic exposure to trichloroethylene and other chemicals in well water. Environ Res 1992 Feb;57(1):1–9. Kardestuncer T, Frumkin H. Systemic lupus erythematosus in relation to environmental pollution: An investigation in an African-American community in North Georgia. Arch Environ Health 1997 Mar–Apr;52(2):85–90.

64   *TCE is regularly detected in breast milk:* National Institute of Environmental Health Sciences. Substance profile, trichloroethylene. Available from http://ntp.niehs.nih.gov/ntp/roc/eleventh/profiles/ s180tce.pdf (accessed May 18, 2007).

65   *Nevertheless, the Department of Defense:* Magner M. Pentagon blocks EPA; Deadly solvent still threatens millions. Los Angeles Times, 2006 March 29. Available from http://www.storiesthatmat ter.org/index.php?option=com_content&task=view&id=15&Itemi d=39 (accessed May 18, 2007).

65   *As one epidemiologist put it:* The TCE Blog/Trichloroethylene is Everywhere, http://www.tceblog.com/posts/1154029184.shtml (accessed April 12, 2007).

69   *certain signaling molecules:* Zouali M. Taming lupus. Sci Am, 2005 Mar;75.

70   *In 2000, Gilbert and Pumford and colleagues:* Gilbert KM et al. Environmental contaminant trichloroethylene promotes autoim-

mune disease and inhibits T cell apoptosis in MRL+/+ mice. J Immunotoxicol, in press. Blossom SJ, Gilbert KM. Ability of environmental toxicant trichloroethylene to promote immune pathology is strain-specific. J Immunotoxicol, in press. Blossom SJ et al. Chronic exposure to a trichloroethylene metabolite in autoimmune-prone MRL+/+ mice promotes immune modulation and alopecia. Toxicol Sci 2007 Feb;95(2):401–11. Blossom SJ, Gilbert KM. Exposure to a metabolite of the environmental toxicant trichloroethylene attenuates CD4+ T cell activation-induced cell death by metalloproteinase-dependent FasL shedding. Toxicol Sci 2006 July; 92(1):103–14. Pumford NR, Gilbert KM. Autoimmunity hepatitis. In Vohr H, ed. *Encyclopedic reference of immunotoxicology.* New York: Springer Publishing Co., 2005. Blossom SJ et al. Activation and apoptosis of CD4+ T cells following *in vivo* exposure to two common environmental toxicants, trichloroacetaldehyde hydrate and trichloroacetic acid. J Autoimmun 2004 Nov;23(3):211–20. Gilbert KM et al. Environmental contaminant and disinfection by-product trichloroacetaldehyde stimulates T cells *in vitro.* Int Immunopharmacol 2004 Jan;4(1):25–36. Gilbert KM et al. Butyric acid derivative induces allospecific T-cell energy and prevents graft-versus-host disease. Immunopharmacol Immunotoxicol 2003 Feb; 25(1):13–27. Griffin JM et al. CD4+ T cell activation and induction of autoimmune hepatitis following trichloroethylene treatment in MRL+/+ mice. Toxicol Sci 2000 Oct;57(2):345–52. Gilbert KM et al. Potential clinical use of butyric acid derivatives to induce antigen-specific T cell inactivation, J Pharmacol Exp Ther 2000 Sep; 294(3):1146–53. Griffin JM et al. Inhibition of CYP2E1 reverses CD4+T cell alterations in trichloroethylene-treated MRL+/+ mice. Toxicol Sci 2000 Apr;54(2):384–9. Griffin JM et al. Trichloroethylene accelerates an autoimmune response in association with Th1 T cell activation in MRL+/+ mice. Immunopharmacology 2000 Feb; 46(2):123–37. Gilbert KM et al. Trichloroethylene activates CD4+ T cells: Potential role in an autoimmune response. Drug Metab Rev 1999 Nov;31(4):901–16.

71 *one in four people carries a gene variant:* Moore EA. Autoimmune diseases and their environmental triggers. Jefferson, N.C.:

McFarland & Company, 2002;5. Also see Swanberg M et al. MHC2TA is associated with differential MHC molecule expression and susceptibility to rheumatoid arthritis, multiple sclerosis, and myocardial infarction. Nat Genet 2005 May;37(5):486–94. Epub 2005 Apr 10.

74   *Even though they themselves are physicians:* Powell JJ et al. Evidence for the role of environmental agents in the initiation or progression of autoimmune conditions. Environ Health Perspect 1999 Oct;107(Suppl 5):667–72.

74   *Moreover, the sheer volume of particles:* Based on an interview with Tony Ward, research assistant professor at the University of Montana in the Center for Environmental Health Sciences, January 29, 2007. Also see Missoulian.com news online, http://www.missoulian.com/articles/2003/08/19/news/local/news03.txt (accessed May 18, 2007).

74   *Five months after Jan's ordeal:* Ghio AJ and Huang YC. Exposure to concentrated ambient air particles alters hematologic indices in humans. Inhal Toxicol 2003 Dec;15(14):1465–78.

74   *Eighteen months later:* Vermylen J et al. Ambient air pollution and acute myocardial infarction. J Thromb Haemost 2005 Sep;3(9):1955–61.

75   *Individuals with rheumatoid arthritis or lupus:* Laden F et al. Reduction in fine particulate air pollution and mortality: Extended follow-up of the Harvard Six Cities study. Am J Respir Crit Care Med, 2006 Mar 15;173(6):667–72. Epub 2006 Jan 19.

75   *If an estimated 25 percent of people:* Dale E et al. A role for transcription factor NF-kappaB in autoimmunity: Possible interactions of genes, sex, and the immune response. Adv Physiol Educ 2006 Dec;30(4):152–8. Fairweather D, Rose NR. Women and autoimmune diseases. Emerg Infect Dis 2004 Nov;10(11):2005–11.

76   *Today, the National Institutes of Health spends:* National Institutes of Health, Autoimmune Diseases Coordinating Committee. Progress in autoimmune diseases research. Report to Congress, 2005 Mar; ii.

76   *autoimmune disease is the number-two cause of chronic illness:* National Institutes of Health, Autoimmune Diseases Coordinating

Committee, Progress in autoimmune diseases research. Report to Congress 2005 Mar; 9. In this report NIH states that cancer affects approximately 9 million people in the U.S.; heart disease affects approximately 22 million; and autoimmune disease up to 22 million. This suggests that autoimmune disease is at least the second most common cause of chronic illness.

76 *slices fifteen years off a patient's life:* On March 16, 2005, I attended a congressional briefing in Washington, D.C., at which Dr. Bhagirath Singh, scientific director of the Canadian Institutes of Health Research, Institute of Infection and Immunity, presented this statistic.

76 *A report by the Institute of Medicine:* American Autoimmune Related Diseases Association. Autoimmune diseases—are a major health problem! Fact sheet, 2004 Winter. Available from the American Autoimmune Related Diseases Association, 22100 Gratiot Avenue, East Detroit, MI 48021-2227, (586) 776-3900, aarda@aarda.org.

76 *While Japan recently spent $135 million:* Daly G. Hundreds of manmade chemicals—in our air, our water, and our food—could be damaging the most basic building blocks of human development. OnEarth 2006 Winter;27.

76 *First, the success rate for federal research:* Garrison HH, Palazzo RE. What's happening to the new investigator? FASEB Journal 2006 Jul;20(9):1288–9. Available from http://www.fasebj.org/cgi/content/full/20/9/1288 (accessed May 18, 2007).

77 *This makes it less likely that grants:* Correspondence by e-mail with Kathleen Gilbert, May 2, 2007.

77 *The FDA approves about 90 percent:* Duncan DE. The pollution within. Nat Geog 2006 Oct;122.

CHAPTER THREE: DIRTY LITTLE SECRETS

79 *Now watch as your computer monitor:* http://www.epa.gov/enviro/emef (accessed May 18, 2007).

80 *When lupus goes undiagnosed:* http://www.lupus.org/education/stats.html (accessed May 18, 2007).

82   *Three months later a thirty-eight-year-old:* This patient's last name has been changed.

92   *The majority of soil samples:* This information on the Environmental Protection Agency's standards is based on a conversation with Enesta Jones, EPA media office, September 15, 2006. Details regarding East Ferry's lead soil tests are from New York State Department of Environmental Conservation, Division of Environmental Remediation. Environmental restoration record of decision, 858 East Ferry Street site, City of Buffalo, Erie County, site number B-00007-9. 1999 Mar; 7.

98   *After that letter appeared, a piece ran:* Dolan TJ. E. side residents fear site may be causing lupus. Buffalo News, 2000 June 10;1C.

100 *Still, while the coalition's numbers were growing:* It should be noted here that Crystal D. Peoples, state assemblywoman, also worked with Grant and supported her efforts, sending a representative from her office to meetings. Peoples later helped to secure the reinstatement of the Superfund account.

104 *However, in one monitored area:* New York State Department of Environmental Conservation, Division of Environmental Remediation. Record of decision, Vibratech Inc. site, Buffalo (C), Erie County, New York, Site No. 915165. 1997 Mar.

105 *Residents learned that night:* Based on two e-mails from Julien Terrell, Toxic Waste/Lupus Coalition, February 16, 2006.

106 *Indeed, exposure to lead in lab animals:* Farrer DG et al. Lead enhances CD4+ T cell proliferation indirectly by targeting antigen presenting cells and modulating antigen-specific interactions. Toxicol Appl Pharmacol 2005 Sep 1;207(2):125–37.

106 *In the years between 1985 and 1995:* Kilburn KH, Warshaw RH. Prevalence of symptoms of systemic lupus erythematosus (SLE) and of fluorescent antinuclear antibodies associated with chronic exposure to trichloroethylene and other chemicals in well water. Environ Res 1992 Feb;57(1):1–9. Adyel FZ et al. Characterization of autoantibody activities in sera anti-DNA antibody and circulating immune complexes from 12 systemic lupus erythematosus patients. J Clin Lab Anal 1996;10(6):451–7. Silman AJ, Jones S. What is the

contribution of occupational environmental factors to the occurrence of scleroderma in men? Ann Rheum Dis 1992 Dec;51(12):1322–4. Bovenzi M et al. Scleroderma and occupational exposure. Scand J Work Environ Health 1995 Aug;21(4):289–92.

107 *as we have seen in the previous chapter, the science demonstrating:* Yurino H et al. Endocrine disruptors (environmental estrogens) enhance autoantibody production by B1 cells. Toxicol Science 2004 Sep;81(1):139–47. Epub 2004 May 27. Schoenroth L et al. Autoantibodies and levels of polychlorinated biphenyls in persons living near a hazardous waste treatment facility. J Investig Med 2004 Apr;52(3):170–6.

109 *the area cannot be artificially constructed:* Mayes MD. Scleroderma epidemiology. Rheum Dis Clin North Am 2003 May;29(2):239–54.

111 *This information is available to all:* See http://seer.cancer.gov—or, specifically, a document called the "Cancer Statistics Review" at http://seer.cancer.gov/csr/1975_2004 (accessed July 18, 2007). For local and regional state cancer profiles, see http://statecancerprofiles. cancer.gov (accessed July 18, 2007)

112 *The Toxic Waste/Lupus Coalition approached Joseph Gardella:* More information is available about Gardella's work in Gardella J et al. Linking community service, learning and environmental analytical chemistry. Anal Chem 2007;Feb79(3):811–18.

114 *According to the Lupus Foundation of America:* http://www.lupus. org/education/stats.html (accessed May 18, 2007).

116 *one 2004 study conducted in the city of Buffalo:* Rey J. Watchdog group accuses state of environmental racism. Buffalo News, 2004 Mar 12;B22. The study "Environmental Racism in New York State" was conducted by the Citizens Environmental Coalition, a statewide environmental watchdog organization.

116 *Elsewhere in the United States and around the world:* Kilburn KH, Warshow RH. Prevalence of symptoms of systemic lupus erythematosus (SLE) and of fluorescent antinuclear antibodies associated with chronic exposure to trichloroethylene and other chemicals in well water. Environ Res 1992 Feb;57(1):1–9.

117 *Further investigation found that these MS patients':* Agency for Toxic Substances and Disease Registry. Public comment draft final report,

El Paso multiple sclerosis cluster investigation. Available from http://
www.atsdr.cdc.gov/elpaso/pubcom.html (accessed May 18, 2007).

117 *Seven other heavy-metal-based clusters of MS:* Ibid. See section titled
"Environmental Exposures and Multiple Sclerosis."

118 *A combination of chemical exposures:* Ibid. Also see http://www
.rideforlife.com/news/als_research/feds_to_study_possible_als_and_
ms_cluster_in_illinois.html (accessed May 18, 2007). Also see http://
www.mult-sclerosis.org/news/Nov2002/MSClusterinFultonCounty.
html (accessed May 18, 2007).

118 *Likewise, a heightened incidence of lupus:* Kardestuncer T, Frumkin
H. Systemic lupus erythematosus in relation to environmental pollu-
tion: an investigation in an African-American community in North
Georgia. Arch Environ Health 1997 Mar–Apr;52(2):85–90.

118 *Although genetics in the closely related Choctaw population:* Arnett
FC et al. Increased prevalence of systemic sclerosis in a Native
American tribe in Oklahoma. Association with an Amerindian HLA
haplotype. Arthritis Rheum 1996 Aug;39(8):1362–70. Mayes MD.
Scleroderma epidemiology. Rheum Dis Clin North Am 2003
May;29(2):239–54.

118 *Other high rates of scleroderma:* Thompson AE, Pope JE. Increased
prevalence of scleroderma in southwestern Ontario: A cluster analysis. J Rheumatol 2002 Sep;29(9):1867–73.

118 *of a small rural area in the province of Rome, Italy:* Valesini G et al.
Geographical clustering of scleroderma in a rural area in the province of Rome. Clin Exp Rheumatol 1993 Jan–Feb;11(1):41–7.

118 *In the south of Boston:* http://www.sclero.org/medical/research/
causes/clusters/south-boston.html and http://www.thebostonchan
nel.com/print/3999742/detail.html (both accessed May 18, 2007).

118 *Blood serum levels of PCBs:* For more on this see http://www.atsdr
.cdc.gov/HS/anniston-final-report.html (accessed July 18, 2007).

118 *The CDC considers a blood PCB level:* http://www.atsdr.cdc.gov/
hac/pha/solvtia/sol_p2.html (accessed August 2, 2007).

118 *And in Libby, Montana:* American Autoimmune Related Diseases
Association. New study linking asbestos to autoimmunity is pre-
liminary, but promising, says American Autoimmune Related
Diseases Association." Press release, 2005 January 10. Available

from http://www.aarda.org/press_release_display.php?ID=26 (accessed May 21, 2007).

119 *the Environmental Protection Agency's EnviroMapper:* http://www.epa.gov/enviro/emef (accessed May 18, 2007).

119 *Just take a peek at one small community:* http://oaspub.epa.gov/enviro/ef_home3.top_display_zip?p_zipcode=37055 (accessed January 31, 2006, using zip code 37055). Also see Herbert B. Poisoned on Eno Road. New York Times, 2006 Oct 2. Available from http://peaceandjustice.org/article.php?story=20061002104142504&mode=print (accessed May 22, 2007).

120 *In another 2002 assessment, ATSDR:* http://www.atsdr.cdc.gov/annual-reports/2002/2002annualreport.html (accessed May 22, 2007).

120 *The Environmental Protection Agency does not release projections:* Shogren, E. Lawmakers band together to challenge EPA. Morning Edition, National Public Radio, broadcast 2006 Sep 18. Available from http://www.npr.org/templates/story/story.php?storyId=6095913 (accessed September 19, 2006).

CHAPTER FOUR: A POTENT PACKAGE

132 *Since 1997, Harley and James have published:* Harley JB et al. An altered immune response to Epstein-Barr nuclear antigen 1 in pediatric systemic lupus erythematosus. Arthritis Rheum 2006 Jan;54(1):360–8. Harley JB et al. Epstein-Barr virus and molecular mimicry in systemic lupus erythematosus. Autoimmunity 2006 Feb;39(1)63–70.

133 *One recent study supporting the link between Epstein-Barr:* Parks CG et al. Association of Epstein-Barr virus with systemic lupus erythematosus: Effect modification by race, age, and cytotoxic T lymphocyte-associated antigen 4 genotype. Arthritis Rheum 2005 Apr;52(4):1148–59.

134 *Researchers concluded that mounting evidence:* DeLorenze GN et al. Epstein-Barr virus and multiple sclerosis: Evidence of association from a prospective study with long-term follow-up. Arch Neurol 2006 Jun;63(6):839–44. Epub 2006 Apr 10.

135 *Likewise, National Institutes of Health researchers:* Lunemann JD et al. Increased frequency and broadened specificity of latent EBV nuclear antigen-1-specific T cells in multiple sclerosis. Brain 2006 Jun;129(Pt 6):1493–506. Epub 2006 Mar 28.

135 *One particularly provocative study out of the Hospital for Sick Children:* Alotaibi S et al. Epstein-Barr virus in pediatric multiple sclerosis. JAMA 2004 Apr 21;291(15):1875–9.

135 *Scientists can now show the precise process:* Ellis NM et al. T cell mimicry and epitope specificity of cross-reactive T cell clones from rheumatic heart disease. Immunol 2005 Oct 15;175(8):5448–56. Fae KC et al. How an autoimmune reaction triggered by molecular mimicry between streptococcal M protein and cardiac tissue proteins leads to heart lesions in rheumatic heart disease. Autoimmun 2005 Mar;24(2):101–9.

135 *the relationship between the measles virus and multiple sclerosis:* Anlar B. Infection and multiple sclerosis. J Neurol Neurosurg Psychiatry 2003 May;74(5):692–3.

135 *viral outbreaks of measles:* Sumelahti ML et al. Multiple sclerosis in Finland: Incidence trends and differences in relapsing remitting and primary progressive disease courses. J Neurol Neurosurg Psychiatry 2003 Jan;74(1):25–8.

136 *enteroviral infection during pregnancy:* Hyoty H et al. A prospective study of the role of coxsackie B and other enterovirus infections in the pathogenesis of IDDM. Diabetes 1995 Jun;44(6):652–7. Dahlquist G et al. Maternal enteroviral infection during pregnancy as a risk factor for childhood IDDM: A population-based case-control study. Diabetes 1995 Apr;44(4):408–13. Dahlquist G et al. Indications that maternal coxsackie B virus infection during pregnancy is a risk factor for childhood-onset IDDM. Diabetologia 1995 Nov;38(11):1371–3.

136 *Other studies tie mumps infection:* Sultz HA et al. Is mumps virus an etiologic factor in juvenile diabetes mellitus? J Pediatr 1975 Apr;86(4):654–6. Prince GA et al. Infection of human pancreatic beta cell cultures with mumps virus. Nature 1978 Jan 12;271(5641):158–61. Sinaniotis CA et al. Letter: Diabetes mellitus after mumps vaccination. Arch Dis Child 1975 Sep;50(9):749–50.

137 *Even some psychiatric conditions:* O'Connor S et al. Infectious etiologies of chronic diseases: Focus on women. Emerg Infect Dis 2004 Nov;10(11):2028–9.

137 *And scientists are now finding tentative links between viral infections and obesity:* Henig RM. Microbesity? Biology researchers are looking beyond diet and genes—to intestinal microbes, viruses and other bugs—in a quest to understand more clearly what makes so many of us so fat. New York Times Magazine, 2006 Aug 13;28.

138 *These new potential plagues:* Cunningham AA. A walk on the wild side—emerging wildlife diseases. BMJ 2005 Nov 26;331(7527): 1214–15.

139 *That's how researchers came to understand that "cold" viruses:* Interview with DeLisa Fairweather, PhD, assistant professor at the Bloomberg School of Public Health's Department of Environmental Health Sciences Division of Toxicology, via e-mail correspondence, October 16, 2006.

140 *Whether those with a predisposition to autoimmunity:* Brown D. Scientists race to head off lethal potential of avian flu. Washington Post, 2005 Aug 23;A1. Chase M. Avian-flu death rate may be tied to overkill by immune systems. Wall Street Journal, 2005 Dec 16;B1.

141 *Initially, nearly 1 million Americans were vaccinated:* Laitin EA, Pelletier EM. The influenza A/New Jersey (swine flu) vaccine and Guillain-Barré syndrome: The arguments for a causal association. Harvard School of Public Health, Drugs and Devices Information Line. Available from http://www.hsph.harvard.edu/Organizations/DDIL/swineflu.html (accessed May 22, 2007).

142 *Later calculations showed:* Ibid.

142 *Epidemiologists wondered if the cause:* Not all scientists today agree that autoimmunity is triggered by molecular mimicry. DeLisa Fairweather, PhD, assistant professor at the Bloomberg School of Public Health's Department of Environmental Health Sciences Division of Toxicology, for example, believes that what may have happened in the swine flu and GBS epidemic is slightly different and the result of "the adjuvant effect" rather than molecular mimicry. According to Fairweather, all animal models of autoimmune disease that are not

induced by genetic mutations are induced by inoculation of mice with self-peptides (like myelin from the myelin sheaths) along with adjuvant, or peptides from a bacteria or virus. This same sort of adjuvant may have been in the swine-flu vaccine. Thus, the innate immune response takes the self-information (a string of amino acids, or peptides, from the myelin) and foreign information (a string of amino acids, or peptides, from the virus) and interprets it as if there were an actual infection in the myelin sheaths of the nervous system. So it launches an antibody and immune-cell response to clear the infection and sends out autoantibodies against the myelin. Because there is no actual infection or damage caused by infection to the nerves, this response actually causes damage in genetically susceptible individuals, causing the damage to myelin and Guillain-Barré syndrome. Fairweather believes that this is how autoimmunity is initiated—a slightly different theory from molecular mimicry. She believes that autoimmune disease develops because both the self and foreign peptides are presented to the immune system at the same time. But exactly how this occurs in patients remains a mystery.

143 *People developed Guillain-Barré:* Lasky T et al. The Guillain-Barré syndrome and the 1992–1993 and 1993–1994 influenza vaccines. N Engl J Med 1998 Dec 17;339(25):1797–802.

143 *In 1994, the* Journal of the American Medical Association: Stratton KR et al. Adverse events associated with childhood vaccines other than pertussis and rubella. Summary of a report from the Institute of Medicine. JAMA 1994 May 25;271(20):1602–5.

143 *Similarly, a correlation has been reported:* Herroelen L et al. Central-nervous-system demyelination after immunisation with recombinant hepatitis B vaccine. Lancet 1991 Nov 9;338(8776):1174–5. Nadler JP. Multiple sclerosis and hepatitis B vaccination. Clin Infect Dis 1993 Nov;17(5):928–9.

144 *Other evidence links the measles:* Shoenfeld Y, Aron-Maor A. Vaccination and autoimmunity-"vaccinosis": A dangerous liaison? J Autoimmun 2000 Feb;14(1):1–10.

144 *Many scientists also believe strong anecdotal evidence:* Alter M. Is multiple sclerosis an age-dependent host response to measles?

Neurol Neurocir Psiquiatr 1977;18(2–3 Suppl):341–55. Shoenfeld Y, Aron-Maor A. Vaccination and autoimmunity-"vaccinosis": A dangerous liaison? J Autoimmun 2000 Feb;14(1):1–10.

144 *Like Epstein-Barr, however, the Hib vaccine:* Classen JB, Classen DC. Clustering of cases of insulin dependent diabetes (IDDM) occurring three years after hemophilus influenza B (Hib) immunization support causal relationship between immunization and IDDM. Autoimmunity 2002 Jul;35(4):247–53.

144 *reports have emerged linking the new human papillomavirus:* http://www.nvic.org/PressReleases/PR081507HPV.htm (accessed September 5, 2007).

144 *Yet as researchers begin to delve more into this troubling correlation:* Regner M, Lambert PH. Autoimmunity through infection or immunization? Nat Immunol 2001 Mar;2(3):185–8.

146 *particularly concerned about mercury:* Pollard KM et al. Xenobiotic acceleration of idiopathic systemic autoimmunity in lupus-prone bxsb mice. Environ Health Perspect 2001 Jan;109(1):27–33. Pollard KM et al. Murine susceptibility to mercury. I. Autoantibody profiles and systemic immune deposits in inbred, congenic, and intra-H-2 recombinant strains. Clin Immunol Immunopathol 1992 Nov;65(2):98–109. Hultman P, Hansson-Georgiadis H. Methyl mercury–induced autoimmunity in mice. Toxicol Appl Pharmacol 1999 Feb 1;154(3):203–11. Silbergeld EK et al. Mercury and autoimmunity: Implications for occupational and environmental health. Toxicol Appl Pharmacol 2005 Sep 1;207(2 Suppl):282–92.

147 *Since the advent of the industrial age:* "The Madison Declaration on Mercury Pollution," a report from the Eighth International Conference on Mercury as a Global Pollutant, summarizes the scientific conclusions presented by four expert panels at the Eighth International Conference on Mercury as a Global Pollutant, on August 6–11, 2006. The 1,150 registered participants in this conference constituted a diverse, multinational body of scientific and technical expertise on environmental mercury pollution. This declaration conveys the panels' principal findings and their consensus conclusions on policy-relevant questions concerning atmospheric sources of mercury, methylmercury exposure, and its effects on humans and

wildlife. Available from http://www.allenpress.com/pdf/i0044-7447-036-01-0062.pdf (accessed May 23, 2007). Wright K. Our preferred poison: A little mercury is all that humans need to do away with themselves quietly, slowly, and surely. Discover 2005 Mar;26(3). See http://discovermagazine.com/2005/mar/our-preferred-poison (accessed July 18, 2007).

147 *Dry particles of mercury travel:* Harris R. Studies find high mercury levels in the wild. Morning Edition, National Public Radio, broadcast 2005 Mar 8.

147 *Today, the National Library of Medicine's* TOXMAP: http://toxmap .nlm.nih.gov/toxmap/main/index.jsp enter "mercury" or "mercury compounds" (accessed July 18, 2007).

148 *in 2004, a study conducted jointly by the Environmental Quality Institute:* http://www.washingtonpost.com/wp-dyn/articles/A49896-2004Oct20.html (accessed May 23, 2007).

148 *Meanwhile, a 2007 New York City Health:* http://www.eurekalert .org/pub_releases/2007-07/nych-oif072207.php (accessed September 7, 2007).

148 *researchers know that mercury can cross the placenta:* Eilperin J. Women in coastal areas are found to have higher mercury levels. Washington Post, 2005 Sep 23;A3.

148 *a newborn's mercury level:* Lee J. E.P.A. raises estimate of babies affected by mercury exposure. New York Times, 2004 Feb 10. Available from http://query.nytimes.com/gst/fullpage.html?sec=health& res=9B07E3DA173AF933A25751C0A9629C8B63 (accessed May 23, 2007).

148 *Recently, researchers found that low levels of mercury:* Li Z et al. Chemically diverse toxicants converge on Fyn and c-Cbl to disrupt precursor cell function. PLoS Biol 2007 Feb;5(2):e35.

149 *Panel members complained that the report:* Parker-Pope T. Metal mouth: Do you need to worry about the mercury in dental fillings? Wall Street Journal, 2006 Sep 12, D1.

150 *Meanwhile, in the field of autoimmune-disease research:* Casciola-Rosen L et al. Scleroderma autoantigens are uniquely fragmented by metal-catalyzed oxidation reactions: Implications for pathogenesis. J Exp Med 1997 Jan 6;185(1):71–9.

150 *other research relating having a high number of dental fillings:* Thompson AE, Pope JE. Increased prevalence of scleroderma in southwestern Ontario: A cluster analysis. J Rheumatol 2002 Sep;29(9):1867–73.

150 *One recent case-control study:* Arnett FC et al. Urinary mercury levels in patients with autoantibodies to U3-RNP (fibrillarin). J Rheumatol 2000 Feb;27(2):405–10.

150 *some of that methyl mercury is converted:* Wright K. Our preferred poison: A little mercury is all that humans need to do away with themselves quietly, slowly, and surely. Discover 2005 Mar;26(3): 1. See http://discovermagazine.com/2005/mar/our-preferred-poison (accessed July 18, 2007).

150 *Inorganic mercury is the major form of mercury:* Hultman P et al. Xenobiotic acceleration of idiopathic systemic autoimmunity in lupus-prone bxsb mice. Environ Health Perspect 2001 Jan;109(1):27–33. Pollard KM et al. Murine susceptibility to mercury. I. Autoantibody profiles and systemic immune deposits in inbred, congenic, and intra-H-2 recombinant strains. Clin Immunol Immunopathol 1992 Nov;65(2):98–109. Hultman P, Hansson-Georgiadis H. Methyl mercury–induced autoimmunity in mice. Toxicol Appl Pharmacol 1999 Feb 1;154(3):203–11.

150 *Even low-dose mercury exposure:* Silbergeld EK et al. Mercury and autoimmunity: Implications for occupational and environmental health. Toxicol Appl Pharmacol 2005 Sep 1;207(2 Suppl):282–92.

153 *Pollard and his colleagues concluded:* Pollard KM et al. Xenobiotic acceleration of idiopathic systemic autoimmunity in lupus-prone bxsb mice. Environ Health Perspect 2001 Jan;109(1):27–33.

153 *And then there is that one lucky mouse:* Interviews with both Kenneth Michael Pollard, associate professor in The Department of Molecular and Experimental Medicine at the Scripps Research Institute, and Dwight Kono, associate professor in the Department of Immunology at the Scripps Research Institute, explain that one of the most important lessons to come from studying mercury-induced autoimmunity in the mouse has been the identification of an area in the mouse genome that allows certain mice to resist developing autoimmunity despite environmental exposures. As Pollard explained to

me in an e-mail correspondence in March 2007, "Important clues to preventing environmental exposures from leading to autoimmune disease lie in identifying the gene or genes responsible for making mice resistant to the development of disease. If we can uncover the mechanisms involved in resistance then we may be able to develop appropriate interventions to treat human disease." For more on this see Kono DH, Theofilopoulos AN. Genetics of SLE in mice. Springer Semin Immunopathol 2006 Oct;28(2):83–96. Epub 2006 Sep 14.

154 *This was at a time when new thimerosal-containing vaccines:* Rock A. The tipping point. Mother Jones 2004 Mar–Apr;29(2):70.

155 *Researchers believe that the genetic background:* Goth SR et al. Uncoupling of ATP-mediated calcium signaling and dysregulated interleukin-6 secretion in dendritic cells by nanomolar thimerosal. Environ Health Perspect 2006 Jul;114(7):1083–91.

155 *Their findings, published in 2006, indicate that thimerosal does induce:* Havarinasab S, Hultman P. Alteration of the spontaneous systemic autoimmune disease in (NZB x NZW)F1 mice by treatment with thimerosal (ethyl mercury). Toxicol Appl Pharmacol 2006 Jul 1;214(1):43–54. Epub 2006 Jan 27.

155 *Another recent study caused a stir within the scientific community:* Wallis C. Inside the autistic mind. Time, 2006 May 15;45.

155 *Even so, if there is an interplay with mercury:* Mundell EJ. Major gene study points to causes of autism. Health Day News. 2007 Feb 18;A3.

156 *The working hypothesis is that these antibodies:* Wallis C. Inside the autistic mind. Time, 2006 May 15;46–7.

156 *A number of scientists are now investigating:* Pardo CA et al. Immunity, neuroglia and neuroinflammation in autism. Int Rev Psychiatry 2005 Dec;17(6):485–95.

158 *More than half of Americans test positive:* Arbes SJ Jr. et al. Prevalences of positive skin test responses to 10 common allergens in the US population: Results from the third National Health and Nutrition Examination Survey. J Allergy Clin Immunol 2005 Aug;116(2):377–83.

159 *Twenty million Americans now suffer from asthma:* http://www .asthmainamerica.com/children_index.html (accessed May 23, 2007).

159 *The number of people suffering from asthma:* Arbes SJ Jr. et al. Prevalences of positive skin test responses to 10 common allergens in the US population. Results from the third National Health and Nutrition Examination Survey. J Allergy Clin Immunol 2005 Aug;116(2):377–83.

160 *The theory is that having younger siblings:* Ponsonby AL et al. Exposure to infant siblings during early life and risk of multiple sclerosis. JAMA 2005 Jan 26;293(4):463–9.

160 *By contrast, someone who is experiencing a true trauma:* Lesher A et al. Increased IL-4 production and attenuated proliferative and pro-inflammatory responses of splenocytes from wild-caught rats (*Rattus norvegicus*). Immunol Cell Biol 2006 Aug;84(4):374–82. Epub 2006 Apr 3.

164 *The innate immune response:* Fairweather D et al. Viruses as adjuvants for autoimmunity: Evidence from coxsackievirus-induced myocarditis. Rev Med Virol 2005 Jan–Feb;15(1):17–27. Fairweather D et al. Cutting edge: T cell Ig mucin-3 reduces inflammatory heart disease by increasing CTLA-4 during innate immunity. J Immunol 2006 Jun 1;176(11):6411–15. Frisancho-Kiss S et al. Cutting edge: Cross-regulation by TLR4 and T cell Ig mucin-3 determines sex differences in inflammatory heart disease. J Immunol 2007, in press.

165 *The immune system must now decide whether:* Coxsackievirus B3 was named after Coxsackie, New York, where the virus was first isolated from a patient.

166 *The way in which mast cells:* Fairweather D, Rose NR. Women and autoimmune diseases. Emerg Infect Dis 2004 Nov;10(11):2005–11.

167 *All gas, no brakes:* To bring home how different hits can combine to overwhelm the immune system, we might look to Ellen Silbergeld's work in several communities in Amazonian Brazil. Silbergeld charted three communities where they had differing levels of mercury exposure (some from gold mining, some from high fish consumption) coupled with malaria exposure. Her findings suggested that mercury exposure can alter immune function and increase circulating levels of autoantibodies. A significantly higher number of subjects with detectable autoantibodies had hair mercury levels greater than the

norm. In a fascinating finding, those with higher hair mercury levels who also reported malaria infection were more likely to have detectable concentrations of autoantibodies as compared to those with low mercury levels. In other words, high mercury exposure and malaria exposure together meant more likelihood of autoimmune disease. For more on this see Silva IA et al. Mercury exposure, malaria, and serum antinuclear/antinucleolar antibodies in Amazon populations in Brazil: A cross-sectional study. Environ Health 2004 Nov 2;3(1):11.

167 *We already know that some environmental triggers:* Criswell LA et al. Smoking interacts with genetic risk factors in the development of rheumatoid arthritis among older Caucasian women. Ann Rheum Dis 2006 Sep;65(9):1163–7. Epub 2006 Aug 3.

CHAPTER FIVE: THE AUTOIMMUNE DISEASE DETECTIVES

187 *over the next ten years:* McCune AB et al. Maternal and fetal outcome in neonatal lupus erythematosus. Ann Intern Med 1987 Apr;106(4):518–23.

188 *In 2003, they published a landmark study:* Scofield RH. Autoantibodies as predictors of disease. Lancet 2004 May 8;363(9420): 1544–6.

188 *Typically, one or two autoantibodies:* Ibid.

190 *About half the patients had autoantibodies:* O'Connor A. On the trail of diseases, years before they strike. New York Times, 2004 May 11;F5. Nielen MM et al. Specific autoantibodies precede the symptoms of rheumatoid arthritis: A study of serial measurements in blood donors. Arthritis Rheum 2004 Feb;50(2):380–6.

191 *the largest surveillance effort on diabetes:* SEARCH for Diabetes in Youth Study Group. The burden of diabetes mellitus among US youth: Prevalence estimates from the SEARCH for Diabetes in Youth Study, American Academy of Pediatrics. Pediatrics 2006 Oct;118(4): 1510–18.

191 *Worldwide studies confirm:* EURODIAB ACE Study Group. Variation and trends in incidence of childhood diabetes in Europe. Lancet 2000 Mar 11;355(9207):873–6.

193 *scientists may be able to develop a blood test:* Avasarala JR et al. A distinctive molecular signature of multiple sclerosis derived from MALDI-TOF/MS and serum proteomic pattern analysis: Detection of three biomarkers. J Mol Neurosci 2005 Jan;25(1):119–25.

193 *Other breakthroughs in MS diagnostics:* Marta CB et al. Pathogenic myelin oligodendrocyte glycoprotein antibodies recognize glycosylated epitopes and perturb oligodendrocyte physiology. Proc Natl Acad Sci U S A 2005 Sep 27;102(39):13992–7. Epub 2005 Sep 19.

193 *state-of-the-art eye exams:* Carmichael A. Eye exams detect early signs of MS. Wall Street Journal, 2007 Jan 2, D6.

196 *Ultimately, understanding how small differences:* In one recent study that sheds light on this, researchers at the Rockefeller University found that reversing the defects in certain genes that play into the autoimmune disease lupus can restore health in animals with lupus. Although lupus clearly results from a combination of genetics that varies from person to person, nevertheless it may be that a common "gatekeeper" gene—called FCRgIIB—is critical to preventing the disease in many cases. If you can reverse the defect in that gatekeeper gene you can reverse disease in animals with lupus by preventing the accumulation of autoantibodies that are responsible for the progression of the disease. It works like this: if a mouse is deficient in this particular FCRgIIB gatekeeper gene it will produce a genetically reduced level of what are known as Fc receptors. Fc receptors are critical, because they work to inhibit the immune-system cells from becoming activated and producing the rogue autoantibodies that go on to attack the body's own tissue. When researchers placed bone marrow in mice that expressed additional copies of the Fc receptor gene, those mice did not develop autoimmune disease. The difference between healthy immune function and autoimmune dysfunction turned out to be surprisingly small: researchers only had to increase the Fc receptor's activity by about 40 percent. Doing so allowed the increased Fc receptors to halt the formation of the autoantibodies associated with lupus. Such a finding suggests that

adjusting the level of Fc receptors could provide a promising future means of preventing and treating lupus.

For more on this see Ravetch JV et al. Restoration of tolerance in lupus by targeted inhibitory receptor expression. Science 2005 Jan 28;307(5709):590–3 and Ravetch JV et al. The inhibitory Fcgamma receptor modulates autoimmunity by limiting the accumulation of immunoglobulin G+ anti-DNA plasma cells. Nat Immunol 2005 Jan;6(1):99–106. Epub 2004 Dec 12.

Also see Ambrose SG. Dallas scientists make gains in lupus research: Genes that set off autoimmune disease in mice identified. Dallas Morning News, 2006 Jun 18;26A. Wakeland EK et al. Tlr7 translocation accelerates systemic autoimmunity in murine lupus. Proc Nat Acad Sci 2006 Jun 27;103(26):9970–5. Epub 2006 June 15.

196 *Likewise, a 2007 genome study:* International Multiple Sclerosis Genetics Consortium et al. Risk alleles for multiple sclerosis identified by a genomewide study. N Engl J Med 2007 Aug 30;357(9):851–62. Epub 2007 Jul 29.

196 *The idea that a gene might be protective:* An international team from the University of Montreal, Massachusetts Institute of Technology, and Harvard have just unveiled a detailed map of human genetic variation within what is known as the major histocompatibility complex, or MHC, a critical region of the human genome that encodes how we respond to infection and whether or not we develop autoimmune disease. The MHC—specifically the genes that constitute it—is associated with more diseases than any other region of the human genome, including rheumatoid arthritis, type 1 diabetes, lupus, multiple sclerosis, and Crohn's disease. The MHC, not surprisingly, is also where our allergy genes are located. This area of the genome may provide critical clues as to why both autoimmunity and allergies are simultaneously on the rise, since they work through similar immune pathways. However, pinpointing the specific genetic differences in humans that cause these diseases is complex, given the extremely high degree of genetic diversity that exists in the MHC among different individuals.

To look at the variability of genetic patterns of the MHC, researchers analyzed its DNA sequence in more than 350 individuals from diverse geographic regions, including Africa, Europe, China, and Japan, providing data that other researchers can begin to use to identify the broader patterns that point to increased genetic risk for autoimmune diseases. Duerr RH et al. A genome-wide association study identifies IL23R as an inflammatory bowel disease gene. Science 2006 Dec 1;314(5804):1461–3. Epub 2006 Oct 26. de Bakker PI. A high-resolution HLA and SNP haplotype map for disease association studies in the extended human MHC. Nat Genet 2006 Oct;38(10):1166–72. Epub 2006 Sep 24.

197 *Women account for nearly 80 percent:* Dale E et al. A role for transcription factor NF-kappaB in autoimmunity: Possible interactions of genes, sex, and the immune response. Adv Physiol Educ 2006 Dec;30(4):152–8.

197 *Yet the precise ways in which sex hormones:* Ibid.

199 *Physicians can then warn patients:* In the Netherlands researchers are using a connect-the-dot approach to determine which patients who show signs of early joint pain and stiffness should be treated prophylactically for rheumatoid arthritis and which should not. Among those who seek out a doctor's help for joint pain and stiffness, the most common diagnosis is undifferentiated arthritis (UA), or arthritic symptoms that do not add up to any specific arthritic disease. Spontaneous remission occurs in 40 to 50 percent of UA sufferers, while about 30 percent develop rheumatoid arthritis, a much more serious disease. A wealth of research supports early aggressive treatment for those with rheumatoid arthritis, or RA, showing that treatment is integral in preventing joint damage and severe disability, but the drugs of choice bring a substantial risk of liver damage and other serious complications. Physicians often face a tough choice of whether to initiate aggressive drug therapy immediately in patients presenting with early signs of arthritis or to wait and see if they are actually going to develop RA. To help inform these individual decisions to treat or not to treat, researchers at Leiden University Medical Center in the Netherlands have found a formula to help determine whether patients who present with UA are, in fact, going to progress to RA. Through a combination of

questionnaires, physical examination, and blood samples, the team identified nine clinical variables that, when combined, have a strong ability to predict rheumatoid arthritis versus undifferentiated arthritis. Looking at gender, age, specific location and duration of symptoms along with specific autoantibodies and other key blood biomarkers, researchers were able to give each patient a score ranging from zero to fourteen and predict quite accurately who would develop the more debilitating of the two diseases. Using such evidence-based predictions promises to be enormously helpful to clinicians who are trying to muddle through the cost-benefit analysis of which patients should be treated with early drug intervention. Van der Helm-van Mil AH et al. A prediction rule for disease outcome in patients with recent-onset undifferentiated arthritis: How to guide individual treatment decisions. Arthritis Rheum 2007 Feb;56(2):433–40.

200 *These drugs do help to stave off joint destruction:* Enbrel (etanercept) "important information" available from http://www.enbrel .com:80/index.jsp?f=7 (accessed May 24, 2007).

201 *Also used in the treatment of Crohn's:* Dale E et al. A role for transcription factor NF-kappaB in autoimmunity: Possible interactions of genes, sex, and the immune response. Adv Physiol Educ 2006 Dec;30(4):152–8.

202 *On June 5, 2006, the U.S. Food and Drug Administration:* http:// www.tysabri.com/tysbProject/tysb.portal (accessed May 24, 2007).

202 *Investigators suspect:* Johannes L. Where drug's setback leaves patients: Withdrawal of Tysabri reshapes options for those with multiple sclerosis, Crohn's, severe arthritis. Wall Street Journal, 2005 Mar 1;D1.

203 *Rituxan works by preventing signals:* Rituxan works by altering the body's production of B cells. B cells, or B lymphocytes, normally respond only to foreign antigens such as bacteria and viruses. But in people with autoimmune disease the cells react to the body's own molecules, generating antibodies that bind to those "self-antigens" and then accumulate—in lupus for example—in their tissue, where they create tissue damage. Rituxan aids autoimmune-disease patients by blocking one of the molecular interactions that lead to an-

tibody production and tissue injury. It works like this: T cells peruse different foreign antigens to decide whether or not they're harmful to the body. If T cells decide that the antigen is a foreign agent that the body needs to fight against, they then send out signals that cause T cells to proliferate—and to also produce B cells. The idea is that if we can prevent these signals from being transmitted, we can prevent B cells from attacking tissue. The train will never leave the station, much less reach its target destination. Rituxan stops the train by targeting a specific protein, known as CD20, on the surface of B cells. Rituxan binds to CD20 and is believed to work with the body's own immune system to attack and kill the marked B cells, although the exact mechanism by which this happens is still unclear. Typical treatments for those with MS, for example, involve one infusion, followed by a second infusion two weeks later and infusions every six months thereafter, a happy improvement over drugs that require daily or even monthly injections.

203 *Rituxan not only helps to stop MS:* http://www.utsouthwestern.edu/utsw/cda/dept37389/files/219222.html (accessed May 24, 2007). Stuve O et al. Clinical stabilization and effective B-lymphocyte depletion in the cerebrospinal fluid and peripheral blood of a patient with fulminant relapsing-remitting multiple sclerosis. Arch Neurol 2005 Oct;62(10):1620–3.

204 *their disease went into remission:* Data presented at the 2006 American College of Rheumatology Congress show that patients receiving repeat treatment with MabThera/Rituxan (rituximab) achieved continued improvement in both physical and mental aspects of quality of life measures. A press release detailing these findings, "Repeat treatment with MabThera provides continuous improvement in quality of life in RA patients: Benefit of B cell therapy confirmed in patients who respond inadequately to one or more TNF inhibitors," is available from http://www.eurekalert.org/pub_releases/2006-11/cwl-rtw111006.php (accessed May 24, 2007).

204 *Doctors and analysts are unsure:* Won Tesoriero H. Drugs in testing show promise for lupus: New treatments target disease, not just symptoms; first big advances in 50 Years. Wall Street Journal, 2007 Jan 23;D1.

204 *These include Orencia:* Ibid.

211 *Over time, such technology:* American Autoimmune Related Diseases Association. Who we are. Press release; 1. Available through the American Autoimmune Related Diseases Association, 22100 Gratiot Avenue, East Detroit, MI 48021-2227, (586) 776-3900, aarda@aarda.org.

211 *compared to the yearly health-care burden:* http://www.cdc.gov/nccdphp/publications/factsheets/Prevention/cancer.htm (accessed May 24, 2007).

212 *One paper in the journal* Science: Kodoma S et al. Islet regeneration during the reversal of autoimmune diabetes in NOD mice. Science 2003 Nov;302(5648):1223–7.

214 *The researchers also apologized to patients with diabetes:* Based on an interview with Denise Faustman, associate professor of medicine at Harvard Medical School, October 21, 2006.

215 *All three labs followed Dr. Faustman's procedures:* Begley S. After initial rejection, scientists back work on cure for diabetes. Wall Street Journal, 2006 Mar 24;B1.

CHAPTER SIX: SHIELDING YOUR IMMUNE SYSTEM

222 *He consulted several other like-minded physicians:* Gerard Mullin consulted Dr. Leo Galland in New York, Loren Marks, a holistic board-certified nutritionist in New York, and John McCorrie in the United Kingdom.

223 *"Yet we have clear data":* Cantorna MT. Vitamin D and its role in immunology: Multiple sclerosis and inflammatory bowel disease. Prog Biophys Mol Biol 2006 Sep;92(1):60–4. Epub 2006 Feb 28. Mark BL, Carson JA. Vitamin D and autoimmune disease—implications for practice from the multiple sclerosis literature. J Am Diet Assoc 2006 Mar;106(3):418–24. van Meeteren ME et al. Antioxidants and polyunsaturated fatty acids in multiple sclerosis. Eur J Clin Nutr 2005 Dec;59(12):1347–61.

223 *Today, 21 percent of patients:* Bensoussan M et al. Complementary and alternative medicine use by patients with inflammatory bowel

disease: Results from a postal survey. Gastroenterol Clin Biol 2006 Jan;30(1):14–23.

223 *Consumers in general in the United States:* http://dietary-supplements. info.nih.gov/pubs/fnce2005/M%20F%20Picciano-Who%20Is%20 Using%20Dietary%20Supplements%20and%20What%20are%20 They%20Using.pdf (accessed May 24, 2007). Also see Eisenberg DM et al. Trends in alternative medicine use in the United States, 1990–1997: Results of a follow-up national survey. JAMA 1998 Nov 11;280(18):1569–75.

224 *$4 billion more than what they spend:* Americans spend roughly $5 billion a year at the movies and $12 billion a year on videos. See http://www.hollywoodmuseum.com/whoweare/whoweare_history. html (accessed May 24, 2007).

224 *Even so, the vast majority:* Eisenberg DM et al. Trends in alternative medicine use in the United States, 1990–1997: Results of a follow-up national survey. JAMA 1998 Nov 11;280(18):1569–75.

224 *a 2007 study of fifty-six second-year gastrointestinal fellows:* Scolapio JS et al. First Annual Fellows' Nutrition Training Course: Outcome of nutrition support, obesity and basic and clinical nutrition training. Gastroenterology 2007 April;132(4):A519.

226 *Patient studies show that higher intake:* Longnecker MP, Daniels JL. Environmental contaminants as etiologic factors for diabetes. Environ Health Perspect, 2001 Dec;109(Suppl 6):871–6.

226 *There is also evidence it may trigger lupus:* Hess EV. Environmental chemicals and autoimmune disease: Cause and effect. Toxicology 2002 Dec 27;181–182:66.

226 *Today, only 10 percent of all American adults:* See the USDA Healthy Eating Index: 1999–2000 at http://www.cnpp.usda.gov/publica tions/HEI/HEI99-00report.pdf (accessed May 24, 2007).

226 *When you look at recent studies on what Americans do get in their diet:* Nielsen SJ, Popkin BM. Changes in beverage intake between 1977 and 2001. Am J Prev Med 2004 Oct;27(3):205–10.

226 *75 percent of preschoolers in America:* Kranz S et al. Dietary fiber intake by American preschoolers is associated with more nutrient-dense diets. J Am Diet Assoc 2005 Feb;105(2):221–5.

226 *fewer than 11 percent of Americans:* Casagrande SS et al. Have

Americans increased their fruit and vegetable intake? The trends between 1988 and 2002. Am J Prev Med 2007 Apr;32(4):257–63.

226 *junk foods such as chips, snacks, desserts, and soft drinks:* http://www.berkeley.edu/news/media/releases/2004/06/01_usdiet.shtml (accessed May 24, 2007).

227 *One reason is that farmers tend to select:* Davis DR et al. Changes in USDA food composition data for 43 garden crops, 1950 to 1999. J Am Coll Nutr 2004 Dec;23(6):669–82.

227 *Acid rain has taken its toll:* Tang RH et al. Coupling diurnal cytosolic Ca2+ oscillations to the CAS-IP3 pathway in *Arabidopsis.* Science 2007 Mar 9;315(5817):1423–6.

228 *Immigrants to America also fall under the spell:* Akresh IR. Many new immigrants to US change diet—and not for the better. University of Illinois at Urbana-Champlaign, study not yet published. See EurekAlert! press release, February 9, 2006, at eurekalert .org.

228 *But what is especially striking:* Farrokhyar F et al. A critical review of epidemiological studies in inflammatory bowel disease. Scand J Gastroenterol 2001 Jan;36(1):2–15.

230 *These villi are covered in cells:* Quigley EM, Quera R. Small intestinal bacterial overgrowth: Roles of antibiotics, prebiotics, and probiotics. Gastroenterology 2006 Feb;130(2 Suppl 1):S78–90.

230 *In healthy individuals, as the villi are renewed:* Watson AJM et al. Epithelial barrier function in vivo is sustained despite gaps in epithelial layers. Gastroenterology 2005 Sept;129(3):902–12.

230 *If food components or bacteria:* Glade M. Certification Board for Nutrition Specialists examination study guide, third edition. Clearwater, Fla.: American College of Nutrition, 2003;17–19.

231 *The first step is to work with your physician:* According to Gerard Mullin, director of Integrative GI Nutrition Services at Johns Hopkins Medical Institutions, the best stool analysis to request your doctor to order is the Comprehensive Digestive Stool Analysis from Genova Diagnostics, available at http://www.gdx.net/home/assessments/findsystems/gastro.html (accessed May 25, 2007). The lactulose breath test is conducted in the gastroenterologist's office.

231 *Interestingly, laboratory studies show that when rats:* Sellon RK et

al. Resident enteric bacteria are necessary for development of spontaneous colitis and immune system activation in interleukin-10-deficient mice. Infect Immun 1998 Nov;66(11):5224–31.

231 *Mullin recommends beginning:* Ask your physician for suggestions on rice or whey protein powders from reliable companies.

232 *In research on those with Crohn's disease:* Giaffer MH et al. Long-term effects of elemental and exclusion diets for Crohn's disease. Aliment Pharmacol Ther 1991 Apr;5(2):115–25. Suzuki H et al. An elemental diet controls inflammation in indomethacin-induced small bowel disease in rats: The role of low dietary fat and the elimination of dietary proteins. Dig Dis Sci 2005 Oct;50(10):1951–8.

232 *In one study, 75 percent of patients with irritable bowel syndrome:* Atkinson W et al. Food elimination based on IgG antibodies in irritable bowel syndrome: A randomised controlled trial. Gut 2004 Oct;53(10):1459–64. O'Mahony L et al. *Lactobacillus* and *Bifidobacterium* in irritable bowel syndrome: Symptom responses and relationship to cytokine profiles. Gastroenterology 2005 Mar;128(3):541–51.

233 *IgE allergic reactions are immediate:* For more information on IgE food allergy testing, see http://www.foodallergy.org (accessed May 27, 2007).

233 *T-cell mediated food allergies:* Ferguson A et al. T-cell mediated immunity in food allergy. Ann Allergy 1983 Aug;51(2 Pt 2):246–8.

233 *With IgG food sensitivities:* Shanahan F, Whorwell PJ. IgG-mediated food intolerance in irritable bowel syndrome: A real phenomenon or an epiphenomenon? Am J Gastroenterol 2005 Jul;100(7):1558–9. However, although the concept of IgG allergies is becoming increasingly accepted, not all doctors agree that IgG allergies exist.

233 *In fact, in one new study at Children's Hospital:* Astrakhan A et al. Local increase in thymic stromal lymphopoietin induces systemic alterations in B cell development. Nature Immunol 2007 May;8(5):522–31. Epub 2007.

233 *Studies confirm that for some patients:* Panush RS. Food induced ("allergic") arthritis: Clinical and serologic studies. J Rheumatol 1990 Mar;17(3):291–4.

234 *For this reason, Mullin recommends:* http://www.usbiotek.com/. US BioTek Laboratories offers "Serum IgG & IgE Antibody Panels for Foods, Indoor/Outdoor Inhalants, Spices & Herbs" as well as "Serum or Finger Stick IgG Antibody Panels for Foods, Spices & Herbs, Inhalants."

234 *What follows is a short list of foods:* For more information, especially on how special diets may help in arachnoiditis, see *Arachnoiditis: The Silent Epidemic,* by J. Antonio Aldrete, MD, MS, at www.arachnoidtitis.com/book.asp. In this book, Gerard Mullin and Loren Marks, DC, DACBN, a certified nutritionist in New York City who frequently works with patients with autoimmune disorders, cowrote a chapter in which they discuss some of the dietary guidelines and supplements that can help in fighting the disease.

234 *consider eating a low-inflammatory diet:* In *Arachnoiditis: The Silent Epidemic,* nutritionist Loren Marks suggests consuming one of the following: smoked salmon on brown rice cakes; a two- to three-egg omelet from hens fed flaxseed, with sweet potatoes and rosemary and black beans on the side; hot brown rice cereal with cinnamon; unsweetened yogurt (if you are not allergic to or sensitive to milk) with flaxseed oil and a half cup of blueberries mixed in; or poached eggs with smoked salmon. Lunch or dinner might consist of a large mixed green salad with sardines and chopped yellow and green and red peppers; broiled red snapper with steamed broccoli and baked yams; four ounces of wild salmon with brown rice pasta and tomato sauce with extra oregano, thyme, and garlic with a side dish of grilled vegetables; or one chicken breast with rosemary, with a half cup of black-eyed peas, roasted onions or garlic, and a spinach salad.

234 *In one recent study of seven hundred children:* Chatzi L et al. Protective effect of fruits, vegetables and the Mediterranean diet on asthma and allergies among children in Crete. Thorax, in press. Epub 2007 Apr 5.

236 *In looking at infants born to Latinas:* Furlong CE et al. PON1 status of farmworker mothers and children as a predictor of organophosphate sensitivity. Pharmacogenet Genomics 2006 Mar;16(3): 183–90. Duramad, P et al. Early environmental exposures and

intracellular Th1/Th2 cytokine profiles in 24-month-old children living in an agricultural area. Environ Health Perspect 2006 Dec; 114(12):1916–22.

236 *This is particularly frightening:* Young JG et al. Association between in utero organophosphate pesticide exposure and abnormal reflexes in neonates. Neurotoxicology 2005 Mar;26(2):199–209.

236 *Combined exposure to mixtures of pesticides:* Duramad P et al. Early environmental exposures and tracellular Th1/Th2 cytokine profiles in 24-month-old children living in an agricultural area. Environ Health Perspect 2006 Dec;114(12):1916–22.

236 *Most to the point:* Sobel ES et al. Acceleration of autoimmunity by organochlorine pesticides in (NZB x NZW)F1 mice. Environ Health Perspect 2005 Mar;113(3):323–8.

236 *farmers who mix their own pesticides:* Rosenberg AM et al. Prevalence of antinuclear antibodies in a rural population. J Toxicol Environ Health A 1999 Jun56(4):225–36. Cooper GS et al. Occupational risk factors for the development of systemic lupus erythematosus. J Rheumatol 2004 Oct;31(10):1928–33.

237 *During the five days in which children ate an organic diet:* Lu C et al. Organic diets significantly lower children's dietary exposure to organophosphorus pesticides. Environ Health Perspect 2006 Oct;114(10):A572; author reply A572–3.

237 *According to new data from the Centers for Disease Control and Prevention:* Zhang J. When eating your vegetables makes you sick. Wall Street Journal, 2005 Nov 30;D1. FDA reviews response to food safety concerns. Sunday Capital, 2007 Mar 18;A3.

237 *Unlike the meat, egg, milk, and processed-food industries:* FDA reviews response to food safety concerns. Sunday Capital, 2007 Mar 18;A3.

238 *In May 1981, for instance, food product:* Posada de la Paz M et al. Toxic oil syndrome: the perspective after 20 years. Epidemiol Rev 2001;23(2):231–47.

238 *FDA inspectors are responsible for visiting:* http://www.washington post.com/wp-dyn/content/article/2007/04/22/AR2007042201551. html (accessed April 25, 2007). In this article ("FDA Was Aware of Dangers to Food"), Elizabeth Williamson quotes the FDA's food

safety chief, Robert E. Brackett: " 'We have 60,000 to 80,000 facilities that we're responsible for in any given year.' Brackett said. Ex-
plosive growth in the number of processors and the amount of
imported foods means that manufacturers 'have to build safety into
their products rather than us chasing after them.' "

239 *In 1989 with an outbreak of eosinophilia-myalgia:* Posada de la Paz
     M et al. Toxic oil syndrome.

239 *in 1998, hundreds of Haitian children:* Epidemic of pediatric deaths
     from acute renal failure caused by diethylene glycol poisoning.
     JAMA 1998 Apr 15;279(15):1175–80.

239 *The FDA itself has rather lax regulations:* Ibid.

241 *Oxidative damage has been linked:* Kurien BT et al. Oxidatively
     modified autoantigens in autoimmune diseases. Free Radic Biol Med
     2006 Aug 15;41(4):549–56. Epub 2006 May 23.

241 *one recent study that followed the diet of twenty-five thousand indi-
     viduals:* Pattison DJ et al. Dietary beta-cryptoxanthin and inflam-
     matory polyarthritis: Results from a population-based prospective
     study. Am J Clin Nutr 2005 Aug;82(2):451–5.

241 *Another study found low levels of antioxidants:* Vipartene D et al.
     [Pro- and antioxidant blood system in patients with rheumatoid ar-
     thritis and systemic lupus erythematosus.] Ter Arkh 2006;78(6):
     10–4.

241 *One particular antioxidant currently under study:* Yadav V et al.
     Lipoic acid in multiple sclerosis: A pilot study. Mult Scler 2005
     Apr;11(2):159–65.

241 *has also been found to help lessen symptoms:* Bregovskii VB et al.
     [Predictors of alpha-lipoic acid treatment efficacy in diabetic poly-
     neuropathy of the lower limbs.] Ter Arkh 2005;77(10):15–19.

241 *Alpha lipoic acid has such a profound effect:* Schreibelt G et al. Li-
     poic acid affects cellular migration into the central nervous system
     and stabilizes blood-brain barrier integrity. J Immunol 2006 Aug
     15;177(4):2630–7.

242 *A growing number of studies show omega-3:* Macdonald A. Omega-
     3 fatty acids as adjunctive therapy in Crohn's disease. Gastroenterol
     Nurs 2006 Jul–Aug;29(4)295–301; quiz 302–3. Cleland LG et al.
     Reduction of cardiovascular risk factors with longterm fish oil treat-

ment in early rheumatoid arthritis. J Rheumatol 2006 Oct;33(10):1973–9.

242 *In one fascinating study, investigators at the Cleveland Clinic:* Seidner DL et al. An oral supplement enriched with fish oil, soluble fiber, and antioxidants for corticosteroid sparing in ulcerative colitis: A randomized, controlled trial. Clin Gastroenterol Hepatol 2005 Apr;3(4):358–69.

242 *Other research shows that higher dietary intake of omega-3:* Omega-3 polyunsaturated fatty acid intake and islet autoimmunity in children at increased risk for type-1 diabetes. Norris, J. JAMA Sept 2007;298(12):1420–1428.

243 *A striking body of data shows:* Munger KL et al. Serum 25-hydroxyvitamin D levels and risk of multiple sclerosis. JAMA 2006 Dec 20;296(23):2832–8.

243 *Other studies show that vitamin D:* Cantorna MT. Vitamin D and its role in immunology: Multiple sclerosis and inflammatory bowel disease. Prog Biophys Mol Biol 2006 Sep;92(1):60–4. Epub 2006 Feb 28.

243 *There is growing evidence that vitamin D:* Mullin GE, Dobs A. Vitamin D and its role in cancer and immunity: A prescription for sunlight. Nutr Clin Pract 2007 Jun;22(3):305–22. Mullin GE. Inflammatory bowel disease mucosal biopsies have specialized lymphokine mRNA profiles. Inflamm Bowel Dis 1996;2(Spring): 16–26.

243 *One provocative investigation:* Willer CJ et al. Timing of birth and risk of multiple sclerosis: Population based study. BMJ 2005 Jan 15;330(7483):120. Epub 2004 Dec 7.

244 *NIH researchers found that curcumin:* Funk JL et al. Turmeric extracts containing curcuminoids prevent experimental rheumatoid arthritis. J Nat Prod 2006 Mar;69(3):351–5.

244 *Other investigations show that two grams of curcumin:* Hanai H et al. Curcumin maintenance therapy for ulcerative colitis: Randomized, multicenter, double-blind, placebo-controlled trial. Clin Gastroenterol Hepatol 2006 Dec;4(12):1502–6. Epub 2006 Nov 13.

244 *In one set of tests using blood samples:* Beeton C et al. Kv1.3 chan-

nels are a therapeutic target for T cell-mediated autoimmune diseases. Proc Natl Acad Sci U S A 2006 Nov 14;103(46)17414–19. Epub 2006 Nov 6.

245 *Ironically, many of the same factors:* Ibid.

246 *therapy with the probiotic* Lactobacillus reuteri: Pena JA et al. Probiotic *Lactobacillus* spp. diminish *Helicobacter hepaticus*–induced inflammatory bowel disease in interleukin-10-deficient mice. Infect Immun 2005 Feb;73(2):912–20.

246 *a recent paper published in the* American Journal of Gastroenterology: Bibiloni R et al. VSL#3 probiotic-mixture induces remission in patients with active ulcerative colitis. Am J Gastroenterol 2005 Jul;100(7):1539–46.

247 *Using nontraditional, ancient medical information:* Buenz EJ et al. Searching historical herbal texts for potential new drugs. BMJ 2006 Dec 23;333(7582):1314–15.

247 *At other institutions around the country:* Ahmed S et al. Regulation of interleukin-1beta-induced chemokine production and matrix metalloproteinase 2 activation by epigallocatechin-3-gallate in rheumatoid arthritis synovial fibroblasts. Arthritis Rheum 2006 Aug;54(8):2393–401. Authors of this study recently presented further research on April 29, 2007, at the Experimental Biology 2007 meeting in Washington, D.C.

247 *If you are concerned about a particular nutrient:* http://ods.od.nih.gov (accessed May 28, 2007).

247 *You can also download the USDA's free nutrient database software:* http://www.ars.usda.gov/main/site_main.htm?modecode=12354500 (accessed May 28, 2007).

248 *Even stressful events that happened in our childhood:* Danese A et al. Childhood maltreatment predicts adult inflammation in a life-course study. Proc Natl Acad Sci U S A 2007 Jan 23;104(4):1319–24. Epub 2007 Jan 17.

248 *those who had suffered more serious, negative life events:* Lantz PM et al. Stress, life events, and socioeconomic disparities in health: Results from the Americans' Changing Lives Study. J Health Soc Behav 2005 Sep;46(3):274–88.

248 *Stressful events are associated with an increased risk:* Buljevac D et al. Self-reported stressful life events and exacerbations in multiple sclerosis: Prospective study. BMJ 2003 Sep 20;327(7416):646.

248 *periods of high stress are linked to the onset:* Gio-Fitman J. The role of psychological stress in rheumatoid arthritis. Medsurg Nurs 1996 Dec;5(6):422–6. Straub RH, Harle P. [Stress, hormones, and neuronal signals in the pathophysiology of rheumatoid arthritis. The negative impact on chronic inflammation.] Med Klin (Munich) 2005 Dec 15;100(12):794–803.

248 *One startling study bears this out all too starkly:* Li J et al. The risk of multiple sclerosis in bereaved parents: A nationwide cohort study in Denmark. Neurology 2004 Mar 9;62(5):726–9.

250 *Stress hormones and chemicals travel to the immune system:* Eskandari F et al. Neural immune pathways and their connection to inflammatory diseases. Arthritis Res Ther 2003;5(6):251–65. Gold SM et al. The role of stress-response systems for the pathogenesis and progression of MS. Trends Immunol 2005 Dec;26(12):644–52.

251 *This increases the likelihood that the immune system:* Viswanathan K, Dhabhar FS. Stress-induced enhancement of leukocyte trafficking into sites of surgery or immune activation. Proc Natl Acad Sci U S A 2005 Apr 19;102(16):5808–13.

251 *One research study found that those experiencing chronic stress:* Ranjit N et al. Psychosocial factors and inflammation in the multiethnic study of atherosclerosis. Arch Intern Med 2007 Jan 22;167(2):174–81.

251 *But those who experience chronic physical illness:* Lucas RE. Long-term disability is associated with lasting changes in subjective well-being: Evidence from two nationally representative longitudinal studies. J Pers Soc Psychol 2007 Apr;92(4):717–30.

252 *Some nuns were in their nineties:* For more on the Nun Study, see http://www.mc.uky.edu/nunnet/faq.htm (accessed May 28, 2007). Or see Danner DD et al. Positive emotions in early life and longevity: findings from the nun study. J Pers Soc Psychol 2001 May;80(5):804–13.

253 *By staying primarily at a low baseline:* Parker-Pope T. The secrets of successful aging. Wall Street Journal, 2006 Jun 20;R1,R3.

253 *areas of the brain that have to do with sensory processing:* Lazar SW et al. Meditation experience is associated with increased cortical thickness. Neuroreport 2005 Nov 28;16(17):1893–7.

254 *Did winning an Oscar:* Redelmeier DA, Singh SM. Survival in Academy Award–winning actors and actresses. Ann Intern Med 2001 May 15;134(10):955–62.

254 *Likewise, exercise can stimulate injured neurons:* Molteni R et al. Voluntary exercise increases axonal regeneration from sensory neurons. Proc Natl Acad Sci U S A 2004 Jun 1;101(22):8473–8.

254 *Other reports show that children with type 1 diabetes:* Herbst A et al. Effects of regular physical activity on control of glycemia in pediatric patients with type 1 diabetes mellitus. Arch Pediatr Adolesc Med 2006 Jun;160(6):573–7.

254 *exercise can improve muscle strength:* Rietberg MB et al. Exercise therapy for multiple sclerosis. Cochrane Database Syst Rev 2005 Jan 25;(1):CD003980.

255 *Each day an average of five new chemicals:* Seventeen hundred new chemicals are put on the market each year, which averages to about five newly approved chemicals a day.

258 *These domestic emissions:* Halpern S, McKibben B. The enemy within: The air in our cities can be less toxic than the carcinogens, hormone disrupters, and neurotoxins in household cleaners. House & Garden, 2006 Oct;741.

258 *Other states may soon encourage similar changes:* Fischler MS. A safe house? New York Times, 2007 Feb 15. Available from http://www.nytimes.com/2007/02/15/garden/15clean.html?ei=5088&en=5feb7ca43ebbOa32&ex=1329195600&partner=rssnyt&emc=rss&pagewanted=print (accessed July 18 2007).

259 *Instead, look for organic products:* Naturally Rockford: Four tips for finding safe, organic alternatives. Rock River Times, 2007 Mar 21. Available from http://www.rockrivertimes.com/index.pl?Cmd=viewstory&cat=6&id=15979 (accessed July 18 2007).

260 *Viruses left on surfaces:* EurekAlert! UVA researchers find that hotel guests with colds can leave their germs behind after checkout. Press release, 2006 Sept 29. Shared at the forty-sixth annual Interscience Conference on Antimicrobial Agents and Chemotherapy, September

29, San Francisco, CA. http://www.eurekalert.org/pub_releases/2006–09/uovh-urf092806.php (accessed May 28, 2007).

260 *The average American washes his or her hands:* Hitti M. America's clean-hands grade sullied. WebMD Medical News, 2006 Sep 22. Available from http://www.webmd.com/news/20060922/americas-clean-hands-grade-sullied (accessed May 28, 2007).

APPENDIX I

263 *Autoimmune and Related Diseases:* This list was compiled with the help of Ahmet Hoke, MD, PhD, Director, Neuromuscular Division, Johns Hopkins Medical Institutions.

ACKNOWLEDGMENTS

This book exists because of the help of three key people in my life. My agent and friend, Elizabeth Kaplan, who once again pushed me to report and write about what I live and then held my hand all along the way when the living got tough. My dear friend Stephanie von Hirschberg, who, lucky me, just happens to be a brilliant editor, and who helped cajole, shape, and edit every page into what you see before you now. Without her, this book would be but a pale rendition of what you hold in your hands. And my husband, Zenji, who has always been there through the hellish ups and downs of my health challenges and by being there has made all the difference. I am also indebted to my editors at Touchstone—Trish Todd, who first recognized the importance of this project, and Trish Grader, who saw it through—both of whom did much to make this project a reality. I also want to thank Doris Cooper for sharing her vision for this project at its inception.

In the beginning of reporting this book I met with several researchers who, although they are not profiled between these covers, played a central role in shaping this project: Kenneth Olden, PhD, ScD, then director of the National Institute of Environmental Health Sciences; Frederick Miller, MD, PhD, chief of the Environmental Autoimmunity Group at the National Institute of Environmental Health Sciences; and Glinda Cooper, PhD, and Dori

Germolec PhD, epidemiologists at the National Institute of Environmental Health Sciences, all spent time with me at their National Institutes of Health offices to help point me in the right direction. I am also particularly indebted to the following scientists and physicians whose names you will find in these pages: DeLisa Fairweather, Denise Faustman, Kathleen Gilbert, John Harley, Ahmet Hoke, Douglas Kerr, Gerard Mullin, Michele Petri, Mike Pollard, Noel Rose, Hal Scofield, and Allen Silverstone. These researchers spent precious hours helping me to understand their research and ensuring that my translation of their work into lay reader terms did not impinge upon the science. I'm grateful for having had what I liken to a two-year course in Immunology 101 at the hands of some of the brightest scientific minds of our time, and any mistakes I have made with their subject matter are purely my own. It is only right that I doubly thank Ahmet Hoke and Gerard Mullin, both of whom, as my physicians, have played a paramount role in helping me to achieve stability with the autoimmune conditions I face. I would also like to thank Dr. Savely Yurkovsky for his help.

My gratitude also goes to Virginia Ladd for her help throughout this project, to Joyce Miller, for tracking down elusive studies, to Dayna Meyers for her stellar research assistance, and to Priscilla Hart and Shannon Brownlee for their comments on the first chapters of this book when it was in an early draft form. A special thanks to the people of Buffalo, who opened their hearts, doors, and files to help me to piece together the history of the lupus cluster in their area, especially Judith Anderson, LaShekia Chatman, Carlos Crespo, Rhonda Lee Dixon, Joe Gardella, Betty Jean Grant, Laurene Tumiel-Berhalter and Julien Turell.

Finally, there was a long period of time in my life when I couldn't do much for myself, physically, due to my own autoimmune crisis, and there were a few amazing women who came each and every day to help me through. Tracy Greenfield, Stephanie von Hirschberg, Sarah Judd, Kimberly Minear, and Valerie Rogers, there are not enough words to thank you for being here every day for me—and for my children.

INDEX

Note: * = name changed to protect privacy